1988
YEAR BOOK OF
SURGERY®

The 1988 Year Book® Series

Year Book of Anesthesia®: Drs. Miller, Kirby, Ostheimer, Roizen, and Stoelting

Year Book of Cancer®: Drs. Hickey and Saunders

Year Book of Cardiology®: Drs. Schlant, Collins, Engle, Frye, Kaplan, and O'Rourke

Year Book of Critical Care Medicine®: Drs. Rogers, Allo, Dean, McPherson, Michael, Miller, Traystman, and Wetzel

Year Book of Dentistry®: Drs. Cohen, Hendler, Johnson, Jordan, Moyers, Robinson, and Silverman

Year Book of Dermatology®: Drs. Sober and Fitzpatrick

Year Book of Diagnostic Radiology®: Drs. Bragg, Hendee, Keats, Kirkpatrick, Miller, Osborn, and Thompson

Year Book of Digestive Diseases®: Drs. Greenberger and Moody

Year Book of Drug Therapy®: Drs. Hollister and Lasagna

Year Book of Emergency Medicine®: Dr. Wagner

Year Book of Endocrinology®: Drs. Bagdade, Braverman, Halter, Horton, Korenman, Kornel, Metz, Molitch, Morley, Robertson, Rogol, Ryan, and Vaitukaitis

Year Book of Family Practice®: Drs. Rakel, Avant, Driscoll, Prichard, and Smith

Year Book of Geriatrics and Gerontology: Drs. Beck, Abrass, Burton, Cummings, Makinodan, and Small

Year Book of Hand Surgery®: Drs. Dobyns, Chase, and Amadio

Year Book of Hematology®: Drs. Spivak, Bell, Ness, Quesenberry, and Wiernik

Year Book of Infectious Diseases®: Drs. Wolff, Barza, Keusch, Klempner, and Snydman

Year Book of Medicine®: Drs. Rogers, Des Prez, Cline, Braunwald, Greenberger, Wilson, Epstein, and Malawista

Year Book of Neurology and Neurosurgery®: Drs. DeJong, Currier, and Crowell

Year Book of Nuclear Medicine®: Drs. Hoffer, Gore, Gottschalk, Sostman, Zaret, and Zubal

Year Book of Obstetrics and Gynecology®: Drs. Mishell, Kirschbaum, and Morrow

Year Book of Ophthalmology®: Drs. Ernest and Deutsch

Year Book of Orthopedics®: Dr. Coventry

Year Book of Otolaryngology–Head and Neck Surgery®: Drs. Bailey and Paparella

Year Book of Pathology and Clinical Pathology®: Drs. Brinkhous, Dalldorf, Grisham, Langdell, and McLendon

Year Book of Pediatrics®: Drs. Oski and Stockman

Year Book of Perinatal/Neonatal Medicine: Drs. Klaus and Fanaroff

Year Book of Plastic and Reconstructive Surgery®: Drs. McCoy, Brauer, Haynes, Hoehn, Miller, and Whitaker

Year Book of Podiatric Medicine and Surgery®: Dr. Jay

Year Book of Psychiatry and Applied Mental Health®: Drs. Freedman, Lourie, Meltzer, Talbott, and Weiner

Year Book of Pulmonary Disease®: Drs. Green, Ball, Menkes, Michael, Peters, Terry, Tockman, and Wise

Year Book of Rehabilitation®: Drs. Kaplan and Szumski

Year Book of Sports Medicine®: Drs. Shepard and Torg, Col. Anderson, and Mr. George

Year Book of Surgery®: Drs. Schwartz, Jonasson, Peacock, Shires, Spencer, and Thompson

Year Book of Urology®: Drs. Gillenwater and Howards

Year Book of Vascular Surgery®: Drs. Bergan and Yao

1988

The Year Book of SURGERY®

Editor
Seymour I. Schwartz, M.D.
Professor and Chairman, Department of Surgery, University of Rochester, School of Medicine and Dentistry

Associate Editors
Olga Jonasson, M.D.
Professor and Chair, Department of Surgery, Ohio State University, Columbus

Erle E. Peacock, Jr., M.D.
Chapel Hill, North Carolina

G. Tom Shires, M.D.
Professor and Chairman, Department of Surgery, New York Hospital— Cornell Medical Center

Frank C. Spencer, M.D.
George David Stewart Professor of Surgery; Chairman, Department of Surgery, New York University; Director, Department of Surgery, New York University Medical Center and Bellevue Hospital

James C. Thompson, M.D.
John Woods Harris Professor and Chairman, Department of Surgery; Chief of Surgery, University Hospitals, The University of Texas Medical Branch, Galveston

Year Book Medical Publishers, Inc.
Chicago • London • Boca Raton

Editorial Director, Year Book Publishing: Nancy Gorham
Sponsoring Editor: Cara D. Suber
Manager, Medical Information Services: Laura J. Shedore
Assistant Director, Manuscript Services: Frances M. Perveiler
Assistant Managing Editor, Year Book Editing Services: Wayne Larsen
Production Manager: H.E. Nielsen
Proofroom Supervisor: Shirley E. Taylor

Table of Contents

The material covered in this volume represents literature reviewed through November 1987.

Journals Represented

Year Book Medical Publishers subscribes to and surveys more than 700 U.S. and foreign medical and allied health journals. From these journals, the Editors select the articles to be abstracted. Journals represented in this YEAR BOOK are listed below.

Acta Chirurgica Scandinavica
American Heart Journal
American Journal of Medicine
American Journal of Physiology
American Journal of Roentgenology
American Journal of Surgery
American Surgeon
Annals of Emergency Medicine
Annals of Internal Medicine
Annals of Plastic Surgery
Annals of the Royal College of Surgeons of England
Annals of Surgery
Annals of Thoracic Surgery
Archives of Dermatology
Archives of Surgery
British Journal of Plastic Surgery
British Journal of Surgery
British Medical Journal
Burns
Canadian Journal of Surgery
Cancer
Cancer Research
Chest
Circulation
Circulatory Shock
Current Problems in Cancer
Diseases of the Colon and Rectum
European Journal of Plastic Surgery
Gastroenterology
Injury
International Journal of Cancer
International Surgery
Journal of the American College of Cardiology
Journal of the American Medical Association
Journal of Applied Physiology: Respiratory, Environmental
  and Exercise Physiology
Journal of Clinical Endocrinology and Metabolism
Journal of Clinical Gastroenterology
Journal of Clinical Investigation
Journal of Experimental Medicine
Journal of Hand Surgery
Journal of Heart Transplantation
Journal of Immunology
Journal of Laboratory and Clinical Medicine
Journal of Parenteral and Enteral Nutrition
Journal of Pediatric Surgery
Journal of the Royal College of Surgeons of Edinburgh
Journal of Surgical Research

Journal of Thoracic and Cardiovascular Surgery
Journal of Trauma
Journal of Vascular Surgery
Lancet
Laryngoscope
Mayo Clinic Proceedings
Nature
New England Journal of Medicine
Nuclear Medicine Communications
Orthopedics
Plastic and Reconstructive Surgery
Radiology
Scandinavian Journal of Clinical Laboratory Investigation
Scandinavian Journal of Thoracic and Cardiovascular Surgery
Science
Southern Medical Journal
Surgery
Surgery, Gynecology and Obstetrics
Thorax
Transplantation
Transplantation Proceedings
World Journal of Surgery

Annual Overview

General Considerations

There has been an increasing emphasis on the complication of heparin-induced platelet activation and thrombocytopenia. The complications occur with either low doses of heparin or therapeutic doses. Thus, any patients receiving heparin should be monitored for thrombocytopenia, and if it develops, aggregation tests should be performed. The prognostic utility of dipyridamole thallium scintigraphy for predicting cardiac events has been compared with exercise testing and clinical variables in patients admitted for elective peripheral vascular surgery. The scanning technique is superior to exercise testing and provides a method of evaluating the cardiac risk in these patients. Refinement of radiographic technique has improved the success rate for percutaneous drainage of subphrenic abscesses. An 85% success rate has been reported, and failure is generally dependent on the presence of multiple noncontiguous collections of pus.

A report of the largest experience in this country emphasizes the effectiveness of thymectomy for patients with myasthenia gravis. The patients with milder disease and without coexisting thymomas did best. Although the authors advocate a transcervical approach, most surgeons prefer a transthoracic approach. Assessment of patients with thymomas undergoing resection indicates that 75% with encapsulated thymomas and about 50% with invasive thymomas survive 10 years. It is felt that in patients with invasive tumors, even with low total resection, postoperative radiation should be administered.

Fluid, Electrolytes, and Nutrition

Most of the investigations this year are related to studies on nutritional support of patients sustaining some form of trauma. These studies dominated the field, with a few other studies indicating more support for replacement of the third space losses of fluid and electrolytes in response to definable areas of trauma.

It is interesting that several specific cell defects, including membrane defects, can be shown to develop in response to starvation. It is equally fascinating, however, that the maintenance of nitrogen balance with intravenous feeding for 10 days to 2 weeks following starvation injury was unable to reverse the cellular injury from a starvation state. Similarly, a defined formula enteral diet also maintained nitrogen balance but allowed continuation of cellular membrane function. Furthermore, total parenteral nutrition failed to improve a liver function, immune functions, and even mortality in thermally injured patients. It is consequently apparent that it takes far more than caloric and nitrogen repletion to repair the damage invoked by starvation and serious injury.

It is quite apparent that the mechanism of protein synthesis interference must be much better defined before adequate prevention or reversal of the metabolic responses to injury can be achieved. Protein malnutrition impairs synthesis and release of mediators as well as specific protein reconstitution. Many studies are aimed at understanding the total amino

1

acid fluxes and synthesis in response to injury. Certainly, the addition of sepsis to starvation and injury is a further and devastating cumulative injury that is not as yet totally understood.

Shock

Literature during the past year in the field of shock has changed rather dramatically. The forms of shock that are being studied most extensively are still those forms most commonly seen in surgical patients, that is, hemorrhagic shock and septic shock. However, the focus on hemorrhagic shock has changed largely to assessment of measurable responses to resuscitation. The most striking change has been the enormous increase in interest in septic shock. The current work on septic shock is focusing sharply on the mediators. It is now clear that these mediators produce the injury and tissue damage as well as the signs and symptoms that have heretofore been attributed to the lipopolysaccharide coming from endotoxin producing the septic shock. This is particularly exciting since specific monoclonal antibodies can be produced against the recombinant human pure proximate mediators.

Insofar as resuscitation of hemorrhagic shock is concerned, there is continuing interest in the use of a hypertonic sodium solution with or without colloid for initial resuscitation in the field in order to use smaller volumes of resuscitative fluid. Critical looks at these data, however, indicate that the volumes used are only relatively smaller than those normally used with isotonic solutions, and, furthermore, the complications, such as the effects on incipient renal failure that have been established prior to the intravenous infusions, have yet to be determined. Apparently this is another one of those efforts that appears periodically with the use of solutions to produce a more rapid hemodynamic response in resuscitation from shock. The complications resulting from such efforts invariably outweigh the gain from use of a smaller volume with a little more rapid response.

Good prospective studies have established what has been universally used in times of war and conflict: for example, the safety of type O uncrossed matched blood as immediate resuscitative oxygen-carrying fluid when combined with crystalloid. Additional studies have shown that if the shock preparation was produced by large protein loss, such as occurs with total intestinal ischemia, then additional replacements, in addition to red blood cells and crystalloid solution, may include albumin solutions.

The most exciting studies on the cytokine mediators that have been discovered to be endogenously produced by macrophages include extensive studies on human cachectin (tumor necrosis factor). Following the recent identification of cachectin as a proximate mediator of the shock and tissue injury induced by lipopolysaccharide, it is clear that the cachectin alone can elicit all of the effects of administered endotoxin. The availability of highly purified endotoxin free recombinant human cachectin has been infused into several species of animals now with the induction of hypotension, metabolic acidosis, hemoconcentration, shock, multiple organ injury, multiple organ failure, and death within hours. Autopsy revealed tissue injury indistinguishable from that caused by the administration of lipopolysaccharide.

Further studies have shown that monoclonal antibody blockade of the mediator cachectin can prevent all of the effects from the injection of endotoxin or live *Escherichia coli* organisms long enough to permit survival.

While cachectin will surely not be the only proximate mediator identified, it is of significant importance that the blockade of this mediator prevents the development of all of the subsequent influences of lipopolysaccharide, including neutrophil degranulation, white cell production of superoxide and hydroxyl anion release, and the cascade development of release of interleukin I, interleukin II, interferon gamma, and other monokines. Consequently, the white cell deterioration and production of toxic intermediates are blocked by the inactivation of mediator.

Other exciting studies this past year included the description of translocation of bacteria from the bowel by the injection of endotoxin. This may well be where the mediators arise in patients who have bowel dysfunction from either disuse of bowel or from systemic sepsis.

One additional prospective randomized study published this year demonstrates rather conclusively that the use of high dose corticosteroids in the treatment of severe sepsis and septic shock is of no value whatsoever. This was the first prospective, randomized, double-blind, placebo-controlled trial involving almost 400 patients with severe sepsis and septic shock. This study should go a long way in dissuading against the use of high dose cortisone, with its known ill effects in patients with sepsis and septic shock.

Trauma

It is interesting to see again this year a tremendous volume of good clinical research concerning improved care of the severely injured patient. It is also encouraging to see assessments of the usefulness of trauma management in training surgical residents as well as the relationship of the roles for diagnostic-related groups to those for others, including the radiologist and basic scientist, in the improved management of the traumatized patient. Similarly, there are continuing studies on all phases of trauma management, including initial transportation, diagnosis, and definitive surgical care of specific injuries.

As mentioned in 1987, more attention is being paid to the experience of a resident on a trauma service and the fact that this experience may not necessarily be reflected in operative load. Pleas are again being made to the American Board of Surgery not to use index cases as a major measurement of management of trauma, but rather that only the patients who receive intensive care or operations by a component surgical specialty should be included.

Specific figures are now available documenting the underreimbursement of hospitals for the severely injured trauma and burn patients. In fact, it appears that the diagnosis-related group reimbursement will frequently be less than a third of actual cost of the critical care necessary to adequately take care of a severely injured or burned patient.

Once again this year we are beginning to see which patients can and will benefit from the use of acute computed tomography (CT) in the delineation of traumatic injuries. The increasing role of CT scan of head injury has become quite obvious. The use of abdominal CT scan is now better understood and, when confined to the stable patient, may be extremely helpful.

Another study of a randomized trial using pneumatic shock garments in prehospital management of penetrating abdominal injuries appeared. It was again shown that there was no advantage in using the antishock garment and that, in short transport time, there was certainly no gain and considerable loss by the delay occasioned when the antishock garments were used.

Better definition of presumptive antibiotic therapy in the injured patient is appearing. It would appear that, with low-risk patients, presumptive antibiotics can be discontinued quite safely in 12 hours, whereas with high-risk patients, antibiotics still need to be given for only about the first 72 hours. Additional studies are showing that the safe, second-line broad spectrum antibiotics given as single agents were quite appropriate in the presumptive antibiotic management of the injured patient.

Additional studies this year document the efficacy of high-frequency jet ventilation in the management of the injured patient. However, these authors conclude that high-frequency jet ventilation has no real therapeutic effect as such, compared to more conventional mechanical ventilation.

Continuing to appear are papers documenting quite clearly that the immediate fixation of long bone fractures is a remarkable advance in the prevention of respiratory distress syndrome, which is almost certainly due to sepsis from the patient who had conservative management. The development of sepsis in patients who are put in traction rather than having fixation may well come from bacteria in the bowel, although it may also come from bacteria arising in the lung when the patient is on prolonged bed rest.

It is interesting to see further refinement of the management of extremely difficult abdominal injuries. For example, most duodenal injuries can be managed quite satisfactorily with simple repair and drainage. More complex procedures, including Roux-en-Y repair, diverticularization, and pancreative pancreaticoduodenectomy, are quite useful when severe injury to the duodenum occurs, particularly when associated with combined pancreatic or common bile duct injury.

Insofar as bowel trauma is concerned, the tried and true conservative managements still produce the lowest morbidity and mortality. For example, rectal trauma still most often requires colostomy with fecal diversion as well as presacral drainage. Right colon injuries can be safely closed only if the injury is minor and usually involving one wall; otherwise some form of decompression or diversion produces the best result. It is interesting that the effects of renal trauma on renal function are additive. That is, patients with renal injury have a higher instance of renal failure than those who have abdominal injury without the kidney being directly involved.

Further delineation of the alteration of function in the phagocytes and lymphocytes continues to emerge. Up regulation or down regulation of the immune response to injury is now undergoing active study.

There are more and more papers documenting the gut theory in the development of sepsis following multiple injury. Several studies indicate the absorption of endotoxin with subsequent possible activation of mediators. It has also generally been found that survival after major abdominal trauma is higher since the advent of immediate jejunostomy feeding, which also supports the gut origin septic theory.

Wound Healing

Enough experience has now accumulated for it to appear unnecessary to graft denuded areas of perineum and buttocks following fairly radical excision of hidradenitis suppurativa. The same recommendations appeared for management of axillary wounds. Practical considerations may make secondary healing in the axilla less desirable than primary healing following rotation or advancement flap coverage. Free skin grafting should not be utilized in any area of changing dimensions such as the axilla and perineum, however. Enthusiasm for injecting bovine collagen to eliminate dermal depressions continues, in spite of increasing warning about the temporary effect of such injections and the possible disadvantages of crossing a major histocompatibility locus to correct a cosmetic defect.

Although the effects are not catastrophic in properly managed patients, studies showed a measurable inhibition of wound healing associated with some severe preoperative illness and the length of preoperative illness prior to surgical intervention. The effect of local heat and moist dressings was studied again; the effect on wound healing is small, but heat apparently can exert some benefit in some wounds. Theoretically, wet heat, more penetrating than dry heat, is slightly better. Animal data were presented that support the clinical impression that nicotine reduces capillary flow and significantly impairs viability of skin flaps. It seems appropriate now to do all that can be done to reduce preoperatively nicotine consumption in patients who require transplantation of skin flaps. In spite of earlier studies to the contrary, it is clear now that acute hemorrhage producing acute oligemia can affect significantly the rate of gain in tensile strength of healing wounds. The difference between data reported this year and previous data probably can be explained on the basis of acute rather than chronic anemia.

Studies comparing suturing and stapling techniques in wound closure showed that the only real advantage in utilizing staples is speed in putting them in the skin. Scar tissue in stapled wounds is no different from scar tissue in sutured wounds; patients report more pain during removal of staples than removal of sutures. Improvement in the appearance of hypertrophic scars was reported following a new technique of crosshatching the surface of the scar and applying a free thin skin graft. It was also reported that the circumferential scar surrounding free full-thickness skin grafts can be improved by dermabrasion. There still is enthusiasm for utilizing meshed grafts rather than solid sheets of skin in burned patients even when conservation of skin is not a factor. Some surgeons apparently do not recognize the major cosmetic differences over the long run between meshed and solid sheet grafts.

Infections

Emphasis on accuracy in diagnosing various forms of cutaneous gangrene and multiorganism symbiotic infections also reminded surgeons of the danger of overlooking acute necrotizing fasciitis, which may have no overlying skin diagnostic features. In patients with septicemia and toxemia more severe than explained by surface inflammatory signs, and particularly in patients who do not respond dramatically to proper antibiotic therapy, acute necrotizing fasciitis must be considered. A biopsy of deep fascia and frozen section interpretation are mandatory if treatment is to be successful. Nomenclature has been a problem in understanding synergistic soft tissue infections. For example, Fournier's gangrene, by definition, is limited to the scrotum, but the actual disease process and the need for early diagnosis and aggressive débridement are the same as for numerous other synergistic infections. Wound exudate contains many active enzymes and other biologically active substances that inhibit healing. Mechanical removal of exudate until the physical properties are typical of a transudate may be all that is required to start secondary healing or prepare wounds for secondary closure. In spite of the mechanical difficulties surgeons despise in paper drapes, bacteriologic and epidemiologic data reveal that paper drapes are probably here to stay. The incidence of infection and the control of costs argue strenuously now for utilization of disposable drapes. The incidence of wound infection following colon anastomoses has been shown to correlate with the thickness of subcutaneous fat in the abdominal wall. The reasons are not clear, but an obese individual has a significantly greater chance of developing abdominal wall infection following gastrointestinal surgery than a person of normal body weight. A new drug, ketoconazole, was reported to be less dangerous and just as effective as amphotericin B in the treatment of *Candida* sepsis. A report showing protection against generalized peritonitis by tetracycline peritoneal lavage raises questions that were thought to have been settled in the past. It is not clear whether the experimental and theoretical advantages of peritoneal lavage outweigh the disadvantages that have been accumulating over the years. Another reason to reduce to an absolute minimum the number of transfusions patients receive is that the immune response is measurably diminished in some patients following a blood transfusion. A high rate of postoperative infection was reported in patients with AIDS undergoing elective and emergency surgery. Finally, tetanus as a postoperative infection must not be overlooked. The medical and medicolegal implications of ignoring tetanus infection in even elective surgical procedures was emphasized.

Burns

Hypomagnesemia, although relatively rare in burned patients, continues to occur and is often not recognized simply because it is not thought of. Although glucose still is the most rapid source of energy, conservative administration of fat, particularly linoleic acid, provides even nutritional support that may be superior to infrequent meals, particularly in children. Rapid expenditure of energy in severely burned patients is still not understood completely, but there seems little doubt that work reported in 1987 supports the old concept that burned tissue elaborates some substance that drives metabolism mercilessly. Early excision of burned tissue, therefore, although not the complete answer to thermally induced hypermetabolism, still seems to be the most effective therapeutic measure available. Attention was called to fever in burned children, particularly the fact that, in children, fever is more labile and apparently a more nonspecific response to injury or illness than elevated temperature in adults. A report emphasizes the importance of not overtreating burned children who have high fever, particularly when physical examination does not reveal infection. Certainly in children, the physical examination has proved more accurate in diagnosing infection than has the temperature chart. Control of common infections in burned patients still seems to lead to eventual sepsis from *Candida,* particularly when antibiotics are continued for prolonged periods. *Candida* must be kept in mind and anti-*Candida* therapy, even amphotericin B, must be instituted early. Other anti-*Candida* drugs are available now but amphotericin B is becoming recognized as not nearly so dangerous as previously thought. The leukopenia occasionally seen following application of sulfadiazine silver to burn eschar is not considered serious in most patients today, but it can be avoided entirely by utilizing other topical silver salts, some of which actually appear more effective in preventing eschar infection. When a long bone such as tibia is burned and exposed, rapid coverage is mandatory if osteomyelitis is to be prevented. The unique muscle fiber arrangements in the tibialis anterior muscle were shown to be useful in splitting the muscle so that half of it could be utilized to cover exposed tibia while leaving the remainder to function normally. Conservative management of facial burns was emphasized again. Even badly damaged skin following a mixture of deep second degree and spotty third degree burns may heal on the face with a cosmetic and functional result superior to a free split or full thickness skin graft. Combination autologous and allogenic skin grafts were shown to provide useful adjuvants to healing that neither graft alone provides. Emphasis upon early recognition and treatment of respiratory tract thermal injury is still timely. Although no new therapy was advanced in 1987, early recognition and treatment was emphasized as necessary if fatal complications are to be avoided.

Transplantation

Speaking at a plenary session of the Transplantation Society at its 1986 Biennial International Meeting, Dr. Ronald Guttmann from Montreal detailed an analysis of the long-term (10 years or longer) outcomes of organ transplantation. The sobering statistics related to continued attrition in the recipient population are important realities to motivate continued research into improved methods of specific immunosuppression. While the field of organ transplantation has greatly expanded and begun to demonstrate its potential for treating large segments of the population with end-stage organ failure since the development of the immunosuppressant cyclosporine, the very encouraging short-term results achieved in all vascularized organ grafts to date must be weighed against the possibilities of long-range complications of the drug.

Cyclosporine nephrotoxicity, its major clinical drawback, is the subject of numerous investigations. Especially interesting are the experimental protocols addressing modification of prostanoid synthesis in the renal cortex during the administration of cyclosporine. Long-term examination of the histology of kidneys of patients receiving heart transplants indicates quite worrisome permanent histologic changes, although functional studies show reversion to normal after stopping the drug for even as long as 1 year.

Cytomegalovirus (CMV) infection remains one of the most serious complications of systemic immunosuppression. Gastrointestinal hemorrhage has now been attributed to CMV infection of GI tract mucosa; the elegant multicenter study of CMV immune globulin to prevent disease in renal transplant recipients, therefore, is viewed with great interest. Transplantation in individuals from tropical climates may also be complicated by parasitic infections such as strongyloides. In interesting studies of patients with strongyloides infection following immunosuppression, bacterial translocation appeared to play an important role in establishing systemic sepsis once the host mucosal defense barrier has been broken down.

For these reasons the investigations into the manipulation of the immune response to cause tolerance of the allograft have always been of great interest to those in the transplantation field. Monaco's group in Boston and Strober's group at Stanford have expanded their work into large-animal models and even to man. The use of recipient preparation with donor bone marrow and either total lymphoid irradiation (Strober) or antilymphocyte serum (Monaco) following establishment of an allograft with minimal immunosuppression holds great promise.

The studies of antigen expression and antigenicity of the donor tissue are also appealing for many of the same reasons. The roles of various lymphokines in inducing antigen expression, and especially the role of the interferons during viral infections, are likely to be found to be of major importance in initiating rejection phenomena.

The old controversy of donor-recipient matching through HLA testing has not gone away. Starzel has proposed a point system for objective allocation of renal allografts that deemphasizes the histocompatibility matching between donor and recipient. Other data, especially from Terasaki's and Sanfillipo's groups, continue to demonstrate significant improvement in outcome when no antigens are mismatched between donor and host. National organ sharing criteria are being adapted to these data.

Interest has persisted in hepatocyte transplantation for experimental subjects with liver failure. We also have an excellent report of the practical use of total artificial heart systems as bridges to transplantation in patients with end-stage heart failure. Small bowel transplantation has shown essentially no progress in terms of control of rejection and is no closer to practical application than it seemed a year ago.

Ethical problems in organ donation continue to need careful and reasoned analysis. As cardiac transplantation in infants has become a reality, anencephalic neonates as a source of donors has again been the subject of considerable thought.

Oncology and Tumor Immunology

It has long been assumed that the development of human tumors is associated with an immune response on the part of the host, although the nature of this immune response has been very difficult to pinpoint. Some of the most powerful evidence that host defenses play an important role in surveillance against the development of malignancies is to be found in the study of patients immunodepressed with pharmacologic or acquired diseases, most notably transplant recipients. In another of the fine series of reports from a voluntary tumor registry of transplant recipients maintained for years by Penn (reviewed in the transplantation section of this volume), the high risks for skin cancers in conventionally immunosuppressed patients and for lymphomas and Kaposi's sarcoma in cyclosporine-treated patients lend credence to the hypothesis that a normal immune system protects the host. The incidence of non-Hodgkin's lymphoma in cyclosporine-treated recipients of heart or liver allografts is especially high.

However, studies of the peripheral blood in search of either antibodies or cells mediating protection have generally been nonproductive. We do understand that certain cells appear to maintain general surveillance functions, such as the NK cells, but mononuclear cells, either in the circulating blood or in the region of the tumor itself, which have direct specific cytotoxic activity for the tumor, have been difficult to identify. In the papers reviewed in this year's section, evidence is provided that human tumors can be induced, perhaps by oncogenes, to express antigens of both the histocompatibility and tumor-specific varieties. These antigens are subject to regulation by lymphokines of various sorts: tumor necrosis factor, epidermal growth factor, and other lymphokines have been implicated. Mononuclear cells, particularly those in tumor-infiltrating lymphocyte populations, have also been shown to produce specific antitumor cytolytic activity and are capable of proliferating, when stimulated by interleukin-2, into large populations of cells with the potential for tumor cell lysis. The use of lymphokine-activated cells and interleukin-2 in clinical trials is proceeding slowly, largely because of the toxicity of systemically administered interleukin-2, but the use of this agent intraperitoneally or in smaller doses may permit a better cost-benefit ratio.

Studies of antigenicity of tumors and regulation of antigen expression, as well as functional capabilities of cells in surveillance or even in the facilitation of tumor growth, are proceeding rapidly. So are investigations in identification of oncogenes and point mutations occurring in hyperplastic states that appear to proceed to the development of tumors. These are especially exciting avenues of research; work to date in these fields must be considered preliminary.

Skin, Subcutaneous Tissue, and the Hand

A plea was made for less complex procedures for closing fingertip amputation wounds. Sacrifice of a few millimeters of length is a small price to pay for quick, uncomplicated healing and minimum time away from work. It is rarely necessary to perform local or distant flaps and free grafts. Experimental data showed that composite soft tissue grafts in the hand can be perfused from the venous side successfully. In 1988, it seems time to stop talking about reconstructive procedures for hands affected by cerebral palsy. Each cerebral palsy patient is so distinct that past experience with a large number of patients provides little insight as to what should be or even could be done for an individual problem. Treatment of neuromas by performing a centrocentral union via an autogenous nerve graft was reported to be an excellent way of controlling neuroma symptoms. Neurorrhaphy in patients with neuromas was performed by microepineural technique. The need for electrical conduction studies when evaluating patients with carpal tunnel syndrome seems even less clear than in previous years. Most experienced hand surgeons are decompressing the median nerve at the wrist because of the symptoms and physical findings, not because of electroneuromyographic results. Conduction studies probably are most needed for patients who are having difficulty deciding between surgical relief and continuation of conservative treatment. It was shown that flexor tendon grafts and repairs passed through an artificial or artificially induced fibrous sheath have reduced blood supply and delayed healing. Immobilization, therefore, should last for at least 4 weeks. Enthusiasm for early motion following repair of tendon lacerations continues. The need for a rubber band is not as definite now: the realization that good judgment in the extent of motion allowed is the important issue. Tenodesis, often overlooked as a method of reconstructing complicated tendon injuries, has the advantages of being simple, reliable, and usually permanent. Because many complex tendon restorations finally and unintentionally become tenodesis with an often less than optimal position, an intentional tenodesis, placing the joint in ideal functional position, is a major accomplishment. At least, attention was drawn to the morbidity of forearm donor sites for composite soft tissue grafts. Use of the forearm as a donor site for a distal or distant reconstructive procedure is almost never necessary. Attention was also drawn to treatment of malignant fibrous histiocytoma in digits. It should be remembered that evaluation of the degree of malignancy is more important in devising treatment than the name of the tumor. It is seldom, if ever, necessary to destroy function by amputation and radiation in patients who have only a low-grade malignancy.

The Breast

A recent report has shown that xeromammographic diagnosis of breast carcinoma was 36% accurate. This is a slight improvement over the 20% positive biopsy data reported following conventional mammographic techniques resulting in needle localization and excisional biopsy. In my judgment, a 36% positivity rate for biopsies is still too low for an effective cost-benefit analysis. It should not be necessary to subject 65% of women to an unnecessary operation because of a radiologic interpretation. Bone scintigraphy is not considered necessary as a preoperative examination for all women undergoing mastectomy for carcinoma. Only when experimental protocols require scintigraphy to evaluate new treatment regimens should bone studies be performed routinely. The cost of remnant preservation in patients undergoing lumpectomy for breast carcinoma still is being explored. Considerable restorative surgery frequently is necessary to make lumpectomy in some breasts an acceptable procedure. The question of the need for postoperative radiation following lumpectomy also is suspect. It may be that once it is more clear which patient should have lumpectomy and how wide lumpectomy should be, postoperative radiation may not be uniformly administered. The term *lumpectomy* itself is a fetish now; critical evaluation of data has not been completed. Another problem that surfaced in 1987 is what extent of axillary dissection should be performed when it is known that radiation will be administered. Again, if lumpectomy is truly sufficient, removal of immunologically active tissue such as axillary lymph nodes may be more valuable to the surgeon during this exploratory period than it ultimately will be to the patient with cancer in the affected area. The psychologic effects of mastectomy are changing. Particularly with the advent of limited excision, immediate or delayed reconstruction, and fewer side effects from expertly administered radiation, fear of mastectomy has been replaced by fear of chemotherapy. The psychologic damage caused by horror stories about complications of chemotherapy has replaced similar psychologic problems based on body image. The most elegant method for reconstructing the cosmetic disaster produced by radical mastectomy, skin loss, and radiation dermatitis is autogenous transfer of abdominal skin and fat on a rectus muscle pedicle. The procedure is a difficult and unforgiving one but has produced the best results reported so far. Fortunately, most women who have had modern modified radical mastectomy or local extirpative surgery do not require a transverse abdominal flap for reconstruction of the breast. Immediate restoration with a submuscular Silastic gel implant is gaining popularity. Most bad results have been from using too large a prosthesis or putting the prosthesis in a subcutaneous position where subsequent migration is more likely. A tissue expander is not usually required. A prosthesis of at least 300 cc can be inserted as a first procedure, and if it is not large enough, replacement with a larger prosthesis or reduction of the contralateral breast can be performed by only one additional procedure. Since two procedures are required when an expander is utilized, it is usually best to start with the largest prosthesis and wait to see if a second procedure is needed.

The Head and the Neck

The old question of what to do when metastatic carcinoma is found in the neck, but no primary lesion is detectable, resurfaced last year. Highly specialized diagnostic techniques are available now, and consultation with specialists is required to find the primary tumor in many patients. Most generalists apparently are no longer able to perform all of the highly specialized studies that can be utilized to locate obscure primary lesions. One new technique applied to head and neck oncology is magnetic resonance imaging. Magnetic resonance imaging has been shown effective in determining whether a parotid tumor is superficial or deep to the facial nerve. Questions were raised again about the need for radical extirpative surgery for a thyroglossal duct cyst as opposed to a sinus in the same location. No new evidence was presented to contradict the Sistrunk concept that even a cyst is only one representation of an area developmental defect and that a central core literally has to be removed to eliminate the high recurrence rate of cysts and sinus tracts in the thyroglossal duct area. Although a recommendation was made not to delay re-excision of an entire area when there is microscopic evidence of tumor at the margins, no new procedures were presented to eliminate the known errors of cutting, fixation, and misrepresentation of borders that often make it seem that a tumor has been incompletely excised when actually it was removed with a margin of normal tissue.

With increasing interest in complex methods of local destruction of tumors by various types of lasers, it was interesting to see reports reaffirming the excellence of local tumor destruction by skilled use of electrocautery. The combined use of megavoltage radiation and various other agents and modalities, such as cisplatin and chemotherapeutic drugs, continued to complicate evaluation of where we stand in the nonsurgical management of advanced head and neck carcinoma. There also seems to be a danger of overlooking past results of radical surgery and reconstruction of hypopharyngeal and oropharyngeal cancer. It is still possible, of course, to excise the lateral and posterior walls of the oropharynx and reconstruct the area with free or pedicle flaps even after radiation and chemotherapy have failed to control the local lesion. It is still not certain, even in 1988, that radiation combined with other agents is significantly better in treating head and neck cancer than expert administration of high voltage radiation alone. Cisplatin given with radiation may be an exception to this statement. Reconstruction of the anterior mandible is clearly best done by free transplantation of a composite tissue bone and soft tissue graft. Several new composite tissue grafts were reported, but donor site complications are not inconsequential. Finally, a plea was made for better tracheostomy scars that are not adherent to the trachea.

This can be accomplished by interposition of muscle and subcutaneous fat between the skin and tracheal wounds.

The Thorax

The review by Haskell defines the importance of lung cancer, which causes 28% of all cancer deaths. The importance of tobacco is most impressive, as it is thought to have a significant influence on etiology in over 90% of all lung cancers. Similarly impressive is a survey that found that 90% of American smokers would supposedly like to stop but only 10%–30% were able to do so. The report of bronchoplastic and angioplastic procedures in 248 pulmonary resections over a period of 10 years must be one of the largest in the world. It seems significant that a 5-year survival of 35% was obtained, even with this type of reconstructive operation. The improved survival reported by Shahian in treating 18 patients with Pancoast tumors is most encouraging. Only two late deaths occurred from local recurrence, documenting the efficacy of combining radiotherapy with surgical excision. Wright proceeded with an even more radical resection in 21 patients, resecting the subclavian artery in four and a portion of the vertebral body in five. Five-year survival was 27%. The review article by Korvick concerning legionnaires' disease is a timely one. As with many diseases, the key to diagnosis is considering the possibility. This is especially important with this disease because the progressive pneumonia can be fatal unless specific treatment with intravenous erythromycin is begun.

The dread complication of postpneumonectomy esophagopleural fistula was successfully treated in two patients by Mud by combining a muscle flap with a thoracoplasty. With the impressive results obtained with large muscle flaps for a variety of thoracic problems, the prompt use of an appropriate muscle flap should significantly decrease the mortality of this rare but lethal complication.

The report of successful lung transplantation in five patients, with four long-term survivors, is a landmark accomplishment. The magnitude of this achievement is illustrated by the fact that in the previous 20 years throughout the world only one patient was discharged from the hospital following a lung transplantation.

A report describes experiences with 18 patients with chylothoraces treated in London over a period of 25 years. Eleven of these developed chylothoraces after thoracic operations; seven were subsequently operated upon. Chylothorax is an unusual but serious complication of thoracic surgery. For the past few years, several reports have emphasized a nonoperative approach, utilizing a special low-fat diet or even hyperalimentation. Experience with modern surgical techniques shows that patients in whom drainage has not stopped within a few days should be promptly reoperated upon; almost always a large lacerated lymphatic, visibly leaking chyle, can be found and ligated to promptly cure the problem. When chylothorax follows a thoracic operation, nonoperative therapy for more than a few days would seem rarely justified.

Congenital Heart Disease

The classic report by Trusler describes experiences with 329 patients in whom Mustard's operation for transposition of the great vessels was employed. The report is from the hospital in Toronto where Mustard performed his first operation in 1963. The operative mortality for the last 10 years has been near 1%. A most important point is that significant right ventricular dysfunction has been uncommon, even in patients followed for over 15 years.

The widening applicability of Fontan's operation for different congenital defects is well documented in the report by Kirklin describing experiences with 102 patients. With current techniques, young age is no longer associated with an increased risk of operation.

A paper from Lyon, France, clearly states that traumatic tricuspid insufficiency is far more common than reported, for the authors were able to collect 12 cases from their own city over a period of years. The ease with which diagnosis can be made by echocardiography, combined with the probability that reconstruction can be performed in most patients, makes this prophetic paper an important one.

Another significant paper from the University of Alabama describes experiences with 127 patients with a double-outlet right ventricle. The importance of the anatomical type of double-outlet was clearly documented; long-term survival was nearly 98% in one group but only 22% in another.

A significant report from Vanderbilt University describes good results with an emergency closed pulmonic valvulotomy for critical pulmonic stenosis in neonates. In recent years, more than one group have described performing valvulotomy with a 3- to 4-minute period of circulatory arrest without bypass, a surgical feat that seems unduly hazardous if a simpler approach is equally satisfactory.

A particularly significant report from the Children's Hospital in Boston describes excellent results in 11 patients in whom the Takeuchi procedure was performed for anomalous origin of the left coronary artery. There was no early or late mortality, a most impressive result.

Finally, the hazard of phrenic nerve paralysis in operations on infants, especially with repeat operations, was clearly indicated in a report from Toronto describing experiences with 125 patients on whom over 7,000 cardiac operations were performed. Traction must be the primary cause, because the majority ultimately recovered. This, in turn, indicates that awareness of the vulnerability of the phrenic nerve to traction should significantly decrease the frequency of this potentially serious complication.

Valvular Heart Disease

The increasing popularity of reconstructive operations for mitral insufficiency, rather than replacement, is well reflected in the review by Bashour. At New York University, over 90% of patients with nonrheumatic mitral insufficiency have been treated by reconstruction over the past 3 to 5 years with excellent results. The successful repair of posterior left ventricular disruption in two patients is particularly significant because this type of repair is usually unsuccessful. Because posterior wall disruption is a highly lethal complication following mitral valve replacement, the keynote is clearly prevention. I have not seen this complication since the policy of preserving a few chordae to the mural leaflet annulus was adopted in 1981. The report by Barratt-Boyes of long-term results with antibiotic-sterilized aortic homograft valves is particularly significant, describing results with 248 patients followed for 9 to 16 years following operation. Seventy-eight percent were free of incompetence 10 years after operation. Recent reports describing a different method of valve preservation suggest that even better results may be achievable.

Coronary Heart Disease

A major question discussed previously is whether the remarkable long-term patency of internal mammary grafts is due to the internal mammary itself or the use of a pedicle. The report by Loop of experiences with 156 patients with complicated free grafts is quite significant; the long-term patency was significantly less than in standard internal mammary operations. If the internal mammary could be consistently used as a free graft, its applicability would be much enhanced.

The applicability of complex internal mammary bypasses is further documented in the report by Rankin, who performed 841 anastomoses in 207 patients. There was a remarkable 99% patency with 338 internal mammary anastomoses.

Additional data confirming the impressive longevity with double mammary grafts were reported by Geha. Of 43 patients with double mammary grafts, 100% survived 5 years and 98%, 10 years.

The serious problem of cardiogenic shock following myocardial infarction was discussed in a report by Guyton: only two deaths occurred.

Cardiogenic shock following a massive myocardial infarction is highly lethal. Unless thrombolytic therapy is applicable, emergency bypass is probably the only chance of survival. Because muscle may become irreversibly infarcted within 3 to 4 hours, the time interval within which bypass must be done is very short.

The report from Switzerland of the long-term follow-up of the first 133 patients undergoing angioplasty is quite significant. Coronary angioplasty began in that country. It was particularly impressive that stenosis occurred in 30% of patients within the first 6 months but was seldom seen thereafter. Only 19 of the 133 patients ultimately required bypass. It should be remembered, however, that these were some of the most favorable patients with coronary disease, for many had predominantly single-vessel disease.

Miscellaneous Cardiac Conditions and the Great Vessels

The report of myocardial preservation studies in neonatal piglet hearts is most significant; the findings are different from those found in experimental studies in adult animals or patients. Specifically, simple topical hypothermia was more effective than crystalloid cardioplegia. Also, normocalcemic blood cardioplegia with potassium was far better than blood cardioplegia with a lowered calcium. These findings indicate that many of the theoretic concepts of myocardial preservation are empirical and are valid only for the experimental model studied. The report by Akins continues to document that, in his hands, intermittent hypothermic fibrillatory arrest for short periods of time can be performed with a high degree of safety. This is an important alternative method if standard cardioplegic techniques cannot be used.

A multi-institutional study of results of temporary cardiac support, with a mortality of 85% among 41 patients, suggests that the type of circulatory assist pump used is not the crucial factor. Probably, the promptness with which the left ventricle is decompressed by some form of circulatory assist is the most crucial factor, because it prevents the progression of myocardial edema to irreversible infarction.

A report from New York University indicates the hazards of ice slush within the pericardium. The 73% frequency of phrenic nerve injury when slush is extensively employed suggests that ice slush should be abandoned. The original Shumway technique of constant pericardial lavage with cold electrolyte is equally effective and far safer. The report from Germany, about disastrous complications in four patients in whom Teflon felt pledgets became infected, is an important one. As the author indicates, frequent use of felt is simply a bad surgical habit that should be corrected. When pledgets are necessary, pledgets of autogenous pericardium or vein are usually safer. A report from Scandinavia documents the effectiveness of treating mediastinitis by operative débridement, sternal closure, and continuous mediastinal irrigation, which was successful in 13 of 15 patients. This point is emphasized because there is a popular tendency to treat all patients by débridement and muscle flap, an effective but unduly complicated procedure for the majority of patients. Certainly, however, in the minority of patients who do not respond to closed mediastinal irrigation, the muscle flap procedure should be employed promptly.

The safety of delayed sternal closure, described by Fanning in a series of 57 patients, is almost astonishing. Infection developed in only two of the 57 patients. Quite probably in the past a postoperative death may have been erroneously diagnosed as "progressive cardiac failure" that was simply caused by compression of an edematous heart by the standard sternal closure. How often one can safely perform open heart surgery with heparinization after a stroke is addressed in the report by Zisbrod. In the 15 patients operated on between 2 and 28 days following onset of neurologic injury, no exacerbation of the injury occurred.

Three different papers describe experiences with the hypothermic circulatory arrest technique for the treatment of aneurysms in the ascending and transverse aortic arch. All six patients operated on with periods of circulatory arrest between 16 and 32 minutes recovered without any neurologic defect. Somatosensory monitoring was done in 38 patients in the series reported by Dasmahapatra. No permanent neurologic problems occurred, although 25% of the patients developed reversible spinal cord ischemia. The somatosensory monitoring was helpful, for the operative technique was modified to avoid complete loss of potentials for more than 14 minutes. Although not yet extensive all available data support the concept that paraplegia following operation for coarctation is extremely rare if somatosensory potentials remain intact, or if the duration of hypotension (below 60 mm Hg) in the aorta distal to the cross-clamp is less than 20 minutes.

Finally, the report by Nakayama is most impressive, describing the results of 15 patients with Wilms' tumors that extended up the vena cava into the heart. These data came from three National Wilms' Tumor Studies. It is quite remarkable that in this group of 15 there were no operative deaths; in 11 patients there was a 2-year actuarial survival of 86%.

The Arteries

The results of a multi-institutional questionnaire indicate that the use of thrombolytic therapy in the treatment of peripheral arterial ischemia is associated with a success rate of about 50% and a morbidity rate of about 20%. In an institutional report, an overall success rate of 20%–38% was reported, but some degree of thrombolysis occurred in 88% of patients. Limb salvage was achieved in 84% of patients. This experience suggests that intra-arterial thrombolysis is best reserved for people with acute limb ischemia caused by an arterial embolus and for those whose femoral or tibial runoff is not likely to require remedial operation. The efficacy of the retroperitoneal approach was compared with the transperitoneal approach. Nasogastric intubation and initiation of oral feeding were significantly prolonged in the transperitoneal group, as was the postoperative hospitalization. These data suggest that the retroperitoneal approach is preferable in routine aortoiliac reconstruction. It was shown that a supraceliac-to-femoral artery bypass is a useful procedure for treatment of patients whose multiple previous aortic reconstructions have failed. Performing this procedure through a thoracoabdominal or flank incision facilitates the operation.

One series of 20 patients with secondary aortoduodenal fistula treated by duodenal repair, excision of the graft, and placement of the new graft in the same location is reported; 83% had no further related problem. Another group reports success with the same procedure and successful direct suture repair of the defect without replacement of the graft. These two articles make a plea for a more conservative approach to the problem.

The natural history of carotid occlusion has been addressed, and the conclusion is that it is of limited value to use the presence or absence of transient ischemia attacks to predict stroke. There is a high mortality related to stroke in patients with carotid artery occlusion, and this should be taken into consideration when therapy is being decided. Neurologic symptoms in the setting of internal carotid artery occlusion may be due to embolic events through the external carotid artery, hemodynamic insufficiency resulting from inadequate collateral development, or the propagation of clot intracranially. In selected circumstances, external carotid artery reconstruction should be considered among the treatment options. In one series of 195 external carotid endarterectomies, resolution was seen in 83% of the patients. Symptomatic thrombosis of the internal carotid artery in the early postoperative period has been managed by emergency operation. Surgical treatment of thrombosis occurring after carotid endarterectomy is associated with clinical improvement in about 60% of patients.

Patency rates were comparable when reversed saphenous and in situ vein grafts were used for infrainguinal reconstruction. The fact that many of the in situ bypasses were anastomosed to vessels at the ankle, whereas none of the reversed bypasses were, suggests that there is a clear superiority of the in situ graft for infrapopliteal reconstruction. It has been shown that reoperation after failure of an infrainguinal bypass graft is associated with long-term limb salvage in most cases without significant compromise in patient safety. Because of the demonstrated safety and efficacy of surgical treatment, repair of popliteal aneurysm is recommended in most patients. There does exist a small group of asymptomatic high-risk patients with small popliteal aneurysms in whom a conservative, nonoperative approach has been shown to be reasonable. A report provides evidence that sympathectomy provides relief in the overwhelming majority of patients with causalgia. It has been shown that involvement of the major arterial circulation does not preclude resection of sarcomas of the extremity with limb salvage.

The Veins and the Lymphatics

A study of the fate of venous repair after civilian trauma demonstrated that a substantial percentage of venous repairs will thrombose in the postoperative period, especially if interposition vein grafting is used. In that series, limb salvage was not adversely affected by venous thrombosis. Noninvasive testing did not provide an accurate assessment of venous patency. The long-term results after venous thrombectomy combined with arterial venous fistula were evaluated. The fistula was closed 3 months after thrombectomy. Good results were obtained in the majority of patients and almost half had a totally patent iliac vein.

Daily has accumulated an impressive series of 41 patients with chronic pulmonary embolism treated by thromboendarterectomy. The operative procedure is a complex one, using multiple periods of circulatory arrest, fortunately without neurologic injury.

The Esophagus

In assessing a large series of infants and children who underwent symptomatic gastroesophageal reflux, it was demonstrated that over half had delayed gastric emptying. Demonstration of delayed gastric emptying indicates that a pyloroplasty should be added to the gastroesophageal fundoplication. In another report, fundoplication successfully controlled symptoms of gastroesophageal reflux in 92% of children. Esophageal replacement by total gastric transposition was performed mainly for esophageal atresia in a group of infants. The results compared favorably with a large previous experience in colon interposition. In an adult population of patients with benign esophageal disease, colon interposition achieved good or excellent results in 75% of patients despite a 30% major complication rate and a 37% late reoperative rate. Isoperistaltic jejunal interposition has also been reported to provide good results in patients with complicated esophageal disease.

Nonmalignant esophageal perforation is best managed by primary closure with drainage regardless of the duration of the perforation, but in selected patients with cervical esophageal perforation, nonoperative management has a role. In one series, most esophageal gunshot wounds were successfully closed primarily. Severe necrosis of the esophagus caused by caustic ingestion may necessitate emergency esophagogastrectomy because of transmural necrosis. A stripping procedure, performed through a cervicotomy and a laparotomy, appears to be safer than open thoracic esophagectomy. One report indicates that over the past 25 years the 5-year survival in patients with carcinoma of the esophagus increased from 2% to 6%. Esophageal resection was accomplished in the more recent group of patients in about 33%. The 5-year survival of patients undergoing resection by the Ivor Lewis technique had a 13% 5-year survival. The survival rate was not improved by adjuvant radiation therapy. In another report, 5-year survival of 86% was reported for patients with stage I carcinoma of the esophagus and 15% for stage III carcinoma of the esophagus. These results support the continued use of the Ivor Lewis esophagogastrectomy for treatment. Yet another group assessed patients in whom combined modality therapy was used. The patients received chemotherapy and radiation therapy preoperatively followed by esophagogastrectomy. Of the 29 patients who completed the integrated therapy, none had residual tumor in the specimen, and 25 of the 29 patients were alive at the time of the report.

The Stomach and the Duodenum

The finding of curved bacilli (now known as *Campylobacter pyloridis*) in the gastric epithelium of patients with chronic gastritis and duodenal ulcer has evoked great interest. Their presence has been known for years, but recent studies strongly suggest an etiologic relationship with gastritis, and perhaps with duodenal ulcer. There do appear to be at least two kinds of gastritis, one associated with chemical injury (alkaline bile reflux) and the other in association with *C. pyloridis*. The relationship may be even more complex since reflux may be sufficiently severe as to injure the antral mucosa and render it inhospitable to see *C. pyloridis*. Operations for duodenal ulcer that permit bile reflux are not associated with postoperative findings of the organism in antral mucosa, whereas after selective proximal vagotomy, which protects against reflux, the organisms persist. Are we all going to have to learn a new concept of the pathogenesis of duodenal ulcer? Time will tell. One idea about the causation of ulcer disease that has waxed and waned is the role of stress. The relationship was clear to our grandmothers, but most recent studies have concluded that ulcer patients have not been subjected to greater stress than their colleagues. There is now strong evidence that ulcer patients are not as well equipped to handle the normal problems of life as are nonulcer patients. Hypochondriasis, a negative perception of life, dependency, and low ego strength appear to occur frequently in duodenal ulcer patients. What about patients who have had their ulcers cured by surgery? Will they continue to have this same set of personality disorders? Are the disorders cause or effect?

What is the best operative treatment for duodenal ulcer? Again there is no consensus, but evidence that selective proximal vagotomy is remarkably free of side effects continues to accumulate. The procedure clearly has a high rate of recurrence (at least 10% in 10 years) but all other postoperative problems are greatly diminished. Proper evaluation will depend upon how easy the recurrences are to manage, and the jury is still out on that question. Efforts to control massive duodenal ulcer hemorrhage by laser photocoagulation have given varying results. Some authorities report success; others, failure. Even though achievement of nonoperative control of ulcer bleeding is the Holy Grail of many endoscopists, there is as yet no clear-cut demonstration that it is safe and effective. How safe is it to operate on patients with perforated duodenal ulcer? If they have a concomitant major medical illness, if they have been in shock preoperatively, and if the perforation is more than 24 hours old, the mortality rate will be devastating. Results after treatment of perforation by simple closure plus proximal gastric vagotomy are excellent, but the problem in teaching hospitals in this country is that there are insufficient numbers of operations for duodenal ulcer to allow training of residents, and in those same hospitals, residents do the majority of emergency operations for perforated ulcer. Perforated gastric ulcers are not common and results after either resection or simple patch closure are difficult to interpret. Retrospective studies of the problem may show that mortality is greatest after patch closure, but doesn't that just mean that the sickest patients were relegated to the simplest procedure? A much higher mortality rate has been reported in duodenal ulcer patients whose perforation was treated by simple closure than in those treated by definitive operation. These results suggest that gastric resection is performed on low-risk patients. Economic issues greatly affect our treatment decisions. The relatively low cost of H_2-receptor blockade treatment has been repeatedly cited as a factor in favor of nonoperative therapy of duodenal ulcer. When viewed from a long-term perspective, however, the high rate of ulcer recurrence after cessation of H_2-receptor blockade (up to 70% in some series) gives strong indications that many patients may receive drug treatment for years, and some for life. After 8 years, maintenance drug therapy may well be more expensive than elective surgery. The only reliable way to cure ulcer disease is by operation.

Resection appears to offer the best results in treatment of gastric lymphoma and the potential additive effects of postoperative radiotherapy are not clear. Survival appears to depend upon size of the tumor and presence of lymph node metastases.

New techniques fascinate surgeons. Leakage from esophagogastric anastomoses in patients with carcinoma of the distal esophagus or proximal stomach can apparently be reduced greatly by wrapping the residual stomach around the esophagus in a manner analogous to a Nissen fundoplication. Percutaneous endoscopic gastrostomy appears to be simple and amazingly safe. Mortality is rare, complications are few, and the method appears to offer a simple and brisk solution to a nagging problem.

The Small Intestine

Experts in bowel function have long hoped that pathologic alterations in small bowel motility might be treated by external electrical pacing, in a manner analogous to treating cardiac dysrhythmias. Particularly attractive is the possibility of slowing rapid intestinal transit in patients with the short bowel syndrome by retrograde pacing. Early attempts at achieving this result have failed, and it is not clear whether the idea is impractical or whether proper instrumentation is not yet available. Although most everyone recognizes that all treatment for Crohn's disease is palliative, now and again surgeons will do a wide resection in order to "get beyond the disease." Results are now clear that surgical treatment should be aimed at local removal of the site of perforation or obstruction or fistulization without an attempt at cure. Accepting this premise, frozen section evaluation of the lines of resection becomes moot and unneeded. The concept of hydrostatic reduction of intussusception in children is well established, but the success rate is often less than half, and bowel infarction is common. The reason for this, of course, is that patients come in late. Recurrent intussusception is not uncommon after hydrostatic reduction but is virtually prevented by operation. Once or twice a year, a surgeon in busy practice will confront a patient who is bleeding occultly from the gut. One of the causes for that frustrating problem is hereditary telangiectasia, a rare lesion that can be diagnosed with regularity by upper and lower endoscopy. Recurrent epistaxis is common and may provide a clue for diagnosis. Patients with systemic lupus erythematosus may develop severe abdominal pains and signs of peritonitis. This development is a signal for high-dose steroid therapy (60–500 mg per day of prednisone). If patients fail to improve, they should be operated on, but prompt initiation of steroid therapy may obviate the need for operation. Although serotonin is the agent we first think of in relationship to the malignant carcinoid syndrome, other agents, such as substance P and tachykinins, may also be secreted. The vast majority of patients with the malignant carcinoid syndrome have midgut tumors, and serotonin receptor antagonist therapy often eradicates the diarrhea. The long-acting somatostatin analogue is effective in blocking the flush and in lowering plasma levels of tachykinin. High rates of 5-year survival can be achieved with the use of interferon and somatostatin. Radiation enteritis is one of the major problems limiting efficacy of the treatment of pelvic malignancies. The terrible consequences of severe irradiation injury to the small bowel may present insoluble problems. Recent experimental studies suggest that keeping the bowel out of the pelvis by means of an absorbable polyglycolic-acid mesh sling may entirely prevent the problem. The sling is readily placed, is completely absorbed within 6 months, causes no adhesions, and allows administration of a full tumoricidal dose to a pelvic organ without small bowel injury. There appears to be no contraindication and the method offers tremendous promise.

The Colon and the Rectum

The outlook for most patients with colovesical fistula is good. The most common etiology is diverticulitis, followed by cancer and Crohn's disease. If the urinary tract has not been greatly damaged by long-standing contamination, most patients respond well to one-stage resection. The diagnostic study of choice is a barium enema. The rate of cell proliferation in colonic crypts of patients at risk for familial colon cancer can be diminished by adding calcium to the diet, and recent experimental studies show that carcinogenesis can also be retarded by dietary calcium. The mechanism is unknown. Should we all be taking daily calcium supplements? Flow cytometric analysis of DNA from human colorectal cells shows better survival in patients with a diploid pattern of DNA than in those with an aneuploid pattern. This pattern is apparently sufficiently homogenous in histologic sections taken from different areas of the tumor that a clinical decision can be made with some confidence from one or two biopsies. In patients who are candidates for local excision of a rectal carcinoma, determination of a diploid pattern in a preoperative biopsy may provide evidence for a better prognosis than if an aneuploid pattern is found. Gastrin clearly appears to stimulate development and growth of colon cancer, and recent studies have shown that this stimulation may be demonstrated in cell culture by application of minute quantities of gastrin that fit the definition of "physiologic." Can we treat colon cancer with agents that block gastrin receptors on colon cells? Current gastrin receptor antagonists are weak and nonspecific, but more potent agents are in the pipeline and deserve clinical trials. Clinical observations have linked gallstones and cholecystectomy to an increased incidence of colon cancer. The relationship has not been shown in a prospective study, and the problem is, who should serve as the control for colon cancer patients?

What should we do with a patient who has had the endoscopic removal of a polyp that shows cancer? Is it safe to leave the colonic segment in place if the stalk is negative? Patients who showed recurrence had incomplete excision, poorly differentiated tumor, invasion of the line of resection, invasion of the stalk, or invasion of venous or lymphatic channels. In the absence of those conditions, local excision appears safe. Intraoperative ultrasonography appears to be the hands-down method of choice in localizing hepatic metastases, and surgeons caring for patients with colon cancer need to learn the method. Sensitivity rates as high as 98% have been reported. How commonly does radiation therapy convert a fixed rectal carcinoma to operability, and what cure rate can be expected after operation? The 5-year survival rate varies from 9% to 28% and clearly depends on patient selection. One problem is whether the tumor is truly unresectable to begin with. Creation of a colostomy and elevation of the small bowel out of the pelvis with a synthetic collagen sling might allow a truly tumoricidal dose to the rectum without injury to the small bowel. All surgeons know that local recurrence of cancer of the rectum follows incomplete resection. Studies from Leeds suggest that whole-mount specimens examined grossly and histologically may provide a method for evaluation of lateral spread. Lateral margins were involved with cancer in 25% of patients, and in those, the incidence of local recurrence was 85%. The outlook for patients with anal carcinoma has been greatly improved by the development of a combined chemotherapy-irradiation regimen followed by local excision. Early results with this method appear to be at least twice as good as those with surgery alone. Most patients with familial adenomatous polyposis (Gardner's syndrome) have in the past been treated by total abdominal colectomy with anastomosis of the ileum to the rectum, followed by careful monitoring of the rectal mucosa for development of further polyps. The question today is whether these patients should be treated by colectomy, mucosal proctectomy, and ileoanal anastomosis. Recent experience gives strong evidence that ileorectal anastomosis is safe, and a policy of colectomy with anastomosis (leaving in 12–15 cm of the rectum) followed by conscientious lifelong follow-up is advocated. The procedure involving proctocolectomy with mucosal proctectomy, pelvic pouch of the ileum, and ileoanal anastomosis appears to be the treatment of choice in young patients who require operation for ulcerative colitis or familial polyposis. Comparison of the J-shaped versus the S-shaped ileal reservoir shows little difference in function. A high frequency of bowel-related symptoms and soilage persists. Are these reservoirs necessary? Would it be legitimate to compare them with a straight ileorectal anastomosis? In the meantime, there is a report from Copenhagen on a plug device that expands to occlude a colostomy to provide for continence. Could this be adapted for ileostomies? Last, good results have been reported with in-office division of the internal anal sphincter while the patient receives local anesthesic.

The Liver and the Spleen

Intraoperative ultrasonography has become an important tool, providing a definition of common duct stones and facilitating hepatic resection. In patients with hepatocellullar carcinoma, ultrasonography helps determine the extent of spread within the liver and also acts as a direct guide for the vascular anatomy, expediting resectional procedures. A report of a large series and a review of the literature demonstrate that most hepatic hemangiomas do not require resection. Resection is performed because of associated pain or tumor size that encroaches on the stomach or puts the liver at risk for trauma. Spontaneous rupture of hepatic hemangioma occurs very infrequently. The effects of pregnancy or of contraceptive medication on tumor growth are inconsistent. The regenerative process of the liver following major resection has been studied histologically. Evidence of active regeneration is found within 10–35 days in patients with normal livers. In livers with cirrhosis or hepatitis, histologic evidence of regeneration occurs during the first 2 months but is substantially less than in the normal liver. Extensive unroofing of a unilocular solitary hepatic cyst minimizes the likelihood of cyst recurrence and obviates the need for resection.

Experience is reported with 225 major hepatic resections for primary carcinoma of the liver; 5-year survival rate was 18%. Another series reported a 25% 5-year survival rate: recurrence of carcinoma was the main cause of death in over half the patients. Yet another series has reported a 5-year survival rate for patients undergoing liver resection for colorectal metastases. Several patients had encouraging results with resection of secondary metastases after the first liver resection. A randomized study compared systemic therapy with hepatic arterial chemotherapy and noted that the latter increased the response rate for hepatic metastases from colorectal carcinoma, but there was no statistically significant difference in survival.

A report details a series of patients with superior mesenteric portal vein obstruction with proved chronic pancreatitis. The splenic vein was included in the majority of these patients. There is continued enthusiasm for the use of endoscopic sclerotherapy; a prospective randomized study concluded that endoscopic sclerotherapy and shunt surgery provided similar results in survival, hepatic function, frequency of encephalopathy, and cost. Endoscopic sclerotherapy is as good as surgical shunting for the acute management of variceal hemorrhage in poor risk patients with massive bleeding. If bleeding continues in these patients, they should be considered for an elective shunt. Endoscopic sclerotherapy also provides control of bleeding in patients with extrahepatic portal venous obstruction. Esophageal varices can be essentially eradicated in these patients.

It has also been shown that under specific conditions, emergency portacaval shunts result in an acceptable long-term survival rate, and the operation should not be abandoned. A mesocaval interposition shunt has also achieved good results; an actuarial survival rate of 70% was achieved for 5 years. Encephalopathy rate was 10%. In time the mesocaval shunt was converted to a total shunt, and this occurrence was not accompanied by increased encephalopathy. The portal hemodynamics after a distal splenorenal shunt have been assessed: morbidity was least when both hepatic portal perfusion and sinusoidal pressures were maintained at near preoperative levels. The Budd-Chiari syndrome has been successfully treated by retrohepatic inferior venacavaplasty in side-to-side portacaval shunt. In the nonalcoholic patients, the Sugiura devascularization procedure has been shown to result in a low operative mortality, a low recurrence rate, and an absence of encephalopathy. The survival rate is also excellent.

Yet another report suggests selective management of blunt splenic trauma. The criteria for nonoperative management should be absolute hemodynamic stability, minimal peritoneal findings, and a requirement of less than two units transfusion. Most patients operated on should have splenic injury repair, but in the presence of associated life-threatening injuries, repair is generally precluded. More late septic complications occur following incidental splenectomy than following splenectomy for trauma. The mortality following major septic complications is reported to be 7%, less than indicated in previous series. Careful follow-up and education after splenectomy may reduce this mortality rate. Pyogenic splenic abscess is noted in patients who are intravenous drug addicts; *Staphylococcus aureus* has been shown to be the predominant bacteriologic agent. A high index of suspicion is warranted in this group of patients if there is fever or abdominal discomfort. Reports continue to indicate that splenectomy results in an immediate and sustained platelet response rate in about three quarters of patients with idiopathic thrombocytopenic purpura; one report suggests that the response rate is lower in older patients. Neither platelet antibody titers nor the measurement of platelet survival or turnover predicts the platelet response to splenectomy in these patients.

The Biliary Tract

A report reveals that conservative management of symptomatic cholelithiasis during pregnancy is often associated with recurrent episodes requiring hospitalization and significant rate of fetal loss; operation performed during the second trimester was associated with little maternal morbidity, no fetal loss, and a substantial reduction in hospital stay. Data have been presented suggesting that a more selective policy of operative cholangiography is appropriate. Such a policy would result in an incidence of unsuspected stones of less than 1%. In a prospective randomized study it was shown that the use of suction drains following cholecystectomy may predispose to the development of subhepatic collections rather than prevent these collections. A series of patients with acute cholangitis who did not respond to conservative therapy has been managed by endoscopic sphincterotomy reserving early operation for those who did not improve following the endoscopic procedure. Elective cholecystectomy following successful endoscopic sphincterotomy was avoided in the elderly and frail patients. Unilateral hepatic duct obstruction is an uncommon lesion usually resulting from operative injury. It is best treated by hepaticojejunostomy rather than repeated dilatations. Patients with biliary obstruction related to malignant disease were randomized to determine whether the endoscopic or percutaneous approach was preferable for insertion of a biliary stent. There was a higher mortality associated with percutaneous stents due to the complication of hemorrhage and bile leak, and the endoscopic technique had a significantly higher success rate for the relief of jaundice.

The Pancreas

Pancreatic transplantation has survived a period of experimental evaluation and is now accepted as a therapeutic procedure for severe diabetic patients. In addition to rejection, the main problem is what to do with the exocrine secretion, and preference appears to have shifted to drainage into the urinary bladder. Such drainage affords an ability to monitor early rejection through urinary measurement of quantitative amylase output. The controversy continues regarding the significance of pancreas divisum in the pathogenesis of pancreatitis. Most recent evidence fails to support a relationship, and pancreas divisum appears to be a normal anatomical variant that only rarely causes pancreatic pain. What should a surgeon do with a patient who is a candidate for a Puestow pancreaticojejunostomy and who also has a pseudocyst? Simultaneous drainage of both the cyst and the duct appears to be safe, provided the cyst is not infected. Metabolic studies with stabile isotopes have shown that abnormalities of glucose metabolism in patients with severe pancreatitis are the same as those in severely septic patients. Pancreatitis patients are heavily dependent upon fats for energy and have a great disability in the utilization of glucose, either endogenous or exogenous.

What is the best way to localize an insulinoma? Different groups tout selective pancreatic vein catheterization for measurement of insulin or intraoperative localization of tumors by ultrasonography. Both methods work, and the results are probably additive. Intraoperative sonography is probably the best method, and resolution is now sufficiently good so as to allow detection of a 3-mm insulinoma. Long experience with patients with gastrinomas show a bewildering spectrum of biologic aggression. Some patients go along for years with little trouble, and others are consumed rapidly by aggressive tumor. A recent report of gastrinoma metastatic to bones suggests that this may not be a rare occurrence, although only seven cases have been reported. It sounds rare to me. All bone metastasis was associated with death, so it must be considered a grave sign. Is it safe to locally excise a benign tumor of the ampulla? It may become malignant, and the safety of local excision is dependent on clear histologic evidence that all the tumor was removed at wide local excision and then upon a mutual decision between patient and surgeon about frequency and diligence of follow-up examination. If the tumor is not fully excised or if there is a recurrence, a Whipple resection must be considered. Estrogen receptors have long been known to be present in the pancreas and in human pancreatic cancer. Recent studies with tamoxifen and with an analog of luteinizing hormone releasing hormone in the treatment of patients with metastatic disease have shown an increase in median survival. This lead should be followed aggressively since the tumor is nearly 100% lethal. Any glimmer of hope merits close and immediate attention. Cystic tumors of the pancreas are potentially curable. Cystadenocarcinomas may have a 5-year survival rate of 20%. These patients often have a prolonged prodrome of symptoms, and ultrasound studies of patients with mild persistent abdominal pain may yield early diagnosis. The question of whether a gastrojejunostomy is a useful addition to biliary diversion in patients with inoperable carcinoma of the head of the pancreas is unsettled. The persuasive evidence against it is the paradox that the more a patient seems to need a gastrojejunostomy (that is, the more imminent duodenal obstruction appears to be), the less likely she or he will have a favorable course. Impending duodenal obstruction is a harbinger of early death. Is any palliative surgical effort worthwhile in these patients? There is great interest in preserving the pylorus in patients undergoing pancreaticoduodenectomy, but whether saving the pylorus compromises the chance for cure in resecting carcinoma of the head of the pancreas seems unsettled and almost ignored. The preservation of the pylorus in patients undergoing pancreaticoduodenectomy for benign disease or for cancer that is not adjacent to the first part of the duodenum seems logical.

The Endocrine Glands

Although the risk of development of carcinoma of the thyroid after irradiation of the head, neck, or upper mediastinum has been well recognized for almost 40 years, the complication was not anticipated after cervical irradiation for Hodgkin's disease because the irradiation dose used was assumed to be sufficient to destroy the thyroid. A few cases of thyroid cancer have developed, and patients irradiated for Hodgkin's disease should be watched carefully. It may be possible to prevent the development by preirradiation suppression of the gland with exogenous thyroxine. The true incidence of thyroid carcinoma in solitary thyroid nodules is one of the great mysteries of the world. Various incidences reflect varying degrees of selection of the population at risk. In all comers, the incidence is probably low. Another variable is the difficulty in accurately assessing solitary nodules by physical examination. Many turn out to be multiple. Recent studies suggest that the incidence of cancer in multinodular goiters approaches that of solitary nodules. Again, the problem is confused by prior selectivity. The high-frequency ultrasonographic apparatus used for detection of small tumors is immensely promising in localizing masses in the neck. In patients with medullary cancer of the thyroid, detection of metastatic cervical lymph nodes was 100% accurate, even though only one third of them were palpable. A study from West Germany reported correct localization in 25 of 29 patients with tumors of the parathyroid. These findings suggest that we should greatly increase our use of the method. Experience with a huge series of patients with hyperparathyroidism has shown that recurrent disease is limited to patients with involvement of more than one gland. Those patients with recurrent disease run a significant risk of surgical hypoparathyroidism. The message is, of course, that all four glands should never be removed or damaged, and that it is far better to reoperate than to render anyone persistently hypoparathyroid. Patients with parathyroid carcinomas seem to have particularly active secretion of parathyroid hormone, with high levels of calcium and frequent involvement of kidney, bone, or the central nervous system. A 60% survival has been reported. Adenomas that are histologically atypical may be premalignant and should be followed.

Elevated levels of vasopressin have been reported at the time of operation for removal of pheochromocytomas. The significance is unknown, but the amounts reported in a recent series in eight consecutive patients are enormous. The long-acting analogue of somatostatin (DMD 201-995) is effective in treating secretory diarrhea in the carcinoid and other syndromes, and in patients with gastrinomas, glucagonomas, and other endocrine tumors of the pancreas. No side effects have been found in patients who have received the agent for as long as 12 months; it was effective for long periods in treating secretory aspects of the Zollinger-Ellison syndrome where its action appears to be twofold; it suppresses gastrin release from tumor cells, and it inhibits the action of gastrin on the parietal cell. No tumoricidal activity of SMS was found, even though clinical and experimental evidence for regression of carcinoid tumors and of endocrine tumors of the pancreas has been reported by others.

1 General Considerations

The Heparin-Induced Thrombocytopenia Syndrome: An Update
Jerry Laster, Dolores Cikrit, Nancy Walker, and Donald Silver (Univ. of Missouri–Columbia Health Sciences Ctr., Columbia)
Surgery 102:763–770, October 1987   1–1

An earlier series of 62 patients with heparin-induced thrombocytopenia carried a morbidity rate of 61% and a mortality of 23%. Twenty-two operations were necessary for thromboembolic complications. Data on a series of 169 more recent cases now are available. Heparin-associated antiplatelet antibody was confirmed by aggregation testing in all cases.

In the more recent series 22.5% of patients had thromboembolic or hemorrhagic complications, or both, and 12% died of complications. Lower platelet counts were associated with a greater risk of complications (table). Twenty-eight surgical procedures were necessary for complications of heparin-induced thrombocytopenia.

Fifteen patients were reexposed to heparin, and 2 of them had devastating thrombotic complications. Five patients continued to receive heparin despite a positive platelet aggregation test. Two of them had serious complications.

Heparin-induced thrombocytopenia occurs in up to 10% of

RELATION OF DURATION OF EXPOSURE AND PLATELET COUNTS
TO MORBIDITY AND MORTALITY

	Duration of heparin exposure (days)	Platelet counts*
Thrombocytopenia (n = 131)	9	A: 239,000/mm³ N: 55,000/mm³ F: 185,000/mm³
Thrombocytopenia and complications (n = 17)	8.2	A: 208,000/mm³ N: 52,000/mm³ F: 158,000/mm³
Thrombocytopenia complications and death (n = 21)	9	A: 208,000/mm³ N: 64,000/mm³ F: 106,000/mm³

*A, admission; N, nadir; and F, final count obtained.
(Courtesy of Laster, J., et al.: Surgery 102:763–770, October 1987.)

---

heparin-treated patients. Close monitoring of platelet counts may minimize complications, but patients with complications still have a high mortality. Heparin should be withdrawn when the syndrome is suspected and should not be readministered until antiplatelet antibodies are no longer present.

▶ The article analyzes the experience from the medical center that has focused surgical attention on this important entity. The discussants point out that complications occur with low dose heparin and intravenous heparin flushes. The message is clear that any patient receiving heparin should be monitored for thrombocytopenia, and if thrombocytopenia develops, aggregation testing should be performed. In response to an important question, the authors indicate that before heparin administration in a patient with previously demonstrated heparin-associated antiplatelet antibodies, the platelet aggregation response to heparin should be studied. If this is negative, heparin can be used cautiously, monitoring the platelet count. If the aggregation response is positive, pretreatment with an antiplatelet aggregation agent, such as aspirin or dipyridamole, is indicated before heparin is administered.—S.I. Schwartz, M.D.

Heparin-Induced Platelet Activation in Sixteen Surgical Patients: Diagnosis and Management
Jeffrey R. Kappa, Carol A. Fisher, Henry D. Berkowitz, Earl D. Cottrell, V. Paul Addonizio, Jr. (Univ. of Pennsylvania)
J. Vasc. Surg. 5:101–109, January 1987   1–2

Heparin-induced platelet activation (HIPA) has been associated with thrombocytopenia, intravascular thrombosis, and arterial emboli. Sixteen patients were evaluated for this syndrome because of the occurrence of thrombocytopenia or a new thrombotic complication during heparin therapy.

Seven men and nine women were referred in an 18-month period for occurrence of thrombocytopenia, heparin resistance, or unexplained thrombotic complications while undergoing appropriate heparin therapy. Sixteen thrombotic events occurred in 10 patients, with a mortality of 18.8%. Diagnosis was confirmed by a demonstration of at least 20% platelet aggregation or 6% ^{14}C-serotonin release, or both, after heparin, 0.1 to 3.0 U/ml, was added to a mixture of patient platelet-poor plasma and aspirin-free, donor platelet-rich plasma. When heparin was discontinued, seven patients continued to have HIPA in their own platelet-rich plasma, although it could no longer be seen in donor platelet-rich plasma. Iloprost, a potent prostacyclin analogue that reversibly inhibits platelet activation, completely prevented HIPA and release in all nine patients tested. Aspirin, an irreversible cyclooxygenase inhibitor, did not prevent HIPA in four of these nine patients.

The HIPA phenomenon has been associated with a very high morbidity and mortality. Evaluation of patient platelet-rich plasma in response to heparin may improve the diagnostic sensitivity of this assay. As aspirin does not reliably prevent HIPA, participation of thromboxane-independent pathways may be involved. If further exposure to heparin is unavoidable, a more effective platelet inhibitor, such as iloprost, is needed to reliably prevent HIPA in vivo.

▶ Increasing emphasis on this newly considered complication appears in the literature. It has been reported by an international committee chaired by Godal (*Thromb. Haemost.* 43:222, 1980) that 0%–6% of patients receiving heparin become thrombocytopenic. The extent of thrombocytopenia is generally more severe in case reports than in prospective studies. The method of administration does not seem to be important. Beef lung heparin was indicted to a greater extent than heart-mucosa heparin. Thrombocytopenia during the first 5 to 7 days in patients who had not received previous heparin is actually a rare event; it is reasonable to monitor platelet counts only when the heparin therapy is continued beyond that period. Delayed onset heparin-induced thrombocytopenia has been reported (Van Der Weyden et al.: *Med. J. Aust.* 2:132, 1983). Silver et al. (*Ann. Surg.* 198:301, 1983) reviewed experience with 62 patients seen over 12 years; 20 of these patients died, 14 of complications of heparin-induced thrombocytopenia.—S.I. Schwartz, M.D.

Noninvasive Evaluation of Cardiac Risk Before Elective Vascular Surgery
Jeffrey Leppo, Joaquin Plaja, Maurissa Gionet, John Tumolo, John A. Paraskos, and Bruce S. Cutler (Univ. of Massachusetts, Worcester)
J. Am. Coll. Cardiol. 9:269–276, February 1987   1–3

Cardiac events, such as infarction and death, are the most significant postoperative complications in patients undergoing vascular surgery, but determination of a patient's cardiac risk profile remains a problem. The prognostic utility of dipyridamole-thallium scintigraphy for predicting cardiac events was compared to that of exercise testing and clinical variables in 100 consecutive patients admitted for elective peripheral vascular surgery. On the basis of these results and clinical evaluation, 11 patients were referred for coronary angiography.

Of the 89 patients who had vascular surgery without catheterization, 15 (17%) had perioperative myocardial infarction, including 1 in whom it was fatal. Of these, 14 had thallium redistribution and three had positive ST segment depression during stress testing. Among the variables tested, the presence of redistribution on serial dipyridamole-thallium images was the most significant predictor of serious cardiac events. The odds of a cardiac event were 23 times greater in a patient with thallium redistribution than in a patient without redistribution. All 11 patients who underwent catheterization had both thallium redistribution and multivessel coronary artery disease. At follow-up, four died, and six underwent coronary artery bypass surgery.

Dipyridamole-thallium imaging is superior to exercise testing and clinical variables for predicting cardiac events in patients undergoing elective peripheral vascular surgery. Because of the increased odds of having a cardiac event in a patient with thallium redistribution, it is strongly suggested that myocardial imaging be used as a primary screening test before elective vascular surgery.

▶ This is a critical consideration because the major complication of peripheral vascular surgery is myocardial infarction. The cardiac risks and complications of noncardiac surgery have been assessed by Goldman (*Ann. Surg.* 198:780, 1983). An increasing percentage of deaths and morbidity from general surgery is related to cardiac complications rather than to surgical problems directly. Multifactorial assessment of the risk distinguishes high risk patients. This present refinement offers an attractive method of improving prediction.—S.I. Schwartz, M.D.

Percutaneous Drainage of Subphrenic Abscess: A Review of 62 Patients
Peter R. Mueller, Joseph F. Simeone, Rodney J. Butch, Sanjay Saini, Susan A. Stafford, Luis Gaston Vici, Carlos Soto-Rivera, and Joseph T. Ferrucci, Jr. (Massachusetts Gen. Hosp. and Harvard Univ., Boston)
AJR 147:1237–1240, December 1986   1–4

Subphrenic abscesses were drained percutaneously under radiologic guidance in 62 patients between January 1981 and December 1985; the diagnosis was usually made with sonography. A combination of sonography and fluoroscopic guidance was used initially, but in the most recent 31 patients drainage was usually done with sonographic guidance alone. Of the 62 catheters placed, 56 (90%) were inserted via an anterior or lateral subcostal access route. Abscess drainage catheters (9–14 F) were used, and follow-up was standard.

In 43 of 61 evaluable patients, successful catheter drainage (defined as no surgical intervention required) was achieved. The cavity was drained completely in nine patients, but in four surgery was performed because it was not believed that percutaneous drainage would be successful; curative surgery was undertaken in five others to treat the underlying process that caused the abscess, including ulcer or acute cholecystitis. Of nine patients in whom percutaneous drainage failed, seven had multiple abscesses in the subphrenic space and other noncontiguous locations.

The time of catheter drainage required for cure of subphrenic abscesses was generally longer than necessary for abscesses in other locations. Twenty patients required catheter drainage for less than 7 days and 32 for at least 10 days. Of the latter group, 24 patients (75%) had a catheter in place for at least 21 days; 11 of these had a low-flow fistulous communication with the biliary tree or small bowel, or an enteric biliary anastomosis. Complications were uncommon. Septicemia, i.e., hypotension with positive blood cultures, developed in two patients after catheter insertion; both were treated successfully with antibiotics and fluid therapy. Another patient had pleural contamination and resulting empyema from the inadvertent entrance of the catheter into the pleural space.

The failure of percutaneous drainage to cure subphrenic abscesses completely is predictable and depends on the presence of multiple non-contiguous collections or the underlying cause of the collection. The patients in this series who had perforated ulcers or gallbladder disease, or both, had complete drainage of their subphrenic collections but still required surgery for the primary problem.

▶ An 85% success rate reported by these authors is commendable. As they point out, the failure of percutaneous drainage is generally predictable and depends on the presence of multiple noncontiguous collections or the cause of the collection. Gerzof et al. (*Arch. Surg.* 120:227, 1985) reported on 125 abscesses drained percutaneously from 113 patients. Cure was achieved by percutaneous drainage in 74% of patients. The technique was effective in 82% of simple abscesses, but only 45% of complex abscesses. Success was achieved in the majority of patients with hepatic abscesses and infected pseudocysts, and also pelvic abscesses.—S.I. Schwartz, M.D.

Effects of Thymectomy in Myasthenia Gravis
Angelos E. Papatestas, Gabriel Genkins, Peter Kornfeld, James B. Eisenkraft, Richard P. Fagerstrom, Jason Pozner, and Arthur H. Aufses, Jr. (Mount Sinai Med. Ctr., New York)
Ann. Surg. 206:79–88, July 1987   1–5

Thymectomy in myasthenia gravis has been observed to lead to remission of symptoms of the disease. But the role of thymectomy is not fully understood. Factors influencing the onset of remission in myasthenia gravis were assessed in 2,062 patients, of whom 962 had had thymectomy.

Follow-up data were obtained by patient examination or questionnaire. In 226 (11%) of the patients with myasthenia gravis, thymomas were observed. Eighty-one (6%) of the 1,254 patients with mild cases had thymomas; 145 (18%) of the 808 with severe symptoms had associated thymic tumors. Only one third of patients without thymomas had severe symptoms, whereas two thirds of those with associated thymomas did. Seventy-two percent of patients who had thymectomy were operated on through the transcervical approach; there was a significant difference in this proportion in relation to presence of thymoma.

Multivariate analysis showed that appearance of early remissions among all patients was significantly and independently affected by thymectomy, milder disease, and absence of coexisting thymomas. Sex and age did not influence the results. Patients with thymomas who had surgery eventually had a higher proportion of remissions than patients without thymomas treated without surgery, although they had considerable delay in remission onset (Fig 1–1). Short duration of disease before thymectomy in mild cases was also associated with earlier remissions. Mortality among all patients was significantly and independently affected by symptom severity, age, associated thymomas, and failure to remove the thymus. Patients without thymectomy and with thymomas were

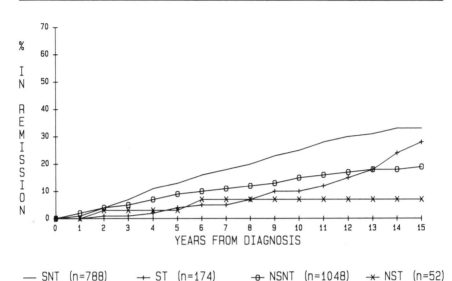

— SNT (n=788)   —+— ST (n=174)   —⊖— NSNT (n=1048)   —✳— NST (n=52)

Fig 1–1.—Intervals from diagnosis to remission in relation to treatment and presence of thymoma. *SNT* = thymectomy, no thymoma; *NSNT,* no surgery, no thymoma; *ST,* thymectomy, thymoma; *NST,* no surgery, thymoma. (Courtesy of Papatestas, A.E., et al.: Ann. Surg. 206:79–88, July 1987.)

found to have an earlier onset of extrathymic neoplasms. Morbidity after the transcervical approach was observed to be minimal.

Early thymectomy by the transcervical approach, when possible, was found to have significant clinical advantages over the transthoracic approach and should be advocated for all patients with myasthenia gravis, including those with ocular disease.

▶ This represents the largest experience in our country. Fischer et al. (*Ann. Surg.* 205:496, 1987) advised external split and extended thymectomy and radical mediastinal dissection rather than the transcervical approach. Our own experience indicates that the transcervical approach may leave thymic tissue; we have had to reoperate on four patients who have had transcervical thymectomy and thymic tissue following a transsternal approach. After removal of this thymic tissue, improvement occurred in the myasthenia. In Fischer's series, drug-free remission was achieved in 46% of the male patients and in 82% of the female patients despite the fact that the mean duration of disease was greater than 3.5 years. A new surgical technique for thymectomy has been presented by Otto and Strugalska (*Thorax* 42:199, 1987). This consists of a small transverse sternotomy that enabled radical thymectomy to be performed with good cosmetic results.—S.I. Schwartz, M.D.

Results of Surgical Treatment for Thymoma Based on 66 Patients
Shigefumi Fujimura, Takashi Kondo, Masashi Handa, Yuji Shiraishi, Nobuaki Tamahashi, and Tasuku Nakada (Tohoku Univ., Sendai, Japan)
J. Thorac. Cardiovasc. Surg. 93:708–714, May 1987   1–6

Progress in thymic tumor morphology and immunology has contributed to the treatment of patients with thymoma. Nevertheless, treatment of patients with autoimmune associated diseases or with invasive thymoma remains controversial. Clinical manifestations and prognosis were assessed in 66 patients with thymoma who underwent surgical treatment at one institution.

Of these patients, aged 13 to 76 years, 31 had encapsulated thymoma, and 35 had invasive thymoma. Six patients with invasive thymoma had superior vena caval syndrome before surgery. Diseases presumed to be associated with thymoma included myasthenia gravis in 5 patients, pure red blood cell aplasia in 3 patients, aplastic anemia in 1 patient, hypogammaglobulinemia in 2 patients, and leukopenia in 1 patient. One patient died of respiratory insufficiency on the fourth day after exploratory thoracotomy for invasive thymoma and was excluded from survival rate calculations. Overall survival rates of the 65 patients assessed were 83.4%, 68%, 61.6%, and 61.6% at 1, 3, 5, and 10 years, respectively (Fig 1–2). For those with invasive thymoma, survival rates were 75.1%, 55.5%, 49.4%, and 49.4% at 1, 3, 5, and 10 years, respectively.

Six of the 31 patients with encapsulated thymoma died within 4 years and 10 months of surgery. Four of the 6 had myasthenia gravis, hypogammaglobulinemia, pure red cell aplasia (PRCA), and PRCA plus hypogammaglobulinemia. Fifteen of 34 patients with invasive thymoma died within 10 years and 1 month of surgery. Nine of the 15 died of local or metastatic tumor, and 6 died of other diseases. The 31 patients with encapsulated thymoma were treated with total resection alone, and none had a postoperative tumor recurrence.

In surgical treatment for invasive thymomas, the tumor should be resected totally, even though adjacent tissues are resected simultaneously. Postoperative radiation should be required, even for patients with total resection of invasive tumor. If residual tumor must be left during surgery, postoperative radiation and anticancer chemotherapy should be aggres-

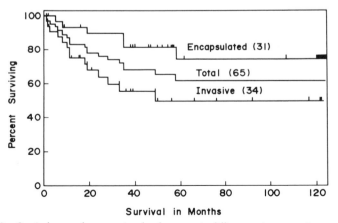

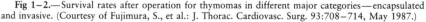

Fig 1–2.—Survival rates after operation for thymomas in different major categories—encapsulated and invasive. (Courtesy of Fujimura, S., et al.: J. Thorac. Cardiovasc. Surg. 93:708–714, May 1987.)

sively scheduled, because distant metastasis may appear in patients with residual thymoma.

▶ It has long been appreciated that the prognosis of thymic tumors can be correlated not with the histology but rather with the extent of invasion. Keen and Libshitz (*Cancer* 59:1520, 1987) stressed the value of computer tomography in the treatment of patients with thymic lesions. The presence or absence of invasion of adjacent structures was predicted in 16 of the 17 patients in whom computed tomographic correlation was available.—S.I. Schwartz, M.D.

2 Fluid, Electrolytes, and Nutrition

Effect of Hormonal and Substrate Backgrounds on Cell Membrane Function in Normal Males
Gary A. Fantini, John P. Roberts, Stephen F. Lowry, James D. Albert, Kevin J. Tracey, Adrian Legaspi, Joseph P. Minei, Jerry Chiao, and G. Tom Shires (New York Hosp.–Cornell Med. Ctr., New York)
J. Appl. Physiol. 63:1107–1113, 1987   2–1

The mechanisms that underlie the changes in cellular membrane function that are associated with shock and ischemia remain incompletely understood. The wide use of intravenous feeding for critically ill and injured patients prompted a study of the roles of substrate availability and the hormonal milieu in cellular membrane function.

The authors studied these effects in 15 healthy men aged 21 to 36 years. Transcutaneous measurements of resting membrane potential were made in the anterior tibialis muscle during intravenous feeding for 10 days and during infusion of epinephrine. Needle biopsy of the vastus lateralis muscle allowed estimates of distribution of transmembrane electrolytes.

Hospitalization and intake of a defined-formula enteral diet for 3 days led to depolarization of the resting membrane potential. Further depolarization was noted after 10 days of intravenous feeding. Intracellular concentration of potassium increased in intravenously fed subjects who were given epinephrine by infusion, and repolarization to normal levels was observed.

Both substrate availability and the hormonal milieu help modulate cellular membrane function in human skeletal muscle. Hormones may facilitate carrier-mediated active solute transport across the cell membrane. Observations of peripheral tissue conservation of amino acids during infusion of epinephrine support this concept.

▶ I have asked Dr. Stephen F. Lowry, Associate Professor of Surgery at Cornell University, whose major interest is metabolism and nutrition, to comment on several abstracts in this chapter.—G.T. Shires, M.D.

▶ This study evaluated the relationship between nutrient background and adrenergic hormonal responses as these variables impact upon somatic cell membrane function. These evaluations were performed in hospitalized, weight-stable, normal volunteers, thereby precluding disease or antecedent malnutrition as confounding variables. Several observations of clinical relevance were made, including that of a progressive decline in skeletal muscle resting

37

transmembrane potential (Em) during the 10- to 14-day course of hospitalization. In addition, weight-maintaining parenteral nutrition was unable to sustain a
normal Em even in the absence of prior or concurrent malnutrition or injury.
The infusion of epinephrine, in a manner designed to mimic those levels
achieved following injury, did acutely improve muscle Em.

These observations raise both teleologic and mechanistic questions regarding the importance of adrenergic responses to injury. It would appear that catecholamines, in addition to increasing energy expenditure and substrate turnover, may also be necessary to counteract the adverse membrane effects of
other local or circulating mediators.—S.F. Lowry, M.D.

**Hyperosmolar Glucose Prevents Stress Ulceration in the Rat Restraint
Model Despite Inhibition of Endogenous Prostaglandins**
Kimberly Ephgrave, Jureta W. Horton, and Dennis K. Burns (Univ. of Texas at
Dallas)
Surg. Gynecol. Obstet. 164:9–16, January 1987   2–2

Stress ulceration still is a problem in critically ill surgical patients, even
when standard prophylaxis is used. Hyperosmolar glucose can prevent
stress ulceration as effectively as antacids in the rat restraint model, possibly by stimulating prostaglandin release. The role of prostaglandin was
studied in stressed rats given intragastric 25% glucose, aspirin to block
cyclooxygenase activity, and both glucose and aspirin.

Restraint-induced ulcers were prevented by intragastric 25% glucose in
water, even when aspirin also was given (Fig 2–1). Focal lesions were
worsened by aspirin alone. Animals given intragastric dextrose had significantly elevated gastric mucosal pH, whether or not aspirin also was
given. The gastric wall water content was reduced by intragastric glucose
and increased by aspirin.

These findings indicate that endogenous prostaglandins, while useful in
gastric mucosal defense, are not necessary for protection against stress ulceration by intragastric glucose in the rat restraint model. The provision
of glucose directly to the stressed gastric mucosa probably enhances several aspects of mucosal defense. Intragastric hyperosmolar glucose may
be useful clinically if volumes small enough not to cause vomiting and
aspiration are effective.

▶ This study further emphasizes the importance of luminal exposure to nutrients as an effective method of mucosal cytoprotection and, in the current
study, as a means of diminishing the incidence of gastric mucosal erosions.
The mechanism underlying this beneficial influence of intragastric hyperosmolar (D25) dextrose upon stress erosin is unclear, but appears to be independent
of, or certainly synergistic to, other clinically useful pharmacologic methods.
While a number of caveats may preclude routine clinical application of this
method in high risk patients, the present study provides additional data to support the use of early enteral feedings in critically ill subjects. When superimposed upon the growing literature suggesting a moderation of metabolic re-

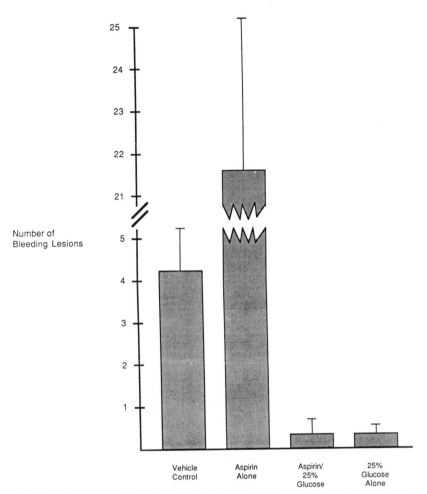

Fig 2–1.—Comparison of the number of bleeding lesions in the four experimental groups. $F = 40.9$, $P < .001$; group 1 was different from groups 3 and 4 and group 2 was different from groups 1, 3, and 4 at $P < .05$. (Courtesy of Ephgrave, K., et al.: Surg. Gynecol. Obstet. 164:9–16, January 1987.)

spones to early enteral nutritional support and of increased rates of enteric derived nosocomial infections in malnourished patients, some degree of enteral nutritional support assumes greater emphasis in the management of critically ill patients.—S.F. Lowry, M.D.

3% NaCl and 7.5% NaCl/Dextran in the Resuscitation of Severely Injured Patients
James W. Holcroft, Mary J. Vassar, James E. Turner, Robert W. Derlet, and George C. Kramar (Univ. of California, Sacramento)
Ann. Surg. 206:279–288, September 1987   2–3

LABORATORY DATA FOR PATIENTS IN FIELD TRIAL AT TIME
OF ARRIVAL IN THE EMERGENCY ROOM*

	7.5% NaCl/Dextran 70	Lactated Ringer's
Serum sodium (mEq/L)	153 ± 4 (144–159)†	142 ± 5 (132–150)
Serum potassium (mEq/L)	3.6 ± 4 (2.9–4.4)	3.9 ± 0.3 (3.5–4.3)
Serum chloride (mEq/L)	119 ± 5 (106–127)	109 ± 6 (98–117)
Osmolaltiy (mOsm/kg)	337 ± 23 (313–358)	315 ± 28 (279–345)
pH	7.27 ± 0.09 (7.10–7.40)	7.34 ± 0.30 (7.06–8.04)
Hematocrit (vol%)	28 ± 7 (16–38)	31 ± 8 (20–41)

*Ranges in parentheses.
†$P < .01$.
(Courtesy of Holcroft, J.W., et al.: Ann. Surg. 206:279–288, September 1987.)

Cardiovascular resuscitation of severely injured patients remains unsatisfactory because the relatively small-bore cannulae used cannot infuse sufficient volumes of fluids to keep up with losses. A previous study showed that a combination of 7.5% NaCl and 6% dextran was effective in resuscitating animals from hemorrhagic shock. Two studies were conducted to determine the effects of hypertonic saline in humans.

In the first study, 20 patients undergoing surgery for severe injuries received infusions of either 3% NaCl or lactated Ringer's solution. Small volumes (≤12 ml/kg) of 3% NaCl restored blood pressure (BP), pH, and urine output with approximately one half of the cumulative fluid requirement of patients who received isotonic fluids. Overall survival rates did not differ between treatment groups. In the second study, 20 severely injured patients in the field were randomized to receive either 7.5% NaCl/4.2% dextran 70 or lactated Ringer's solution in a prospective, double-blind trial. Total fluid administered during helicopter transport was 700 ± 500 ml of 7.5% NaCl/dextran 70 versus 1,300 ± 900 ml of lactated Ringer's solution. Administration of the hypertonic/hyperoncotic fluid resulted in augmented blood pressures during flight and tended to improve survival when compared with the lactated Ringer's group. Serum sodium and chloride concentrations and osmolalities were significantly elevated by time of emergency room admission in those receiving 7.5% NaCl/dextran 70 (table). Except for the sensation of warmth and transient flushing, no other untoward events, e.g., phlebitis or type-matching or cross-matching problems, occurred.

It appears that 7.5% NaCl/dextran 70 solution is particularly promising for field resuscitation of injured patients. The 7.5% NaCl/6% dextran 70 solution has a calculated osmolality of 2,400 mOsm/kg and an oncotic pressure of 75 mm Hg. The immediate beneficial effects of this solution arise from the hyperosmolality per se resulting in plasma volume expansion, enhancement of myocardial contractility, and augmentation of organ blood flow mediated by dilation of precapillary resistance vessels.

► This is another study from the same group of authors who have been investigating the use of smaller volume hypertonic solutions in the initial resuscitation from shock. The present study has been performed as a field study on injured patients.

The data indicate that there is a slightly more rapid volume expansion, enhancement of myocardial contractility, and augmentation of organ blood flow by the use of hypertonic solutions. When one critically looks at this study, however, it appears that the volume used in initial resuscitation in the field is more than half of the volume used with the usual, safer isotonic fluids such as Hartman's solution (lactated Ringer's). Furthermore, as has frequently been the case with other nonphysiologic, nonisotonic resuscitative fluids, there are still no data to indicate what effect the use of hypertonic fluids, such as described here, might have on incipient organ failure induced by the shock state, primarily renal failure. Most such previous efforts to produce a more rapid or better response in resuscitation of shock have eventually proven not useful because the solution used generated more complications than gains. In the past, this has included complications related to clotting mechanism and pulmonary function, as well as renal function.—G.T. Shires, M.D.

Infusion Volumes of Ringer's Lactate and 3% Albumin Solution as They Relate to Survival After Resuscitation of a Lethal Intestinal Ischemic Shock

Ingemar Dawidson, Johan Ottosson, and Joan S. Reisch (Univ. of Texas at Dallas)
Circ. Shock 18:277–288, 1986   2–4

Improved fluid and electrolyte replacement is one reason that mortality from intestinal obstruction has declined to less than 10% from previously much higher levels. The authors compared Ringer's lactate and a 3% colloid solution in Ringer's lactate, given 6–10 hours, in rats subjected to lethal intestinal ischemic shock. Shock was induced by exteriorizing the small bowel for 75 minutes. This form of shock is associated with marked hemoconcentration, with about a 50% reduction in plasma volume and a marked increase in weight of the exteriorized bowel. Extensive mucosal injury is observed.

Plasma volume fell to 57% of baseline in shocked animals. No volume of Ringer's lactate restored the plasma volume to preshock levels, but infusion of 15 ml of 3% albumin per 100 gm of body weight was effective. For a given volume infused, a much greater proportion of 3% albumin remained as plasma volume. Survival was prolonged with both fluid regimens.

Less 3% albumin solution than Ringer's lactate is required for comparable blood volume expansion, in a ratio of 1:4.4. Fluid infusion alone does not assure survival in severe shock. No volume of Ringer's lactate will restore plasma volume to the preoperative level.

► This article shows again the efficacy of crystalloid resuscitation for a specific form of shock produced by intestinal ischemia. The authors point out that in this particular experimental preparation the loss of albumin from circulation is acute and significant, and therefore less crystalloid solution was used if albumin was given in addition. In this highly specific experimental preparation, the data indicate that resuscitation can be accomplished with less volume. However, as the authors point out, replenishment of functional extracellular fluid, both intravascular and extravascular, is the key to resuscitation following even this form of hypovolemic shock.—G.T. Shires, M.D.

Immediate Trauma Resuscitation With Type O Uncrossmatched Blood: A Two-Year Prospective Experience
C. William Schwab, John P. Shayne, and John Turner (Univ. of Medicine and Dentistry of New Jersey, Camden, and Eastern Virginia Med. School, Norfolk)
J. Trauma 26:897–902, October 1986   2–5

The ideal fluid for use in trauma resuscitation would have many of the properties of whole blood but would not have to be crossmatched and would be free from disease-producing organisms. The use of uncrossmatched type O packed red blood cells was evaluated in 83 severely injured and hypovolemic patients seen in 1982–1983. Seventy-four patients received 250 units of group O red cells, averaging 3.3 units per patient, while nine received 27 units of type-specific blood, averaging 3 units per patient. Fifty-three units of blood were given to the former patients before fully crossmatched blood became available. All units of red cells were expanded with warmed normal saline.

No transfusion reactions occurred, and there was no difficulty in subsequent crossmatching. More than one third of patients required more than 10 units within 24 hours. No deaths were ascribed to transfusion reaction or blood incompatibility. Adult respiratory distress syndrome (ARDS) developed in 7% of patients and disseminated intravascular coagulation in 12%. Two patients had positive hepatitis screens, and there was one clinical case of hepatitis. No case of disseminated intravascular coagulopathy (DIC) was caused by incompatible blood transfusion.

The use of uncrossmatched group O packed red cells in trauma patients appears safe, avoiding the problems resulting from transfusion of large amounts of antibody. There seems to be no problem in subsequently administering type-specific blood or fully crossmatched blood, or both.

▶ As the authors of this paper point out carefully, an ideal resuscitative fluid has not yet been perfected. An ideal solution would have the critical properties of whole blood in terms of volume and oxygen-carrying capacity, but also would include no requirement for crossmatching and freedom from all disease-producing organisms or viruses. These authors investigated the group O low titer Rh positive whole blood concept in the sense that group O red blood cells were used for initial resuscitation and in addition to a physiologic isotonic crystalloid fluid. The data indicate that for immediate trauma resuscitation type O red blood cell is safe and has advantages over type-specific blood or type O whole blood transfusion. These advantages include immediate availability, universal application for all recipients, and no risk of transfusing high titer plasma. It would appear in this prospective study of patients that at the present time this resuscitative regimen of type O blood cells with crystalloid fluid is an excellent resuscitative approach.—G.T. Shires, M.D.

Failure of TPN Supplementation to Improve Liver Function, Immunity, and Mortality in Thermally Injured Patients
David N. Herndon, Marshall D. Stein, Thomas C. Rutan, Sally Abston, and Hugo Linares (Shriners Burns Inst. and Univ. of Texas, Galveston)
J. Trauma 27:195–204, February 1987   2–6

After major thermal injury, patients often have hypermetabolism, with negative nitrogen balance and immune deficiency. These patients often have poor gastrointestinal (GI) function, making it difficult to meet nutritional requirements. Patients with burns over greater than 50% of their total body surface area were randomly assigned to treatment in which 13 received total parenteral nutrition (TPN)—and 15 did not receive this supplementation—for the first 10 days following the burn.

Patients receiving TPN exhibited significantly lower helper-to-suppressor T-cell ratios. There was no difference in mortality between the two groups. All patients who died developed hepatomegaly, associated with fatty infiltration cholestasis and liver function abnormalities.

Use of TPN for the first 10 days postburn had no apparent beneficial effect on immune function, liver function, or survival; use of TPN early in the treatment of burn victims should therefore be discouraged. Hepatic cholestasis and fatty infiltration, both present after major burn injury, are not likely related to TPN use.

▶ This study continues to address the important issues of both the route and timing of nutritional intervention following major burn injury. While abnormalities of liver function and of lymphocyte phenotype were observed in most patients following injury, there are clearly trends towards improvements in these parameters in patients receiving a predominance of enteral nutrition. It would appear that the mere provision of more calories or nitrogen by the intravenous route, or both, provided no benefit to the parameters of immune function that were assessed. This data again emphasizes the likely role of enteral nutrition as a modulating influence upon both organ-specific and systemic responses to injury.—S.F. Lowry, M.D.

Aggressive Nutritional Support Does Not Prevent Protein Loss Despite Fat Gain in Septic Intensive Care Patients
Stephen J. Streat, Alun H. Beddoe, and Graham L. Hill (Univ. of Auckland, Auckland, New Zealand)
J. Trauma 27:262–266, March 1987   2–7

Critically ill postoperative patients with sepsis receive intravenously administered nutrition to prevent loss of body protein, but such an effect has not been confirmed by direct body composition estimates. Total body water, protein, and fat were measured before and after 10 days of intravenously administered nutrition in eight critically ill, septic surgical patients, six of whom were discharged from hospital. All patients had both respiratory failure and septic shock syndrome. Neutron activation analysis and tritiated water dilution were used in the study. The mean daily intakes of nonprotein energy and amino acid were 2,750 kcal and 127 gm, respectively. The patients had recovered from septic shock at the start of intravenously administered nutrition, but remained ventilator-dependent.

Most patients lost weight, although not to a significant degree. Loss of water was chiefly responsible. Total body protein decreased by a mean of 12.5% during the 10-day study period. The patients gained fat or glycogen as a group. The estimated mean daily total energy expenditure was 3,263 kcal, assuming that gains in total body fat represented gains in glycogen and that losses were fat.

Critically ill, septic surgical patients gain energy stores when given aggressive nutritional support, but protein loss nevertheless occurs. Most survivors also lose considerable body water during intravenously administered nutrition. Further work is needed to determine the ability of various substrates to suppress proteolysis and to assess the functional consequences of protein loss.

▶ It is increasingly clear that the utility of nutritional support, as currently practiced, may be of limited benefit with respect to preservation of lean tissue stores in surgical patients. Accumulating evidence suggests this to be the case not only in injured or septic patients as reported herein, but in other hospitalized patient populations not subject to severe "stress." The authors of this manuscript have, with sophisticated isotope dilution and neutron activation techniques, determined that progressive erosion of skeletal muscle proteins may continue despite evidence of clinical improvement. While the mechanisms underlying this seeming paradox of homeostasis remain unclear, a number of elements such as enforced immobility, nutrient substrate imbalances resulting from injury, and the influence of local and circulating inflammatory mediators are suspected to contribute. As noted by the authors, the functional consequences of this structural protein loss remains unclear, although the relatively high survivorship in this limited series suggests this not to be an acute problem.—S.F. Lowry, M.D.

Effect of Protein Depletion and Short-Term Parenteral Refeeding on the Host Response to Interleukin 1 Administration
Michael D. Drabik, Frederick C. Schnure, King Tong Mok, Lyle L. Moldawer, Charles A. Dinarello, George L. Blackburn, and Bruce R. Bistrian (Harvard Univ. and Tufts Univ.)
J. Lab. Clin. Med. 109:509–516, April 1987   2–8

Protein malnutrition impairs the synthesis and release of interleukin 1 (IL-1) by monocytes. The authors studied responses to exogenous IL-1, and whether parenteral feeding would stimulate and support the host response in the severely protein-malnourished guinea pig given a 2% casein diet for 1 week. Interleukin 1 was administered intravenously in the postabsorptive state or during total parenteral nutrition. Animals were challenged with *Salmonella enteritidis* endotoxin.

Protein-depleted animals in the postabsorptive state had no fever, granulocytosis, or acute-phase protein response after administration of either IL-1 or endotoxin. Serum zinc and iron levels decreased in animals given IL-1, but not in endotoxin-treated animals. Total parenteral nutrition for 1 day restored positive leucine balance. The body temperature response of malnourished guinea pigs to IL-1 and total parenteral nutrition depended on initial body temperature.

Protein malnutrition is associated with impaired ability to synthesize IL-1 and failure to mount an appropriate acute-phase protein response to exogenous IL-1 in the guinea pig. More than short-term intravenous nutritional repletion appears necessary to restore normal responses to infection and injury.

▶ The current study, which follows upon the authors' previous evaluation of monocyte pyrogen production in protein-malnourished patients, has sought to determine the in vivo influence of short-term intravenous nutritional repletion upon the capacity to respond to a known exogenous pyrogen or pyrogens. Protein malnutrition resulted in a blunting of the acute-phase response to the partially-purified cytokine, IL-1, and 1 week of nutritional support failed to restore responsiveness. While it has previously been proposed by the authors that the inability of the impaired host both to secrete cytokines, such as IL-1, and to mount an appropriate stress response is inherently detrimental, it has yet to be conclusively demonstrated that this down-regulation is maladaptive. Rather, given the increased awareness of potential toxicities inherent to some cytokines, such a response might be viewed as protective to the compromised host. Additional work will be necessary to clarify the purported role that exogenous IL-1 administration might play in the management of critical illness.—S.F. Lowry, M.D.

Recipient Growth and Nutritional Status Following Transplantation of Segmental Small-Bowel Allografts

Wolfgang H. Schraut, Kenneth K.W. Lee, and Michael Sitrin (Univ. of Chicago) J. Surg. Res. 43:1–9, July 1987   2–9

Patients with short-gut syndrome are limited by their dependence on total parenteral nutrition. In addition, a number of serious complications, including sepsis, may occur. Intestinal transplantation is the logical approach to this problem. In previous studies, cyclosporine permitted the acceptance of small-bowel allografts by adult rats. The authors determined whether young immature rats would grow and mature following replacement of the entire small bowel by a segmental ileal or jejunal allograft from an adult donor. Orthotopic small bowel transplantation was done in rats aged 4–6 weeks, and cyclosporine was given for 4 weeks.

All recipients had normal global nutritional parameters 6 and 12 months after transplantation, and had gained weight at a rate similar to that in age-matched control animals. No clinical nutritional deficiencies were apparent. Recipients of segmental grafts had significantly reduced levels of vitamins A and E by 10–12 months. Vitamin B_{12} levels were less markedly lowered. Fecal fat was increased in all grafted rats, particularly those with jejunal grafts. Serum triglyceride levels were reduced, and this effect persisted in animals with segmental grafts. Biopsy specimens of segmental grafts showed villous hyperplasia but normal intestinal architecture.

Adult small bowel allografts allow normal growth of young recipients. Grafts of ileum or jejunum can provide caloric nutritional balance; ileal grafts are preferable. The entire small bowel is preferable, but limited space may mandate a segmental graft.

▶ This study lends additional experimental credence to the concept that segmental small bowel transplantation may permit normal growth. With the exception of subclinical fat malabsorption and of predictable abnormalities of vitamin concentration, adequate nonprotein caloric and nitrogen retention was achieved in these transplanted animals. Additional studies will be necessary to determine the etiology of the transplant-related mechanism for fat malabsorption and the implications of this process for maintenance of immunosuppression via enterally administered cyclosporine.—S.F. Lowry, M.D.

Influence of Injury and Nutrition on Muscle Water and Electrolytes: Effect of Severe Injury, Burns and Sepsis

Jonas P. Bergström, Jörgen Larsson, Hans Nordström, Erik Vinnars, Jeffrey Askanazi, David H. Elwyn, John M. Kinney, and Peter J. Fürst (Huddinge Univ., Stockholm, and Univ. Hosp., Linköping, Sweden; Columbia Univ., New York; and Univ. Hohenheim, Stuttgart, West Germany)
Acta Chir. Scand. 153:261–266, April 1987   2–10

Severe trauma involves sodium and water retention, which are reflected in skeletal muscle changes in the immediate postoperative phase. Tissue changes were assessed by muscle biopsy in 45 Swedish and 17 American patients at varying intervals after injury or infection. The Swedish patients had multiple injuries or burns, while the Americans had major accidental injuries, usually gunshot wounds or extensive abdominal sepsis. Nutrition ranged from brief hypocaloric intake to prolonged high-calorie parenteral nutrition, with and without amino acids and fat.

Total and extracellular water and total sodium and chloride content in muscle increased 2–30 days after trauma. Muscle potassium remained low, and magnesium content declined. Similar changes in muscle water and electrolytes occurred in all patient groups. High- and low-glucose infusions had no significant effects in the four injured and three septic patients studied.

The extracellular volume expands, and intracellular components are lost in severely injured or septic patients. In less severe injury, such as elective surgery, a less marked extracellular volume expansion is seen, without losses of potassium or magnesium. The changes attending severe injury last up to a month and are not closely dependent on the type of nutrition supplied.

▶ A characteristically abnormal pattern of muscle water, electrolyte, and mineral content in moderately to severely injured patients is reported by the authors. The extent to which resuscitation and nutritional support may have influenced both the acute and late-phase water and electrolyte content of muscle biopsy specimens remains unclear. In addition, the calculated distributions of water and electrolytes have utilized an assumed resting transmembrane potential. There is increasing evidence to suggest that this assumption is not valid in hospitalized patients and, as evidenced by the summarized report of Fantini et al. in this volume, may be significantly altered by the hormonal milieu commonly observed in severely injured patients.

Of interest in these studies are both the acuity of the alterations in muscle water and solute content as well as the prolonged nature of these abnormalities despite clinical improvement. Such observations are reminiscent of the extended period of reduced body functional capacity and increased fatigability described by other investigators. While the mechanisms whereby such cellular and body functional changes occur either acutely or during rehabilitation remain poorly defined, it is evident that a number of hormonal, nutritional, and activity components are involved. Additional investigation of methods to promote early recovery of cellular function may have significant impact upon the clinical outcome of critically ill patients.—S.F. Lowry, M.D.

Branched Chain Amino Acid Uptake and Muscle Free Amino Acid Concentrations Predict Postoperative Muscle Nitrogen Balance
Daniel J. Johnson, Michael Colpoys, Robert J. Smith, Zhu-Ming Jiang, C. Raja Kapadia, and Douglas W. Wilmore (Harvard Univ., Boston)
Ann. Surg. 204:513–523, November 1986   2–11

Accelerated release of amino acids from skeletal muscle after major surgery, trauma, or septicemia is associated with increased total-body nitrogen loss. Since visceral amino acid uptake exceeds muscle release, plasma levels decline and intravenously administered amino acids may be required. Skeletal muscle amino acid metabolism was studied after a standard laparotomy and retroperitoneal dissection in dogs given either saline or amino acid formulas containing varying levels of branched-chain amino acids (BCAA). Amino acid nitrogen exchange rates were measured using hindquarter flux techniques.

The rate of BCAA uptake by muscle correlated significantly with decreased total nitrogen release from hindquarter skeletal muscle after operation (Fig 2–2). There also was a significant relation between muscle nitrogen balance and the postoperative change in either total muscle amino acids or glutamine. The BCAA uptake and the change in muscle

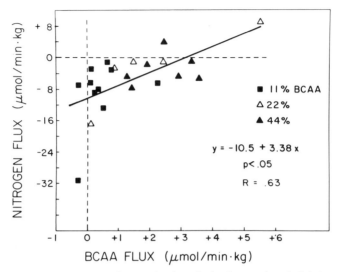

Fig 2–2.—Hindquarter nitrogen flux is related to the hindquarter branched-chain amino acids *(BCAA)* flux 6 hours after operation. (Courtesy of Johnson, D.J., et al.: Ann. Surg. 204:513–523, November 1986.)

free amino acid concentration predicted skeletal muscle nitrogen release with a correlation coefficient of 0.86.

The net turnover of muscle protein, as reflected in skeletal muscle amino acid release, is predicted by the rate of BCAA flux across skeletal muscle and the concentration of nitrogen in the skeletal muscle free amino acid pool. While muscle BCAA uptake is not a function simply of the rate of intravenous infusion of amino acids, the intracellular pool of amino acids can be predictably maintained by infusing amino acid solution.

▶ The current study underscores the complex relationship between skeletal muscle energy and protein balance following injury. When amino acids are infused in the absence of other nutrients, the branched chain amino acids are taken up, possibly to serve as a readily oxidizable source of energy. It has been amply demonstrated in both unstressed and injury conditions that the branched chain amino acids dominate the pattern of skeletal muscle protein uptake, even during total parenteral nutrition.

As is evident from this study of mild injury, some loss of cellular glutamine will also occur in the absence of an exogenous nitrogen source. This loss of glutamine may be abrogated by infusion of standard amino acid sources with enrichment of either glutamine or of branched chain amino acid content. While the signal which induces cellular glutamine loss presumably arises outside the skeletal muscle, the provision of appropriate amino acids can, at least acutely, counteract this characteristic muscle amino acid response to injury. Although clinical trials of branched chain enriched nutritional formula have proven generally disappointing with respect to maintenance of body and lean tissue nitrogen homeostasis, the provision of additional glutamine to IV feeding regimens may prove of benefit to both skeletal muscle and splanchnic integrity. Experimental evidence pointing to such benefit has accumulated, and it will be of interest to determine the clinical utility of such regimens in the future.—S.F. Lowry, M.D.

Effect of Sepsis and Starvation on Amino Acid Uptake in Skeletal Muscle

Brad W. Warner, J. Howard James, Per-Olof Hasselgren, Robert P. Hummel III, and Josef E. Fischer (Univ. of Cincinnati)

J. Surg. Res. 42:377–382, April 1987   2–12

In severe trauma or sepsis, released amino acids are taken up by the liver and other visceral tissues and are used for gluconeogenesis and protein synthesis. Muscle amino acid uptake appears to be inhibited under these conditions. The interaction of sepsis and starvation with respect to muscle amino acid uptake was studied by determining α-aminoisobutyric acid (AIB) uptake in soleus muscle from rats starved up to 72 hours. In addition, the effects of septic plasma on muscle amino acid uptake in vitro were studied.

Addition of septic plasma to the incubation medium significantly inhibited AIB uptake by soleus muscle (Fig 2–3). Uptake of AIB was about halved after 48 hours of fasting. Septic plasma lowered amino acid transport in muscles from fed rats and those fasted for 24 hours, but longer starvation had no added effect. Cellular levels of amino acids transported by system-A, such as serine, glycine, and alanine, were lower in muscle from fasted animals than in muscle from fed rats.

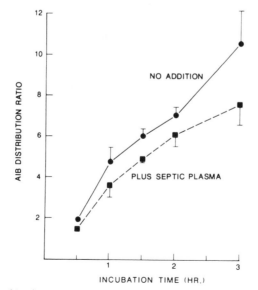

Fig 2–3.—Effect of incubation time on α-aminoisobutyric acid *(AIB)* uptake by normal fed-rat soleus in the presence *(squares)* or absence *(circles)* of septic rat plasma. Septic plasma significantly inhibited AIB uptake: 30 minutes, $P < .001$; 60 and 90 minutes, $P < .01$; 120 minutes, $P < .02$; and 180 minutes, $P < .05$. Standard error bars at 30 minutes are within the circles and squares. (Courtesy of Warner, B.W., et al.: J. Surg. Res. 42:377–382, April 1987.)

Starvation reduces amino acid uptake in skeletal muscle. The nutritional state of muscle is an important part of the response to whatever factor in septic plasma inhibits amino acid uptake. Whether reduced muscle amino acid uptake is mediated by a factor common to both sepsis and starvation remains to be determined.

▶ This experimental study addresses the relative importance of antecedent nutritional status and of circulating factors upon skeletal muscle amino acid transport systems during sepsis. The observed failure of plasma from septic animals to further inhibit the transport of α-aminoisobutyric acid (AIB) in starved animals likely represents a biologic response applicable to several substrates. In addition, mediators derived from endotoxin primed immune cells (cytokines) that have been previously shown by others to alter AIB transport may also be operative in the starvation or malnourished states where enhanced intestinal translocation of bacteria and systemic exposure to endotoxin may be presumed to exist. The clinical implications of this concept suggests that nutritional support, particularly by the enteral route, should be considered an integral component in the management of the septic patient. Although previous reports, including citations in this volume, often fail to document a significant clinical or metabolic benefit to nutritional therapy, it remains likely that critical organ sensitivity to such inflammatory mediators may be exaggerated by malnutrition.—S.F. Lowry, M.D.

3 Shock

Shock and Tissue Injury Induced by Recombinant Human Cachectin
Kevin J. Tracey, Bruce Beutler, Stephen F. Lowry, James Merryweather, Stephen Wolpe, Ian W. Milsark, Robert J. Hariri, Thomas J. Fahey III, Alejandro Zentella, James D. Albert, G. Tom Shires, and Anthony Cerami (New York Hosp.–Cornell Med. Ctr. and Rockefeller Univ., New York)
Science 234:470–474, Oct. 24, 1986   3–1

Cachectin, or tumor necrosis factor, is a protein produced by endotoxin-activated macrophages and implicated as a mediator of lethality from endotoxin. The authors infused recombinant human cachectin into rats to determine whether it alone can elicit the effects of administered endotoxin. Highly purified cachectin (Fig 3–1) was infused into unanesthetized female rats in varying doses.

Infusion of cachectin in amounts similar to those produced endogenously in response to endotoxin led to hypotension, metabolic acidosis, hemoconcentration, and death within hours, due to respiratory arrest. Hyperglycemia and hyperkalemia also were noted. Autopsy showed diffuse pulmonary inflammation and hemorrhage, ischemic and hemorrhagic lesions of the gut, and acute renal tubular necrosis.

The pathophysiologic and histologic sequelae of infused cachectin in the rat resemble the changes induced by lethal doses of endotoxin. Cachectin appears to have a proximate role in the pathogenesis of

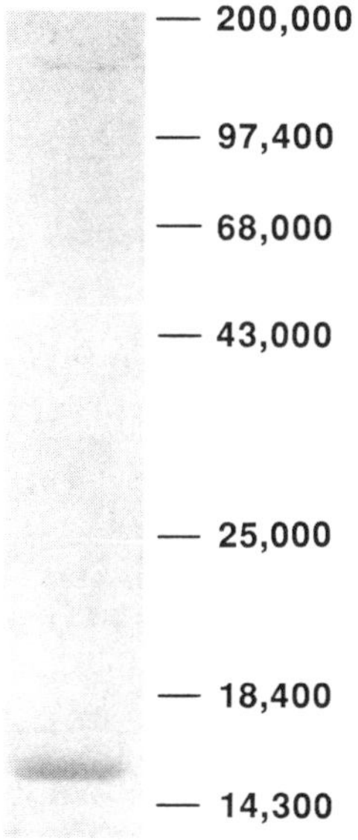

— 200,000

— 97,400

— 68,000

— 43,000

— 25,000

— 18,400

— 14,300

Fig 3–1.—Recombinant human cachetin, purified as described in the text, was subjected to electrophoresis in a 10%–15% polyacrylamide gel under denaturing conditions and was stained with Coomassie blue. Molecular weights are indicated. (Courtesy of Tracey, K.J., et al.: Science 234:470–474, Oct. 24, 1986.)

endotoxin-induced tissue injury. New treatments might involve the interruption of cachectin production or inhibition of its action.

▶ This is the first article to show physiologically that cachectin, a protein produced by endotoxin-activated macrophages, is a mediator of lethality from endotoxin. In this study recombinant human cachectin was infused into rats to determine whether it alone could elicit the effects of administered endotoxin. Infusion of cachectin in amounts similar to those produced endogenously in response to endotoxin led to hypotension, metabolic acidosis, hemoconcentration, and death within hours due to respiratory arrest. Hyperglycemia and hyperkalemia accompanied the autopsy findings of pulmonary damage as well as ischemic and hemorrhagic lesions of the intestine and acute renal tumor necrosis.

The physiologic and histologic sequelae of infused cachectin resembled the changes induced by lethal doses of endotoxin, and therefore cachectin appears to have a proximate role in the pathogenesis of septic tissue injury.—G.T. Shires, M.D.

Cachectin/Tumor Necrosis Factor Induces Lethal Shock and Stress Hormone Responses in the Dog

Kevin J. Tracey, Stephen F. Lowry, Thomas J. Fahey III, James D. Albert, Yuman Fong, David Hesse, Bruce Beutler, Kirk R. Manogue, Steve Calvano, He Wei, Anthony Cerami, and G. Tom Shires (New York Hosp.–Cornell Med. Ctr. and Rockefeller Univ., New York)
Surg. Gynecol. Obstet. 164:415–422, May 1987   3–2

Cachectin/tumor necrosis factor (TNF) has been implicated in the marked changes of metabolic and hemodynamic homeostasis that accompany lethal endotoxemia. In particular, cachectin may account for many of the acute adverse effects of sepsis. Dogs were administered cachectin intraarterially, and their hemodynamic status, along with skeletal muscle transmembrane potential difference and lactate release from the isolated hindlimb, was monitored. Recombinant human cachectin was used.

Infusion of cachectin led to progressive hypotension and shock; animals died within 3 hours. Pulmonary capillary wedge pressure declined, and fluid requirements increased significantly. Circulating stress hormones increased during cachectin-induced hypotension. Peripheral lactate release contributed to the development of metabolic acidosis. Autopsy showed pulmonary hemorrhages, bleeding in the kidneys, and adrenal necrosis. Capillary thrombosis and necrosis were seen in several vital organs. Skeletal muscle transmembrane potential difference decreased when cachectin was infused into the isolated hindlimb (Fig 3–2).

These findings suggest a prominent role for cachectin in the mobilization of host energy stores and the development of shock following infec-

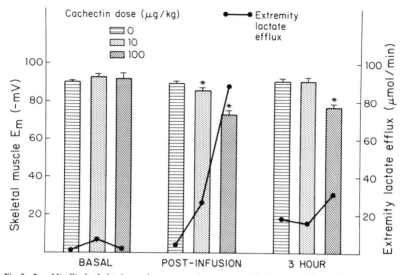

Fig 3–2.—Hindlimb skeletal muscle transmembrane potential difference (E_m) and extremity lactate efflux were determined for each group at several points in time: basal (t = −60 minutes), after infusion (t = 15 minutes), and 3 hours (t = 180 minutes). Extremity lactate efflux for each group during the aforementioned time points is depicted as the line graph. *Asterisk* indicates $P < .05$ as compared with the control group at similar time points. (Courtesy of Tracey, K.J., et al.: Surg. Gynecol. Obstet. 164:415–422, May 1987.)

tion. It might be possible to treat endotoxic shock with antibodies directed against either the circulating peptide or peptide receptor binding.

▶ This is an extension of the cachectin mediator studies into the dog. Once again, cachectin administered intra-arterially produced the hemodynamic in metabolic as well as skeletal muscle membrane derangements as seen in septic shock or pure endotoxin shock. Recombinant human cachectin was administered to animals, and all of the sequelae and sepsis, including the organ damage, both in vivo and at autopsy, were described. This study certainly pointed to the possibility that treatment of sepsis with antibodies directed against the circulating peptide or even the peptide receptor binding, such as cachectin binding sites, might well be feasible for treatment.—G.T. Shires, M.D.

Recombinant Tumor Necrosis Factor/Cachectin and Interleukin 1 Pretreatment Decreases Lung Oxidized Glutathione Accumulation, Lung Injury, and Mortality in Rats Exposed to Hyperoxia

Carl W. White, Pietro Ghezzi, Charles A. Dinarello, Sherrie A. Caldwell, Ivan F. McMurtry, and John E. Repine (Univ. of Colorado, Denver; Inst. di Ricerche Farmacologiche "Marie Negri," Milan, Italy; and Tufts Univ., Boston)
J. Clin. Invest. 79:1868–1873, June 1987   3–3

Endotoxin pretreatment protects against pulmonary oxygen toxicity. It also can stimulate the production of the potent cytokines tumor necrosis factor/cachectin (TNF/C) and interleukin 1 (IL-1). The authors attempted to learn whether treatment with TNF/C or IL-1, or both, might influence susceptibility to lung injury from hyperoxia. Single preexposure parenteral injections of recombinant TNF/C and IL-1 were given to rats, followed by continuous exposure to more than 99% oxygen at 1 atmosphere.

Both TNF/C and IL-1 together prolonged survival of rats exposed to hyperoxia. Interleukin-1 alone was not comparably effective. Animals given combined treatment had less pleural effusion, less morphologic lung damage, and lower pulmonary artery pressure and pulmonary resistance than saline-injected animals. The pulmonary ratio of reduced to oxidized glutathione was higher in treated animals after exposure to hyperoxia for 52 hours.

Exposure to cytokines markedly increases survival in rats exposed continuously to hyperoxia. Endotoxemia and other events that trigger the release of cytokine mediators therefore may have widespread physiologic consequences in protecting against oxidative injury. Pretreatment of rats in the present study with both TNF/C and IL-1 altered lung glutathione redox status favorably and limited lung injury from hyperoxia.

▶ This study is probably the first to show a rational explanation for the often observed phenomenon of protection against sepsis with pretreatment of sublethal doses of endotoxin. It is clear from this study that pretreatment stimulates the production of potent cytokines such as cachectin and interleukin 1. It is also clear that at these levels the cytokine mediators may well protect against oxidative injury such as occurs in response to overwhelming sepsis, although in the present study the enhanced survival was in response only to the stimulus of hyperoxia.—G.T. Shires, M.D.

Neutrophil Function in a Rat Model of Endotoxin-Induced Lung Injury
Richard K. Simons, Ronald V. Maier, and E. Stan Lennard (Univ. of Washington, Seattle)
Arch. Surg. 122:197–203, February 1987   3–4

Chronic endotoxemia may alter the production of cytotoxic oxygen intermediates by polymorphs, thereby inducing acute lung injury in adult respiratory distress syndrome (ARDS). In addition, the microbicidal capacity of polymorphs is depressed, which may contribute to the infectious complications of ARDS. These hypotheses were studied in a model of rat-lung injury induced by chronic endotoxemia, which closely resembles ARDS both clinically and histologically.

Rats infused with *Escherichia coli* endotoxin for 3 days developed interstitial and intraalveolar edema, basement membrane thickening, and intraalveolar polymorph aggregation. Superoxide production was markedly enhanced in circulating polymorphs from endotoxemic animals. My-

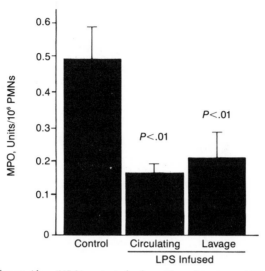

Fig 3–3.—Myeloperoxidase *(MPO)* content of polymorphonuclear neutrophil lymphocytes *(PMNs)* from circulation of normal rats *(control)* and from circulation and bronchoalveolar lavage of rats endotoxemic for 72 hours. Both PMN populations from endotoxemic rats have marked depression of MPO content compared with controls. *LPS* indicates lipopolysaccharide. (Courtesy of Simons, R.K., et al.: Arch. Surg. 122:197–203, February 1987.)

eloperoxidase activity was reduced in both circulating and lavaged polymorphs (Fig 3–3).

Increased superoxide anion release by circulating polymorphs characterizes this model of ARDS. The bactericidal deficit of polymorphs in endotoxic shock might be due in part to a reduction in myeloperoxidase.

▶ This is another of the articles demonstrating endotoxin-induced organ injury, probably mediated largely through monokines. In this particular study, the production of cytotoxic oxygen intermediates by polymorphonuclear leukocytes was described in a model of rat lung injury induced by chronic endotoxemia which closely resembled the form of pulmonary failure seen in septic shock. Superoxide production was markedly enhanced in the circulating polymorphonuclear leuocytes from endotoxemic animals, as well as superoxide anion released by circulating polymorphs.—G.T. Shires, M.D.

Endotoxin Promotes the Translocation of Bacteria From the Gut
Edwin A. Deitch, Rodney Berg, and Robert Specian (Louisiana State Univ., Shreveport)
Arch. Surg. 122:185–190, February 1987   3–5

The intestinal mucosa is a major barrier that prevents bacteria colonizing the gut from invading systemic organs and tissues. The role of endotoxin in promoting the systemic spread of organisms, or bacterial trans-

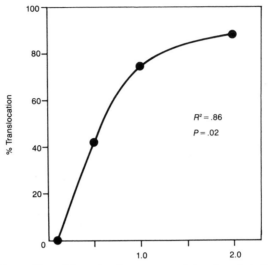

Fig 3–4.—Incidence of bacterial translocation to mesenteric lymph node in CD-1 mice receiving doses of endotoxin ranging from 0.1 to 2 mg, administered intraperitoneally. (Courtesy of Deitch, E.A., et al.: Arch. Surg. 122:185–190, February 1987.)

location, was studied in pathogen-free mice of both genetically endotoxin-resistant and sensitive strains. Lipopolysaccharide from *Escherichia coli* was given intraperitoneally, intramuscularly, or subcutaneously to female mice, aged 2–3 months, with a stable indigenous gastrointestinal tract flora.

Bacterial translocation to the mesenteric lymph nodes was directly related to the dose of intraperitoneally administered endotoxin (Fig 3–4). Spread to the liver, spleen, or blood was not observed. Intramuscularly administered endotoxin also promoted bacterial translocation to the mesenteric nodes, but subcutaneous administration did not. Genetic sensitivity to endotoxin was not associated with spontaneous translocation of bacteria.

These findings suggest that the gut may serve as a reservoir for bacteria, causing systemic infection during endotoxemia. Immunomodulators should not be empirically used to prevent endotoxin-induced bacterial translocation until the mechanisms by which endotoxin induces translocation are understood.

▶ This fascinating study examined the role of the intestinal mucosa as a major barrier to bacterial invasion from the gut invading systemic organs and tissues. The role of endotoxin in promoting the systemic spread organisms or bacterial translocation was studied. *Escherichia coli* lipopolysaccharide was given systemically, and bacterial translocation to the mesenteric lymph nodes was directly related to the dose of such endotoxin. It would appear from studies such as this that the gut may serve as a reservoir for bacteria, causing systemic infection during endotoxemia.—G.T. Shires, M.D.

Effect of Stress and Trauma on Bacterial Translocation From the Gut

Edwin A. Deitch and R. McIntyre Bridges (Louisiana State Univ., Shreveport)
J. Surg. Res. 42:536–542, May 1987   3–6

Both endogenous and other bacteria colonizing the gut can cross the mucosal barrier and spread systemically. The authors studied bacterial translocation from the gastrointestinal tract in healthy pathogen-free mice subjected to cold exposure, femoral fracture amputation, and thermal injury. Necrotic tissue is retained in thermal injury but not in the femoral fracture amputation model. Mice with normal gut microflora and others monoassociated with *Escherichia coli* C-25 were used in the studies.

The incidence and magnitude of bacterial translocation to the mesenteric lymph nodes were not increased by cold exposure. Translocation to the spleen and liver was higher in animals with normal flora who underwent femoral fracture amputation than in those subjected to thermal injury (table). Translocation of bacteria to the liver or spleen was more frequent in burned mice monoassociated with *E. coli* C-25 than in similar mice subjected to femoral fracture amputation.

These findings suggest that stress alone does not promote bacterial translocation. However, trauma, especially when combined with retained necrotic tissue, does promote bacterial translocation in the mouse. More knowledge of the relations among trauma, host defenses, and bacterial colonization of the gut may help in developing treatment for potentially life-threatening opportunistic infections arising from the gastrointestinal tract.

▶ This is another study by the same group studying bacterial translocation under a variety of conditions. It is interesting that stress alone in the form of hypothermia did not promote translocation of bacteria from the bowel to either mesenteric lymph nodes or other organs. However, in severe injury, particularly with retained necrotic tissue such as a burn, the bacterial translocation was promoted quite significantly. Studies such as these may well explain the development of life threatening opportunistic infections arising from the gastrointestinal tract in the face of significant trauma.—G.T. Shires, M.D.

TRANSLOCATION OF *ESCHERICHIA COLI* C-25 FROM THE GASTROINTESTINAL TRACT IN MICE RECEIVING FEMORAL FRACTURE/AMPUTATION (FX/AMP) OR THERMAL INJURY

Group	n	MLN*	Liver	Spleen	Combined liver and spleen	Cecum (CFU/g)†
Control	20	14/20	0/20	0/20	0/40	$2 \pm 2 \times 10^{10}$
Fx/Amp	23	18/23	4/23	4/23	8/46§	$3 \pm 4 \times 10^{10}$
Burn	10	10/10	6/10‡	5/10‡	11/20‖	$6 \pm 16 \times 10^{9}$

*Data expressed as number of organs containing viable *E. coli* C-25, divided by total number of organs tested.
†Means ± SE of enteric bacilli as colony-forming units per gram cecum.
‡$P < .05$ vs. control or Fx/Amp mice.
§$P < .05$ vs. control.
‖$P < .01$ vs. control or Fx/Amp mice.
(Courtesy of Deitch, E.A., and Bridges, R.M.: J. Surg. Res. 42:536–542, May 1987.)

Lethal Toxicity of Lipopolysaccharide and Tumor Necrosis Factor in Normal and D-Galactosamine-Treated Mice

V. Lehmann, M.A. Freudenberg, and C. Galanos (Deutsche Krebsforschungszentrum, Heidelberg, and Max-Planck Inst., Freiburg, West Germany)
J. Exp. Med. 165:657–663, March 1987   3–7

Cachectin, or tumor necrosis factor (TNF), has an important role in mediating the lethal effects of lipopolysaccharides. Studies with human recombinant TNF have shown that lipopolysaccharide and TNF have identical lethal effects in D-galactosamine-treated mice. Mice were made hypersensitive to endotoxin by treatment with D-galactosamine.

Mice treated with D-galactosamine were sensitive to the lethality of submicrogram amounts of TNF. In its absence, TNF caused about 80% lethality at a dose of 500 μg. Sensitization to TNF lasted up to 8 hours after D-galactosamine administration, and sensitization to lipopolysaccharide lasted for up to 4 hours. Sensitization to both substances was inhibited by uridine. In contrast to lipopolysaccharide, toxicity of TNF also was expressed in endotoxin-resistant mice given D-galactosamine. These mice were as susceptible to TNF as were endotoxin-sensitive animals.

These findings support the concept that TNF mediates lethal endotoxin toxicity. As is the case with lipopolysaccharide, the activity of TNF may be enhanced in animals with impaired liver metabolism.

▶ This interesting study once again demonstrates the concept that cachectin mediates lethal endotoxin toxicity. In this particular study, it appears that the activity of cachectin (TNF) may well be enhanced in animals with impaired liver metabolism. In this particular model, that state was produced by treatment with D-galactosamine.—G.T. Shires, M.D.

Effect of Polyethylene Glycol-Superoxide Dismutase and Catalase on Endotoxemia in Pigs

Neil C. Olson, Mary K. Grizzle, and Donald L. Anderson (North Carolina State Univ.)
J. Appl. Physiol. 63:1526–1532, 1987   3–8

Suproxide anion and hydrogen peroxide may be important mediators of endotoxin-induced acute respiratory failure. These toxic oxygen radicals influence pulmonary function and may potentiate lung injury by activating host granulocytes. The role of these radicals was studied by infusing specific scavengers, polyethylene glycol-superoxide dismutase (PEG-SOD) and PEG-catalase (PEG-CAT), in domestic pigs before induction of endotoxemia. *Escherichia coli* endotoxin was infused into anesthetized animals.

Endotoxin decreased cardiac index and pulmonary compliance and increased pulmonary vascular resistance and the alveolar-arterial oxygen gradient. Endotoxemia also led to granulocytopenia and increased the albumin content of bronchoalveolar lavage fluid. Although PEG-SOD failed to significantly alter this course, PEG-CAT attenuated the early fall in cardiac index and the increases in pulmonary vascular resistance and total periphral resistance. In addition, granulocytopenia was less marked when PEG-CAT was given. The scavenger was effective during the first 2 hours but not subsequently.

Superoxide anion does not appear to directly contribute to endo-toxin-related lung injury. However, hydrogen peroxide or a subsequent metabolite does contribute to the early endotoxin-induced changes, including hemodynamic instability, granulocytopenia, and increased permeability of the alveolocapillary membrane.

▶ This interesting study examined the role of superoxide anion and hydrogen peroxide as mediators of endotoxin-induced acute respiratory failure. The role of these toxic oxygen radicals was studied by infusing specific scavengers such as polyethylene glycol-superoxide dismutase and catalase in pigs prior to the induction of endotoxemia. From these studies it appeared that the superoxide anion did not directly cause endotoxin-evoked lung injury; however, hydrogen peroxide or a subsequent metabolite did contribute to the early endotoxin-induced changes of hemodynamic instability, granulocytopenia, and increased permeability of the alveolar capillary membrane, which is the precursor of septic lung injury in the acute respiratory failure of sepsis.—G.T. Shires, M.D.

Superior Mesenteric Artery Occlusion Shock in Cats: Modification of the Endotoxemia by Antilipopolysaccharide Antibodies (Anti-LPS)
P. Gathiram, S.L. Gaffin, M.T. Wells, and J.G. Brock-Utne (Univ. of Durban/Westville and Univ. of Natal Med. School, Durban, South Africa)
Circ. Shock 19:231–237, 1986   3–9

Conventional antibiotic therapy fails in about half of patients with septic shock, partly because of the release of highly toxic lipopolysaccharide (LPS, endotoxin) from killed bacteria. Human anti-LPS antibody has been used effectively to treat gram-negative bacterial infection in human beings. The course of plasma LPS was followed in cats undergoing occlusion of the superior mesenteric artery for 1 hour. Treated animals received an intravenous infusion of anti-LPS hyperimmune plasma in a dose of 1 cc/kg of body weight 1.5 hours before occlusion, immediately after release of occlusion, or 10 or 20 minutes after release. The preparation contained 1,200 µg/ml of LPS-precipitable IgG.

Plasma LPS increased after 20 minutes of occlusion except when anti-LPS was given prophylactically (Fig 3–5). Levels of LPS remained at or below baseline throughout the postocclusion period in the latter animals. When anti-LPS was given just after release of occlusion, the plasma LPS decreased progressively.

Administration of anti-LPS before arterial occlusion prevented a rise in plasma LPS in this study. Treatment in the reperfusion period reversed endotoxemia. Anti-LPS antibodies rapidly lower high concentrations of

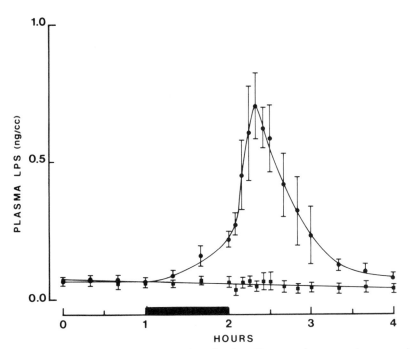

Fig 3–5.—Effect of prophylactic antilipopolysaccharide *(LPS)* on superior mesenteric artery occlusion endotoxemia. Cats intravenously received 1.0 cc/kg of body weight of equine hyperimmune plasma 1.5 hours before occlusion of their superior mesenteric arteries for 60 minutes. In the untreated cats *(circles)*, femoral arteries blood samples showed a small rise in LPS concentration during the occlusion period, but a larger one peaking 20 minutes after release of the occlusion, which returned to baseline levels after an additional 90–100 minutes. In those cats receiving prophylactic anti-LPS *(squares)*, no rise was seen in blood samples either during or after the occlusion period. (Courtesy of Gathiram, P., et al.: Circ. Shock 19:231–237, 1986.)

LPS in the systemic circulation and may thereby improve survival in septic shock.

▶ This study is another attempt to neutralize the endotoxin or lipopolysaccharide which is the cause of organ failure and death in sepsis. In this particular study, human antilipopolysaccharide antibody was used to produce survival when administered prior to superior mesenteric artery occlusion in animals. Even treatment in the reperfusion period reversed endotoxemia so that the antilipopolysaccharide antibodies will rapidly lower higher concentrations of LPS in the systemic circulation.—G.T. Shires, M.D.

A Controlled Clinical Trial of High-Dose Methylprednisolone in the Treatment of Severe Sepsis and Septic Shock
Roger C. Bone, Charles J. Fisher, Jr., Terry P. Clemmer, Gus J. Slotman, Craig A. Metz, Robert A. Balk, and the Methylprednisolone Severe Sepsis Study Group (Rush-Presbyterian-St. Luke's Med. Ctr., Chicago)
N. Engl. J. Med. 317:653–658, Sept. 10, 1987   3–10

The use of high-dose corticosteroids in treating severe sepsis and septic shock remains controversial. In a prospective, randomized, double-blind, placebo-controlled trial, 382 patients with severe sepsis and septic shock received either high-dose methylprednisolone sodium succinate (30 mg/kg body weight) or placebo in four infusions starting within 2 hours of diagnosis. Diagnosis was based on the clinical suspicion of infection plus the presence of fever or hypothermia (rectal temperature $>38.3°C$ [101°F] or $<35.6°C$ [96°F]), tachypnea (>20 breaths per minute), tachycardia (>90 beats per minute), and presence of one of the following indicators of organ dysfunction: change in mental status, hypoxemia, elevated lactate levels, or oliguria.

There were no significant differences between treatment groups in the prevention of shock, the reversal of shock, or overall mortality at 14 days. Patients who had renal insufficiency (serum creatinine level >2 mg/dl) initially and were treated with methyprednisolone had significantly higher incidence of shock development and mortality and tended to have decreased shock reversal. Although the incidence of secondary infection did not differ between groups, the deaths of patients treated with steroids were related to secondary infection significantly more often.

The use of high-dose corticosteroids does not appear to be of any benefit in the treatment of severe sepsis and septic shock.

▶ This fascinating study was the first prospective, randomized, double-blind, placebo-controlled trial of high dose methylprednisolone therapy for severe sepsis and septic shock.

No significant differences were found in the prevention of shock, the reversal of shock, or the overall mortality from sepsis or septic shock. Quite the contrary, mortality rate at 14 days was significantly increased among those having received high dose methylprednisolone compared to the placebo-controls. Those delayed deaths in the group treated with methylprednisolone were related to secondary infection. This is an extremely important randomized study and should lay to rest a lot of data, gathered in a meaningless way, claiming clinical benefits from high dose corticosteroid treatment of severe sepsis and septic shock.—G.T. Shires, M.D.

4 Trauma

The Importance of Nonoperative Trauma Management in Postgraduate Surgical Education
Jonathan R. Hiatt and Ronald K. Tompkins (Univ. of California, Los Angeles)
J. Trauma 27:769–773, July 1987   4–1

Activities of a trauma service in a university hospital and level I trauma center were analyzed to determine whether the operative caseload alone adequately measures the trauma experience of surgical residents. A total of 378 major trauma victims were admitted in a 2-year period. Blunt trauma was responsible in 79% of cases. Patients spent 2.8 days on average in intensive care.

Fifteen senior residents rotated through the service during the review period and averaged 25 patients each. They were supervised by 11 chief residents. Sixty-four percent of patients had blunt multisystem trauma.

Major surgery was done in 156 patients, 126 of whom had laparotomy for intra-abdominal injury. Eighty-three patients had further procedures by specialty services. Another 222 patients had surgery by specialty services only, minor procedures by the trauma service, or no surgery. Critical care was an important part of the management of all groups of patients. There were 18 hospital deaths.

Trauma services manage significant numbers of patients with multisystem injuries who do not undergo general surgery, and these patients are a prominent component of surgical education in trauma. A surgical residency should include adequate training in the critical care of surgical patients. It may be appropriate to have residents document specific areas or disease processes when nonoperative critical care has been given.

▶ This is a very useful study documenting the fact that the measurement of resident experience in trauma management probably should not be confined entirely to operative experience. A plea is made for use of critical care of trauma patients and surgical patients as a measure of the adequacy of the training process.—G.T. Shires, M.D.

Caring for the Major Trauma Victim: The Role for Radiology
James J. McCort (Santa Clara Valley Med. Ctr., San Jose, Calif.)
Radiology 163:1–9, April 1987   4–2

Injuries are the third leading cause of death in the United States. Both the development of emergency medical service systems and the wide use of computed tomography (CT) have contributed to better survival of major trauma victims. Trauma centers require close radiology support, including constant coverage by experienced technologists, and facilities for CT, sonography, and angiography. A radiologist must be promptly available.

Computed tomography first was used to study head injury, reliably demonstrating intracranial hemorrhage; it is especially useful in abused children. Computed tomography is better than other methods in evaluating blunt abdominal trauma and has much reduced the need for exploratory laparotomy. Computed tomography has promoted the nonoperative management of splenic lacerations in both children and adults. Liver lacerations also are managed nonoperatively in hemodynamically stable patients. Computed tomography is able to demonstrate pancreatic transection. Renal trauma is first assessed by intravenous urography, and CT is used for further evaluation where required.

Computed tomography provides accurate information in cases of vertebral trauma and involves less manipulation than conventional radiography. Bone fragments and foreign bodies are visualized within the spinal canal. Computed tomography can show occult acetabular fractures and adjacent soft tissue injuries. The modality is useful in studying facial fractures, including orbital blow-out injuries.

▶ This article documents nicely the increasing role of radiology in the care of the traumatized patient. There is no question that computed tomography, for example, is a necessity in the acute care of patients having sustained head injury. When readily and promptly available, computed tomography is very useful in approximately 20% of the patients with abdominal trauma. Similarly, its usefulness in other areas, such as fractures, is becoming apparent. While the expense for such available radiologic services is significant, the benefits in patient care certainly justify the cost.—G.T. Shires, M.D.

Clinical Indications for Cervical Spine Radiographs in the Traumatized Patient

Ben L. Bachulis, William B. Long, Gerald D. Hynes, and Martin C. Johnson (Emanuel Hosp. and Health Ctr., Portland, Ore.)
Am. J. Surg. 153:473–478, May 1987   4–3

The large expenditure for cervical spine radiographs in injured patients led to a review of spinal radiography in 4,941 trauma patients, 38% for whom cervical spine radiographs were obtained. Cervical spinal injury was detected in 94 (5%) patients of those evaluated.

Ninety study patients had cervical spine fractures, and four had disruption of the cervical longitudinal ligaments without bony injury. The overall incidence of cervical spine injury in trauma patients was 2%. No patient who was neurologically intact at admission developed deficit. Twenty-eight patients were quadriplegic when admitted. Cervical spine or spinal cord injury was diagnosed in the emergency department in 60 patients, and elsewhere in 24 patients. In only one patient was the diagnosis missed altogether. Lateral cervical spinal radiographs were negative

RADIOLOGIC SCREENING FOR CERVICAL SPINE INJURIES
IN THE TRAUMA PATIENT*

Patient Status	Initial Radiographs	Secondary Testing
Physiologically Stable		
Alert, Sober, asymptomatic	None	None
Symptomatic	Lateral, anterior/posterior, odontoid, right & left oblique	CAT scan, tomography, flexion/extension as indicated
Intoxicated, decreased mentation	Lateral, anterior/posterior, odontoid, right and left oblique	CAT scan, tomography, flexion/extension as indicated
Physiologically Unstable		
Alert, sober asymptomatic	None	None
Symptomatic	Lateral†	Complete work-up after resuscitation
Intoxicated, decreased mentation	Lateral†	Complete work-up after resuscitation

*The terms used are defined as alert: normal level of consciousness; asymptomatic: no neck pain or tenderness and no neurologic findings compatible with cervical origin; symptomatic: any complaint of neck pain, tenderness, or neurologic findings compatible with cervical origin; intoxicated: by clinical diagnosis or a blood alcohol level of 0.08 or higher; decreased mentation: Glasgow Coma Score of 13 or less; physiologically stable: blood pressure of 90 torr or higher, respiratory rate of 13 to 29, pulse rate of 60 to 110; physiologically unstable: vital signs outside the limits just mentioned.

†Apply Philadelphia collar and assume patient has an unstable cervical fracture if the lateral radiograph is normal.

(Courtesy of Bachulis, B.L., et al.: Am. J. Surg. 153:473–478, May 1987.)

in the nine patients diagnosed after admission. Five of these patients had altered consciousness. The lateral cervical spine radiograph was diagnostic in 73% of patients. In the 21 patients where this radiograph was not adequate to make a diagnosis, computed tomography was most often diagnostic of bony injury.

The alert, cooperative trauma patient who has no neck pain or tenderness does not require radiographic study of the cervical spine. Computed tomography is of great value where cervical spine injury is suspected but plain roentgenograms are negative. The present scheme of radiologic screening for cervical spine injury is outlined in the table.

▶ This is an interesting new approach designed in an attempt to evaluate the indications for cervical spine radiographs in the traumatized patient. The data presented here indicate that in the alert, cooperative trauma patient who has no neck pain, tenderness, or neurologic deficit, radiographic study of the cervical spine is probably not required, since the overall instance of cervical spine injury of trauma patients is only 2%. This argument is bolstered by the fact that no patient in the study who was neurologically intact at admission developed a neurologic deficit. These authors also pointed out that the computed tomography is of great value where cervical spine injury is suspected following plain x-rays.—G.T. Shires, M.D.

Potentiated Hormonal Responses in a Model of Traumatic Injury
Eric J. DeMaria, Michael P. Lilly, and Donald S. Gann (Brown Univ.)
J. Surg. Res. 43:45–51, July 1987   4–4

Major trauma frequently involves repeated insults, sepsis, and multiple organ system failure, all of which may stimulate hormone release. The authors studied adrenocoticotropin (ACTH) and cortisol responses to repeated hemorrhages in splenectomized dogs. Circulating vasopressin, plasma renin activity, and angiotensin II were estimated to determine whether the release of other trauma-related hormones is influenced by previous hemorrhage. Ten percent of the blood volume was removed. The shed blood was returned at 30 minutes, and the hemorrhage repeated 5 hours later.

Initial bleeding led to a small but significant rise in adrenal cortisol and circulating ACTH, as well as increases in vasopressin, angiotensin II, and plasma renin activity. The ACTH and cortisol responses to the second bleed were exaggerated, as was the vasopressin response. The renin and angiotensin II responses, however, were no greater than those to initial bleeding. The potentiated responses could not be ascribed to differences in blood volume, heart rate, or arterial pressure after the two hemorrhages.

Potentiated hormonal responses were seen in this model of repeated injury. The biologic significance of this phenomenon remains to be determined, but potentiated humoral responses may have important clinical implications. Increased vasopressin release may stimulate the release of ACTH.

▶ This is an interesting study confirming what many have contended from clinical impressions only over a long period of time. These studies show that repeated hemorrhage in animals led to a potentiation of the hormonal responses as seen in this model of repeated injury. It could well be that the potentiated hormonal responses have significant effects insofar as survival is concerned now that it is becoming quite clear that some of the stress hormones, for example, have far more influence on protein metabolism than was previously suspected.— G.T. Shires, M.D.

The Gut Origin Septic States in Blunt Multiple Trauma (ISS = 40) in the ICU
John R. Border, James Hassett, John LaDuca, Roger Seibel, Steven Steinberg, Barbara Mills, Patricia Losi, and Donna Border (SUNY at Buffalo)
Ann. Surg. 206: 427-448, October 1987   4–5

After a period of stability or improvement which lasts 2 to 3 days after initial treatment a critically injured patient may develop a severe septic response with failure of several organs, especially the lung. Evidence of bacterial infection develops at about 10 days. Sepsis then may stabilize, but bacteriologic evidence of infection worsens. The longer the course, the more likely the patient will die. Early management itself may lead to persistence of the pulmonary failure septic state.

Data were reviewed on 66 patients with blunt multiple trauma and an injury severity score (ISS) that exceeded 22. Longer ventilation was closely associated with more severe sepsis. The number of ventilator days was best predicted by delayed operation and positive blood cultures.

A greater number of antibiotics also was associated with more severe sepsis. Only increased enteral protein was consistently associated with a less severe septic state. Patients who died in sepsis tended to receive many antibiotics and to require persistent ventilatory support.

Incomplete early surgical care is the primary determinant of the degree of sepsis in blunt trauma victims and the duration of stay in the ICU. Incomplete surgery leads to the use of more broad-spectrum antibiotics and other drugs, more monitoring and drainage lines, and more prolonged ventilation. Enteral protein is important in limiting clinical sepsis. Many later complications can be avoided by total surgical care, including fracture treatment the night of admission. This will allow the patient to be out of bed and sitting up a day or two afterward.

▶ This is a continuing study by the group that first pointed out that immediate fracture stabilization with early ambulation significantly reduces the ARDS occurring after injury and that this ARDS is virtually always septic in origin. Certainly, the patients who were managed conservatively had longer ventilatory support, more infection, and therefore, more liberal use of antibiotics. To complement this gut origin of the sepsis, the authors also indicated that increased enteric protein was consistently associated with the less severe septic state. While this again is indirect evidence of the gut origin theory of sepsis, it is certainly strongly suggestive and strongly supportive evidence. Enteral protein is increasingly being recognized as a major limiting factor in the development of clinical sepsis.—G.T. Shires, M.D.

Plasma Extracellular-Superoxide Dismutase in the Acute Phase Response Induced by Surgical Trauma and Inflammatory Disorders

Stefan L. Marklund, Per Arne Kling, Stig Nilsson, and Michael Boomhman (Umeå Univ., Umeå, Sweden)
Scand. J. Clin. Lab. Invest. 47:567–570, October 1987   4–6

In the acute-phase response to infection or tissue trauma, activated phagocytic leukocytes produce large amounts of superoxide radicals and other toxic oxygen reduction intermediates, which promote tissue damage. Extracellular-superoxide dismutase (EC-SOD) is the major enzymic protector against superoxide radicals in plasma and other extracellular fluids. Plasma EC-SOD was studied serially in 13 patients following operative trauma and in 15 patients with an acute phase response to various inflammatory disorders.

A decrease in EC-SOD lasted for about 3 days after surgery. Plasma C-reactive protein increased markedly, and levels of α-1-antitrypsin, haptoglobin, and orosomucoid nearly doubled after surgery. These substances increased twofold to threefold in patients with inflammatory disease. Plasma EC-SOD did not change significantly in this group.

This study gave no conclusive evidence of a positive or negative acute phase response of plasma EC-SOD after surgery or in inflammatory disorders. The fall in EC-SOD after operation may be explained by hemodilution and also by replacement of lost blood with administered fluid.

▶ This study measures the extracellular-superoxide dismutase, which is an endogenous enzymic protector against superoxide radicals that would appear free in plasma and extracellular fluids following tissue trauma. It would appear that the trauma investigated was relatively minimal, that is, operative trauma, and consequently no protective enzyme elevation was seen. However, with the degree of trauma studied, this does not seem surprising at all. It is also true that many of the activated phagocytic leukocytes producing superoxide radicals and other toxic oxygen reduction intermediates will show up only in the tissues that are end-organ, such as the lung.—G.T. Shires, M.D.

Alterations in T-Helper and T-Suppressor Lymphocyte Populations After Multiple Injuries

E. Fosse, J.H. Trumpy, and A. Skulberg (Ullevål Hosp., Oslo)
Injury 18:199–202, May 1987   4–7

Infection is a serious problem in multiply injured patients. Two thirds or more of the late deaths among injured patients are due to bacterial infection. Previous studies of the ratio of T helper–T suppressor cells after major surgery have given conflicting results. This ratio was correlated with the Injury Severity Score (ISS) in 18 consecutive patients who were admitted with multiple injuries. Thirteen patients required surgery in the first 24 hours. The median ISS was 25.

Fifteen patients who survived their injuries had a mean white blood cell count of 11.1×10^9/L at admission, with no significant change during observation. Lymphocytes decreased, mainly because of a fall in T lymphocytes from 1.8 to 0.6×10^9/L. Survivors had a median T helper–T suppressor ratio of 1.5 at admission, compared with 2.0 for control subjects. The ratio fell to 0.8 in the nine patients with ISS scores higher than 16. The T helper–T suppressor cell ratio and ISS did not correlate significantly. No surviving patient developed signs of septicemia. The five patients who received methylprednisolone shortly after admission had cell ratios that were similar to those of the other patients.

Patients with multiple injuries and an ISS greater than 16 are severely injured and at risk of complications, including infection and septicemia. Immunity is impaired in these patients.

▶ This article shows once again studies that have been previously reported by Antonacci and others indicating that, following injury, the lymphocyte population is reduced. Furthermore, this population reduction is largely due to a depression in the T lymphocytes. Most investigators believe that most of this suppression is due to T helper cells suppression in patients with significant injuries such as burns.—G.T. Shires, M.D.

Diagnosis-Related Groups and the Salvageable Trauma Patient in the Intensive Care Unit

David J. Kreis, Jr., Debbie Augenstein, Joseph M. Civetta, Gerardo Gomez, James J. Vopal, and Patricia M. Byers (Univ. of Miami)
Surg. Gynecol. Obstet. 163:539–542, December 1986   4–8

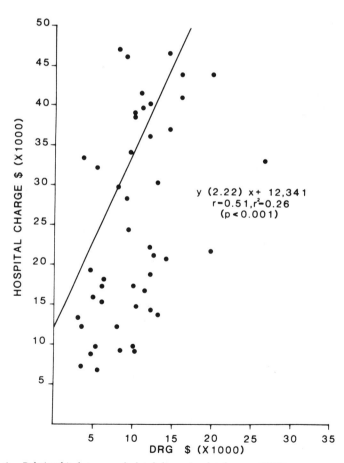

$$y\ (2.22)\ x + 12{,}341$$
$$r-0.51, r^2-0.26$$
$$(p < 0.001)$$

Fig 4–1.—Relationship between calculated diagnosis-related group (DRG) payments and hospital charges. (Courtesy of Kreis, D.J., Jr., et al.: Surg. Gynecol. Obstet. 163:539–542, December 1986.)

A proportion of trauma patients accounts for a disproportionate share of total hospital costs for trauma. The prospective payment system consequently may underestimate charges for these patients, who often are managed in the surgical intensive care unit (SICU). Actual charges for 59 patients treated for multiple injuries in an SICU in 1983 were compared with calculated reimbursement using the diagnosis-related group (DRG) system. An attempt was made by hospital staff to choose the DRG giving the highest payment per patient.

Data on 42 patients with blunt trauma and 17 with penetrating trauma were reviewed. The mean injury severity score was 31, and the mean hospitalization was 31 days. The mean time in the SICU was 5 days. Forty-four patients were operated on, and there was 18 deaths. The DRG payments would have accounted for only 32% of actual hospital charges. A significant relationship between calculated DRG payment and hospital charge was apparent (Fig 4–1). Injury severity score did not correlate significantly with either hospital charge or calculated DRG payment.

Current DRG payment schedules for trauma care do not reflect either the elements of care currently expended or the modifiers required to adjust for acuity and severity. Modifiers are urgently needed for trauma patients in the SICU; otherwise, some hospitals may have to give up trauma care or limit their resources.

▶ This interesting article documents one of the major national threats to improving care of the trauma patient. Using their own patients as controls prior to the diagnosis-related group method of payment, it is clear that the DRG payments would have accounted for only 32% of actual hospital costs incurred in the care of these severely injured patients. Furthermore, the severity of injury did not correlate significantly with the DRG payment, which is calculated as a single diagnosis reimbursement. The authors' conclusions that current DRG payment schedules for trauma care do not reflect either the elements of care currently expended or the modifiers required to adjust for acuity and severity.

This policy of DRG payments, which has now been extended to virtually all payors in the country, is greatly impeding the urgent need for improved care for the severely injured patient. Many hospitals have had to give up trauma care because of this unwarranted governmental restriction.—G.T. Shires, M.D.

Randomized Trial of Pneumatic Antishock Garments in the Prehospital Management of Penetrating Abdominal Injuries
William H. Bickell, Paul E. Pepe, Mark L. Bailey, Charles H. Wyatt, and Kenneth L. Mattox (Baylor College of Medicine, Ben Taub Gen. Hosp., and City of Houston Fire Dept. Emergency Med. Services, Houston, Texas)
Ann. Emerg. Med. 16:653–658, June 1987   4–9

Pneumatic external counterpressure on the lower body may have a tamponade effect on the intraabdominal vessels and elevate central blood pressure. The authors conducted a prospective randomized trial of the pneumatic antishock garment (PASG) in 201 patients seen in a 2½-year period with penetrating anterior abdominal injury and a prehospital systolic blood pressure of 90 mm Hg or less. Patients younger than age 12 were excluded. In the study patients, the PASG was applied to the legs and abdomen and fully inflated.

The two groups were well matched for age and type of injury. Most patients had three or more organ/vessel injuries. The prehospital clinical condition of patients was not significantly altered by the use of the PASG, as determined from trauma scores. Number of transfusions, length of stay in the surgical intensive care unit, and hospital costs were not significantly different in the two groups. Times to death also were similar in the PASG and control groups.

No significant advantage of the PASG was evident in this study of hypotensive patients with penetrating abdominal injuries. The garment should continue to be studied in other settings, such as blunt injury, and where prolonged transport is necessary. Commercial modifications may have lowered the therapeutic benefit observed with the experimental model of the PASG.

▶ This is one of the first prospective randomized studies of the pneumatic antishock garment. This particular study was designed to evaluate the usefulness of this garment in penetrating abdominal injuries. It is clear that the two groups were well matched and that the end points, including a number of transfusions, length of stay in the surgical intensive care unit, and hospital cost, were not significantly different in the two groups. No significant advantage of the pneumatic antishock garment was evident in this study of hypotensive patients with penetrating abdominal injuries. While not examined in this study, one would have to conclude that any usefulness at all of the pneumatic antishock garments may be confined to long-term transport and then only probably under specific circumstances, such as pelvic injury.—G.T. Shires, M.D.

Benefits of Immediate Jejunostomy Feeding After Major Abdominal Trauma: A Prospective, Randomized Study
Ernest E. Moore and Todd N. Jones (Denver Gen. Hosp. and Univ. of Colorado, Denver)
J. Trauma 26:874–881, October 1986   4–10

In the early postinjury period, accelerated substrate mobilization is needed for energy supply, host defense, and wound repair. Excessive substrate requirements not supported by exogenous nutrients may erode visceral protein, compromise immune function, and result in multiple organ failure. A prospective study was done to determine the effect of immediate enteral feeding in critically injured, previously well-nourished patients.

Seventy-five patients undergoing emergent celiotomy with an abdominal trauma index greater than 15 were randomized to a control group— who received no supplemental nutrition during the first 5 days— or to an enteral-fed group. Demographic features, trauma mechanism, shock, co-

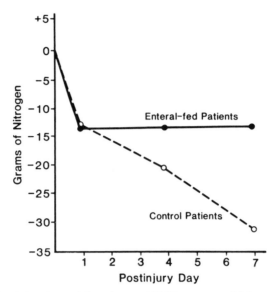

Fig 4–2.—Cumulative nitrogen balance in control (D_5W) versus enteral-fed groups during first week postinjury. (Courtesy of Moore, E.E., and Jones, T.N.: J. Trauma 26:874–881, October 1986.)

lon injury, splenectomy, abdominal trauma index, and initial nutritional assessment were comparable between groups. Enteral-fed patients had a needle catheter jejunostomy placed at laparotomy, with the constant infusion of an elemental diet begun 18 hours afterward and advanced to 3,000 ml/day within 72 hours. Twenty of the enteral-fed patients were maintained on the elemental diet for more than 5 days; 4 needed total parenteral nutrition. Nine of the control patients required total parenteral nutrition. Nitrogen balance was found to be markedly improved in patients fed enterally (Fig 4–2). Septic morbidity was greater in the control group than in the enteral-fed group: in the control group, 7 had abdominal infection, and 2 had pneumonia, whereas 3 enteral-fed patients had abdominal abscess. Visceral protein markers and overall complication rates did not differ significantly between the groups. Analysis of patients with abdominal trauma indexes of 15 to 40 revealed sepsis in 26% of control group patients and in 4% of enteral-fed patients.

These findings indicate that immediate postoperative enteral feedings via needle catheter jejunostomy are feasible after major abdominal trauma. Early nutrition may reduce septic complications.

▶ This interesting study is the first clinical trial to evaluate the feasibility of early enteric feeding following abdominal injury. The authors conclude that early jejunal feeding is feasible following injury and that there may be a significant reduction in the instance of infection.

This article fits well with the currently evolving concepts that the sepsis in many patients with parenteral feeding only may well have its origin in the bowel. Certainly, this can be reduced significantly if bowel feeding is used for support early after injury as opposed to parenteral nutrition.—G.T. Shires, M.D.

Penetrating Abdominal Trauma: The Use of Operative Findings to Determine Length of Antibiotic Therapy

Brian J. Rowlands, Charles D. Ericsson, and Ronald P. Fischer (Univ. of Texas at Houston)

J. Trauma 27:250–255, March 1987

4–11

Antibiotic therapy for trauma patients now often is limited to between 12 and 72 hours, with no apparent increased risk of infectious complications. The authors allocated patients to low and high risk groups, and administered antibiotic therapy for 24 or 72 hours after injury, respectively. Two regimens active against both aerobic and anaerobic enteric organisms were used. Tobramycin was combined with either metronidazole or clindamycin initially. High risk findings included penetration of the bowel, major liver or pancreas injury, a close-range shotgun wound, and deficient hemostasis.

Significantly more trauma-related infections occurred in 102 high risk patients than in the 58 low risk patients. No difference in antibiotic efficacy was seen. One third of patients with large-bowel injuries had infection. There were 16 trauma-related wound infections and seven intra-abdominal infections. One high risk patient died of pseudomonas pneumonia, multiple organ system failure, and septicemia.

Low risk trauma patients may be given antibiotics only perioperatively. Those with high risk operative findings are treated for no more than 72 hours postoperatively, unless the temperature or white blood cell count remains elevated. The use of an aminoglycoside, plus clindamycin or metronidazole, provides adequate coverage against aerobes and anaerobes.

▶ This is another article indicating the value of perioperative antibiotic therapy in the traumatized patient. This study also confirms other recent articles that, if antibiotic therapy is used early, the length of time the antibiotics are necessary is relatively short. The major point of the current study was to indicate that patients with low risk, as determined intraoperatively, can have antibiotic therapy continued for 24 hours or less, whereas high risk groups determined intraoperatively will still need presumptive antibiotics for probably no more than 72 hours postoperatively.

Studies such as these continue to indicate that the use of presumptive antibiotics in the traumatized patient are an absolute necessity. It is also prudent to limit the use of these antibiotics when given appropriately preoperatively.—G.T. Shires, M.D.

Presumptive Antibiotics for Penetrating Abdominal Wounds

Mitchell C. Posner, Ernest E. Moore, Lee Anne Harris, and Maria D. Allo (Univ. of Colorado, Denver)

Surg. Gynecol. Obstet. 165:29–32, July 1987

4–12

The best antimicrobial coverage for patients who have penetrating abdominal injury remains uncertain. One hundred consecutive patients who had celiotomy in a 2-year period were randomized to receive either 4 gm of mezlocillin every 6 hours or a combination of 600 mg of clindamycin every 6 hours and gentamicin, in a loading dose of 2 mg/kg, followed by 1.5 mg/kg every 8 hours.

Septic morbidity occurred in 16% of the mezlocillin group and in 13% of patients who were given combined treatment. There were no significant group differences in major infections. In patients with colonic injury intra-abdominal abscess developed in 29% of those who were given mezlocillin and in 26% of those who were given combined antimicrobial therapy. Aerobic gram-positive organisms predominated at reexploration in the latter group, and anaerobes predominated in mezlocillin-treated patients. No predominance of side effects was associated with either regimen.

The broad-spectrum antibiotic mezlocillin is recommended for use in patients with penetrating abdominal wounds. It is less expensive than combined treatment with clindamicin and gentamicin, and the potential toxicity is less.

▶ This is another article again indicating the striking advantage of presumptive antibiotic usage in patients who have sustained penetrating abdominal injury. Like other recent articles, single-drug therapy with broad-spectrum coverage given in a very early presumptive, preoperative fashion, produces maximal protection. Given in this way, the presumptive antibiotic usage is both helpful and also economical.—G.T. Shires, M.D.

Single GE Cephalosporin Prophylaxis for Penetrating Abdominal Trauma: Results and Comment on the Emergence of the Enterococcus
David V. Feliciano, Layne O. Gentry, Carmel G. Bitondo, Jon M. Burch, Kenneth L. Mattox, Pamela A. Cruse, and George L. Jordan, Jr. (Baylor College of Medicine, Houston)
Am. J. Surg. 152:674–681, December 1986   4–13

A prospective, randomized study was undertaken to determine the efficacy of three single agents—cefoxitin, cefotaxime, and moxalactam—in preventing infection in patients having perforating bowel injuries. Patients seen in 1982–1984 for gunshot, shotgun, or penetrating knife wounds of the abdomen were considered for inclusion in the study. Both cefotaxime and cefoxitin were given in a dose of 2 gm every 6 hours, and moxalactam was given in a dose of 2 gm every 8 hours. Antibiotics were given intravenously (IV) just before and for 48 hours after exploration. Cefotaxime was given to 124 patients; cefoxitin was given to 149, and moxalactam was given to 152 during the 20-month study period.

Organ injuries were comparably frequent in all treatment groups. Ninety-three percent of all patients had uncomplicated recoveries, and only six patients (1%) had sepsis-related deaths. Only three cefotaxime-treated patients had any type of postoperative infection. Cefoxitin-treated patients did less well than in previous studies. Moxalactam-treated patients did relatively well, 94% recovering without complications. Enterococci were isolated in four of seven wound infections and in nine of 15 intraabdominal abscesses.

Patients in this study who received single-agent treatment with cefotaxime or moxalactam generally did well. The reasons for the development of a relatively large number of abscesses in cefoxitin-treated patients are not clear. The isolation of enterococci in many wound infections and abscesses is a disturbing finding.

▶ This additional study evaluates the use of single agent antibiotic therapy as presumptive treatment in patients having sustained penetrating abdominal trauma. As with other studies, several good broad-spectrum, safe, single agent antibiotics were effective as presumptive therapy. The key point once again is that the presumptive antibiotics were given preoperatively and when done so, the time of administration could be shortened in this instance to 48 hours. The emergence of enterococci in wound infections has been reported by other investigators and may present a pathogen variation requiring coverage in presumptive antibiotic therapy.—G.T. Shires, M.D.

Diagnostic and Therapeutic Aspects of Rectal Trauma: Blunt Versus Penetrating

Richard G. Brunner and Clayton H. Shatney (Univ. of Florida, Jacksonville)
Am. Surg. 53:215–219, April 1987   4–14

High morbidity and mortality are associated with both penetrating and blunt rectal injuries. Sixteen patients were seen at University Hospital with penetrating rectal injuries between 1978 and 1985, and nine others were seen with blunt trauma, which was usually caused by vehicular accidents. Ten patients with penetrating injuries had gunshot wounds, and five were sexually abused with foreign objects. Associated injuries were more prevalent in the blunt injury group.

Thirteen patients with penetrating injuries had transmural injuries; three of the five who were sexually assaulted had only mucosal tears. Colostomy and mucuous fistula were used to treat 13 penetrating injuries. Eleven patients also had presacral drainage. Four patients had postoperative morbidity.

The only death in those with penetrating injury occurred in a patient with systemic sepsis in whom the penetrating injury was missed on initial examination. Three patients with blunt injuries died within 24 hours of admission; two died of pelvic exsanguination and one died of systemic sepsis after unsuccessful ureteroureterostomy. All patients with blunt injury had morbidity after operation.

Postoperative complications are especially frequent in patients with blunt rectal trauma. Therefore, different protocols are required for blunt and penetrating rectal injuries. The emphasis is on hemodynamic stabilization, colostomy with mucous fistula, and presacral drainage or perineal packing.

▶ This article points out again the seriousness of rectal trauma, an injury with high morbidity and high mortality. A principle that has been espoused frequently but is too often ignored is reemphasized in this paper. That is, hemodynamic stabilization, diverting colostomy and presacral drainage are hallmarks of treatment of penetrating rectal trauma.—G.T. Shires, M.D.

Penetrating Right Colon Trauma: The Ever Diminishing Role for Colostomy

Manohar N. Nallathambi, Rao R. Ivatury, Pravin M. Shah, Prakashchandra M. Rao, Michael Rohman, and William M. Stahl (Lincoln Med. and Mental Health Ctr., and New York Med. College, Bronx)
Am. Surg. 53:209–214, April 1987   4–15

Ninety consecutive patients were treated for penetrating right colon injuries in 1976–1985. Fifty-nine patients had gunshot wounds and 31 had knife wounds. Most patients were young men aged 20–30 years. Sixty-five patients had definitive treatment, by primary repair in 46 cases and resection-ileocolic anastomosis in 19. Antibiotics were given intravenously after operation for 5 days or longer. The healed exteriorized repair was returned to the peritoneal cavity after 7–9 days, but unhealed repairs were converted to formal colostomies.

No morbidity resulted from colonic repair. Exteriorized repair succeeded in 6 of 8 patients. For 13 patients who had loop colostomy, the mean colon injury score and penetrating abdominal trauma index were comparable to those of the group which had primary repair. Four patients with extensive injuries underwent resection colostomy. Two patients developed intra-abdominal abscess. None of the four deaths was related to the treatment of colon trauma.

Primary repair and resection-ileocolic anastomosis are safe and effective in many patients with penetrating right colon injury, even if associated organ trauma is present. Exteriorized repair is helpful in selected cases. Colostomy is reserved for patients who have established peritonitis and for unstable patients with extensive injury who require colonic resection.

▶ Most surgeons treating penetrating right colon trauma would still take the conservative approach to management. Small isolated injuries can be safely closed as was pointed out again in this study. However, exteriorization as espoused by these authors is frequently not used in favor of decompressing cecostomy with suturing of the cecum to the anterior abdominal wall. The alternative is immediate right colectomy. Most authors would not use diverting colostomy for right colon injuries.—G.T. Shires, M.D.

Intraoperative Endoscopic Retrograde Cholangiopancreatography (ERCP) in Penetrating Trauma of the Pancreas

Raymond D. Laraja, Vincent J. Lobbato, Sebastiano Cassaro, and Sreeranga-palle S. Reddy (Cabrini Med. Ctr., New York)

J. Trauma 26:1146–1147, December 1986   4–16

Pancreatic injury occurs in a small proportion of abdominal trauma cases, usually in those with penetrating trauma. Proper management requires knowledge of the integrity of the pancreatic duct system and of injuries to adjacent structures. Endoscopic retrograde cholangiopancreatography (ERCP) may be done during emergency laparotomy in these patients. The authors describe such a case.

Woman, 36, sustained an epigastric stab wound in an assault. Wound exploration showed penetration of the parietal peritoneum, and blood was seen in the peritoneal cavity. The wound penetrated the left lobe of the liver, and a subcapsular hematoma was noted at the junction of the pancreatic head and body. The knife had penetrated deep into the pancreatic substance. Intraoperative ERCP showed a normal pancreatic duct without extravasation of dye. The lesser sac and liver injury were drained. Fever and leukocytosis persisted after operation; the serum level of amylase rose to 540 U/100 ml. Sonography showed an abscess which communicated with the site of the sump drain in the left upper quadrant. On intravenous injections of antibiotics and total parenteral nutrition the patient became afebrile and did well. Findings were normal at repeat ERCP.

Intraoperative ERCP is an accurate means of evaluating the pancreatic duct system and does not expose the patient to the risks of duodenotomy or resection of the pancreatic tail. Open techniques should be used only when endoscopy is not readily available.

▶ This interesting case report illustrates some significant principles in the management of penetrating trauma to the pancreas. First, it is quite clear that pancreatic injuries not involving the major pancreatic duct can and should be treated conservatively with local control of bleeding and adequate drainage. Usually it is possible to tell when the pancreatic duct has been transected. When this is the case, obviously more definitive therapy, such as distal pancreatic resection, are necessary. In the occasional patient such as the one cited in this article, where it is impossible to determine the degree of pancreatic injury and, more specifically, pancreatic duct integrity, several approaches have been used. One has been extensive débridement, another has been pancreatogram using a duodenotomy and pancreatic cannulation, and a third includes intraoperative ERCP as demonstrated in this study. When expert ERCP is available (intraoperatively, in the unusual situation described here) certainly it would appear to be useful.—G.T. Shires, M.D.

Injuries of the Duodenum

Robert M. Shorr, Gregory C. Greaney, and Arthur J. Donovan (Univ. of Southern California, Los Angeles)

Am. J. Surg. 154:93–98, July 1987   4–17

Management of duodenal injuries was reviewed in 105 patients seen in a 5½-year period with both blunt and penetrating trauma. Gunshot wounds were responsible for half the cases, and stab wounds, for another 40%. Four fifths of patients had associated injuries, most often involving the liver, major blood vessels, pancreas, and large bowel. In 83% of patients, the duodenal wound was sutured and drains were placed. Duodenal diverticulization was performed in 12 patients.

Seventy percent of patients had uncomplicated postoperative courses, including all but two of 21 patients with isolated duodenal injury. Sixteen patients had septic complications, and four developed septic shock. Many patients with sepsis had colonic perforation. Three patients developed overt pancreatitis. Four patients had duodenal fistulas following technically difficult closures. Four patients, two of whom had diverticulization and developed duodenal fistulas, died.

Primary repair with drainage is the preferred approach to duodenal injury. Gastrostomy and feeding jejunostomy are helpful adjuncts. Duodenal fistula continues to be a serious postoperative complication. Pancreaticoduodenectomy is reserved for devastating injuries. Duodenal diverticulization for pyloric exclusion and gastric diversion is appropriate for some cases of severe duodenal injury.

▶ This article is a review of a well-managed group of patients with duodenal injuries. The conclusions, which now seem to be standard, are that most duodenal injuries can be primarily repaired with adequate drainage. Certainly, gastrostomy and feeding jejunostomy are helpful adjuncts, even though no prospective, randomized trial has been studied demonstrating this. As with most centers managing such injuries, a Whipple resection is reserved for devastating and combined injuries usually involving pancreas, duodenum, and common bile duct. Duodenal diverticulization or pyloric exclusion with gastric diversion is appropriate in some cases of severe but isolated duodenal injury.—G.T. Shires, M.D.

Management of Combined Pancreatoduodenal Injuries
David V. Feliciano, Tomas D. Martin, Pamela A. Cruse, Joseph M. Graham, Jon M. Burch, Kenneth L. Mattox, Carmel G. Bitondo, and George L. Jordan, Jr. (Baylor College of Medicine, Houston; Ben Taub Gen. Hosp., Houston, and St. John's Regional Med. Ctr., Joplin, Mo.)
Ann. Surg. 205:673–680, June 1987   4–18

Combined injuries to the pancreas and duodenum are among the most difficult traumatic gastrointestinal (GI) lesions to treat. Late morbidity and mortality are often affected by the type of repairs used. The formation of fistulas leading to breakdown of adjacent repairs and hemorrhage in patients with moderately severe injuries to either organ has often been reported. An 18-year experience with patients with combined pancreatoduodenal injuries is described.

From 1969 to 1985, 129 patients with such injuries were treated at

one urban trauma center. One hundred four (80.6%) had penetrating wounds; multiple visceral and vascular injuries were often associated with the pancreatoduodenal injury. The head of the pancreas and the second portion of the duodenum were the areas injured most commonly. Multiple duodenal injuries were seen in 30 patients. Simple repair and drainage were done in 31 patients; duodenal repair or resection, pancreatic repair, distal resection, or Roux-en-Y, with or without pyloric exclusion, and drainage were done in 79 patients; pancreatoduodenectomy was done in 13; and no procedure was done in 6. Major pancreatoduodenal complications occurring in the 108 patients who survived more than 48 hours included pancreatic fistulas (25.9%); intraabdominal abscess formation (16.6%); and duodenal fistulas (6.5%). Overall mortality was 29.5%.

The acute mortality among patients with such injuries will likely remain high because of injuries to associated organs and vascular structures. Nevertheless, it is recommended that (1) primary repair and drainage should be used for simple perforations or ruptures of the duodenum combined with nonductal pancreatic injuries; (2) more extensive duodenal injuries with pancreatic injuries not involving the duct in the head should be managed with repair or resection, pyloric exclusion with gastrojejunostomy, and drainage; and (3) a Roux-en-Y drainage or Whipple procedure should be considered for stable patients with devascularized duodenum, transected pancreatic duct in the head, or destroyed ampulla of Vater. A conservative resection, pyloric exclusion with gastrojejunostomy, and drainage should be done if the patient's condition is unstable.

▶ This article is a review of current management of pancreatoduodenal injuries. As with other articles in the last several years, primary repair with drainage is used most often for simple injuries of the duodenum and with nonductal pancreatic injuries. More extensive isolated duodenal injuries were managed with pyloric exclusion and gastroenterostomy. More extensive duodenal injuries, with combined pancreatic injuries not involving the duct and the head, can be managed with repair or resection or pyloric exclusion. A Roux-en-Y drainage or Whipple resection can be considered for stabilized patients with multiple organ injuries including duodenum, transected pancreatic duct, and destroyed ampulla of Vater.—G.T. Shires, M.D.

Biomechanics of Liver Injury by Steering Wheel Loading
Ian V. Lau, John D. Horsch, David C. Viano, and Dennis V. Andrzejak (General Motors Research Labs., Warren, Mich.)
J. Trauma 27:225–235, March 1987   4–19

Impact with the lower rim of the steering wheel on the upper abdomen can cause intraabdominal injuries. The authors studied the sequelae of steering wheel contact at a velocity of 32 km per hour in anesthetized swine, using a Hyge sled. The lower rim of the wheel was 5 cm below the xyphoid. Wheel stiffness, orientation, and column angle were varied.

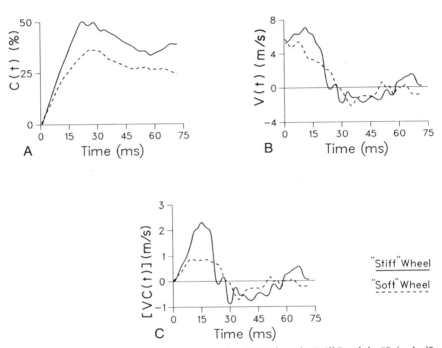

Fig 4–3.—Derivation of the viscous injury criterion *[VC(t)]* from the "stiff-" and the "Soft-wheel" tests. Instantaneous deformation was derived from analysis of high-speed movies of the tests. Velocity of deformation (**B**) was obtained by differentiation. [VC(t)] (**C**) was the product of velocity of deformation (**B**) and compression (**A**, which represents deformation normalized to the initial abdominal thickness). [VC(t)] leveled off at 10 msec for the "soft-wheel" test but continued to increase up to 15 msec for the "stiff-wheel" test. (Courtesy of Lau, I.V., et al.: J. Trauma 27:225–235, March 1987.)

Wheel stiffness was the chief determinant of abdominal injury severity. Injury occurred when the rim impacted the abdomen above a combined velocity and compression sensitive tolerance limit. Injury took place in the first 15 milliseconds of wheel contact. The severity of injury correlated with the peak viscous response, the product of the instantaneous velocity of abdominal deformation and abdominal compression (Fig 4–3). It did not correlate with spinal acceleration. None of the biomechanical responses were correlated with thoracic injury or with minor lung and heart injuries.

Liver injury from the steering wheel rim apparently results from a combined velocity and compression-sensitive tolerance limit, occurring before acceleration or compression limits are approached. A softer wheel may provide better abdominal protection. Spinal acceleration does not correlate with abdominal injury in this setting.

▶ This interesting study proposes a new concept for injuries to the torso produced by blunt injury. The viscus injury criteria, that is, a combination of velocity of deformation and abdominal compression, has been shown to be a better predictor of abdominal injury than the use of velocity alone. This bioengineering concept has been quite useful in the reduction of blunt abdominal injuries resulting from the design of automotive steering devices that reduce wheel stiffness significantly. These authors have been leaders in this field, and this article shows evidence of significant biomechanical rationale for the design alterations that have been made.—G.T. Shires, M.D.

Atrial Caval Shunting in Blunt Hepatic Vascular Injury
Peter F. Rovito (Allentown Affiliated Hosps., Allentown, Pa.)
Ann. Surg. 205:318–321, March 1987   4–20

Control of the hepatic veins and retrohepatic vena cava in patients with blunt liver injury is very difficult. The atrial-caval shunt allows continuous venous return and will maintain ventricular filling pressures while also providing a relatively bloodless field for repairing injured vascular structures. Nine of 51 patients seen at a level I trauma center with major liver injury received an atrial-caval shunt.

All but one of the nine study patients were aged 20–29 years. All patients were in shock when admitted and had major liver injury and multiple trauma. Four patients had major hepatic vein injury, and four had both hepatic vein and retrohepatic vena cava injuries. Four of these eight patients survived. A sternal split approach was used in most cases. Blood was replaced mainly through components. Disseminated intravascular coagulation or "washout" coagulopathy was universal. Hypothermia occurred in all patients who survived.

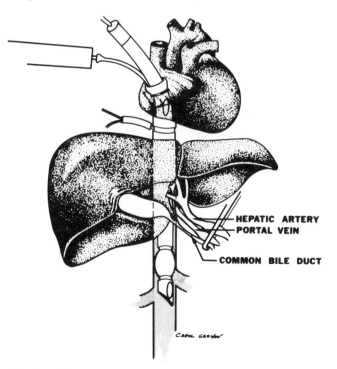

HEPATIC ARTERY
PORTAL VEIN

COMMON BILE DUCT

Fig 4–4.—Atrial caval shunt using endotracheal tube as the shunt. (Courtesy of Rovito, P.F.: Ann. Surg. 205:318–321, March 1987.)

The median sternotomy approach to atrial-caval shunting (Fig 4–4) provides more rapid and better control than the infrarenal approach. Direct intracardial transfusion is possible, as is open heart massage if necessary. Care in catheter insertion will minimize the risk of air embolism. Aggressive use of the shunt can control bleeding in patients with liver trauma before the onset of coagulopathy or hypothermia.

▶ This article indicates that in many instances the atrial-caval shunting of blood through the vena cava in blunt hepatic vein injuries may be extremely useful. This technique has been described by several authors, including your reviewer, and all of us have had survival of patients that we believed would not survive otherwise. This technique is often belittled because the mortality rate is understandably quite high. However, as pointed out by these authors, there are occasions when the caval shunting technique in serious retrohepatic injuries can be very useful and lifesaving.—G.T. Shires, M.D.

The Role of Splenorrhaphy in Splenic Trauma
David J. Kreis, Jr., Nestor Montero, Marcia Saltz, Renato Saltz, Miguel Echenique, Gustavo Plasencia, Roberto Santiesteban, Gerardo A. Gomez, James J. Vopal, and Joseph M. Civetta (Univ. of Miami)
Am. Surg. 53:307–309, June 1987   4–21

Splenectomy has been, until recently, the procedure of choice for splenic injury, but the risk of postsplenectomy sepsis now has prompted splenic salvage in increasing numbers of cases. The management of 85 patients who were seen with splenic trauma from 1981 to 1983 was reviewed. Mean age of the 73 male and 12 female patients was 34 years. Blunt trauma accounted for 51 (60%) cases. Associated injuries were frequent, especially in patients with penetrating trauma.

Splenectomy was done in 43 cases, and splenorrhaphy was done in 42. Twenty-three (67%) patients with penetrating injuries were managed by splenorrhaphy. Six patients (7%) died; only one had penetrating trauma. Two patients developed intra-abdominal abscesses. Two required reoperation for intra-abdominal bleeding. One patient in each of the operative groups had an abscess and required reoperation.

The spleen can be salvaged during laparotomy for splenic trauma in 50% of all cases, particularly in those with penetrating trauma. Splenorrhaphy is a safe operation, and nonoperative management should rarely be elected for adults who are suspected of having isolated spleen injury from blunt trauma. If nonoperative treatment is chosen, great caution is necessary.

▶ This article documents the utility of splenorrhaphy in patients with splenic trauma. The experience reported here indicates that about 50% of patients having splenic injury can have splenic salvage through repair of the injury and that this can be done safely. As expected, it is also easier to perform splenorrhaphy in the patient with penetrating trauma as compared to the more often shattering injuries produced by blunt abdominal trauma. These authors again make the plea that, if nonoperative therapy of splenic injury is elected following blunt trauma, great caution must be used and careful follow-up must be made. Many other papers also point out the significant instance, ranging from 20% to 50%, of associated injuries in these patients.—G.T. Shires, M.D.

The Effects of Treatment of Renal Trauma on Renal Function
Michael D. McGonigal, Charles E. Lucas, and Anna M. Ledgerwood (Wayne State Univ., Detroit)
J. Trauma 27:471–476, May 1987   4–22

Controversy continues regarding the risks and benefits of conservative vs. aggressive operative treatment of renal injuries. The authors assessed renal function in 275 severely injured patients with hemorrhagic shock and requiring massive transfusion. Forty-five patients had renal injury. Nine of these patients had renorrhaphy, and 19 underwent partial or total nephrectomy. Seventeen patients with renal injury were not explored. Forty-five patients without renal injury were matched with the study group for number of blood transfusions and severity of shock. Patients given albumin infusions were excluded from the study.

Patients without renal injury had significantly reduced renal perfusion. Excretory function was affected less than perfusion and filtration. Renal failure occurred in 7% of patients without renal injury and 11% of those with renal injury. Mortality was 8% and 16% in these groups; the increased mortality was chiefly in patients who underwent nephrectomy. The incidence of renal failure in patients who died was 68% in those without renal injury and 29% in those with renal injury.

Preservation of renal parenchyma will assure maximal renal function in severely injured patients. Exploration of Gerota's fascia is best limited to patients with an expanding or uncontained hematoma. Control of the renal pedicle before opening Gerota's fascia lowers the risk of uncontrolled bleeding. Massive hematuria in the postoperative period may be controlled by arteriographic embolization of bleeding vessels.

▶ An interesting principle that is periodically espoused is that the risk of diminution in renal function is higher with abdominal trauma if the kidney itself is involved as one of the injured organs. This premise has been documented previously but seems to go unnoticed. Certainly, these patients sustaining abdominal trauma that includes injury to the kidney require maximal support for detection and prevention of acute renal failure.—G.T. Shires, M.D.

The Role of High-Frequency Ventilation in Post-Traumatic Respiratory Insufficiency
James M. Hurst, Richard D. Branson, and C. Bryan DeHaven (Univ. of Cincinnati)
J. Trauma 27:236–241, March 1987   4–23

The adult respiratory distress syndrome (ARDS) is often associated with multiple organ-system injury. Mechanical ventilation (CMV) with continuous positive airway pressure (CPAP) is the standard therapy. Side effects of this therapy include pulmonary barotrauma, decreased cardiac output, fluid retention, and worsening of ventilation/perfusion matching. High frequency ventilation (HFV) has been suggested as an alternative therapy. The efficacy of two types of HFV were evaluated in 54 patients with multiple–organ system injury who required ventilation.

Initially, CMV was provided with a time-cycled ventilator, delivering 12–15 cc/kg tidal volume and a mechanical rate adjusted to provide Pa_{CO_2} 38–42 torr. The HFV for 33 patients was provided by a solenoid-based jet ventilator (HFJV) or a pneumatic cartridge high frequency pulse generator (HFPG).

All patients on HFJV improved CO_2 elimination. Patients on HFPG had comparable gas exchange and hemodynamic profiles but lower CPAP/PIP. The mean airway pressure (PAW) was significantly lower with HFPG than with CMV.

Another HFV technique, high frequency percussive ventilation (HFPV), is described. It combines features of HFJV and HFO with CMV. In this series, HFPV was most effective when used to treat hypoxemia. The HFPV technique improves Pa_{O_2} and reduces Pa_{CO_2} at lower peak, mean, and end-expiratory pressures and should therefore reduce the risk of barotrauma.

▶ This is another study evaluating the role of high frequency ventilation. As with the other studies, it appears that high frequency ventilation, when used correctly, offers adequate respiratory support. Most studies such as this indicate that there is probably no striking advantage over any other form of mechanical airway support but that the high frequency jet ventilation is an effective form of ventilatory support.—G.T. Shires, M.D.

High-Frequency Ventilation
Blaine L. Enderson and Charles L. Rice (Univ. of Washington)
World J. Surg. 11:167–172, April 1987   4–24

High frequency ventilation (HFV) is reported to be clinically useful in a wide range of settings. The modes include high frequency positive-pressure ventilation, high frequency jet ventilation, and high frequency oscillation. All three systems use high volumes of gas. Humidification is important to prevent drying and damage to the tracheal mucosa. It has proved more difficult to humidify high frequency positive-pressure ventilation systems than the others.

In the intensive care unit, HFV provides adequate gas exchange at lower tidal volumes than conventional mechanical ventilation. Little experience is available in patients with chronic obstructive lung disease. High frequency ventilation has been most widely used in patients with adult respiratory distress syndrome. Other indications are to provide ventilation during bronchoscopy, laryngoscopy, and tracheobronchial suctioning. It has been used to prevent aspiration in patients who do not tolerate a cuffed endotracheal tube. High-frequency jet ventilation may be used to wean patients who cannot be weaned conventionally.

High frequency ventilation, like mechanical ventilation in general, does not cure any disease but is a support system for maintaining gas exchange while giving time for treatments to be effective.

▶ This is another of the recent studies evaluating high frequency ventilation in a wide range of settings. In the intensive care unit, the high frequency ventilation provides adequate gas exchange at somewhat lower tidal volumes than conventional mechanical ventilation. This form of ventilatory support has also been useful in providing ventilation during bronchoscopy, laryngoscopy, or tracheobronchial suctioning.

While there is no unique advantage to high frequency ventilation over mechanical ventilation, the use of ventilatory support such as this does enhance ventilatory exchange while the underlying cause of the pulmonary insufficiency is corrected.—G.T. Shires, M.D.

Pulmonary and Cardiovascular Consequences of Immediate Fixation or Conservative Management of Long-Bone Fractures
Jeffrey Lozman, D. Curtis Deno, Paul J. Feustel, Jonathan C. Newell, Howard H. Stratton, Nell Sedransk, Robert Dutton, John B. Fortune, and Dhiraj M. Shah Albany Med. Ctr., N.Y.; Rensselaer Polytechnic Inst., Troy, N.Y.; and State Univ. of New York, Albany)
Arch. Surg. 121:992–999, September 1986   4–25

The best orthopedic management of long-bone fractures in multiply injured patients remains uncertain. Cardiorespiratory function was assessed in patients seen in 1981–1984 with multiple injuries, including fractures of the femur or tibia. All required insertion of both arterial and balloon-tip pulmonary artery catheters, and all had to be intubated at the outset. Eight patients experienced immediate stabilization of all lower extremity fractures by internal fixation, intramedullary fixation, or external fixation, if a severe open wound was present. Upper limb fractures usually were internally fixed. Ten other patients were managed conservatively. Age and injury severity scores were similar in the two groups.

Intrapulmonary shunt fractions were lower in the immediate fixation group. Cardiac index was higher in this group, and it remained nearly constant in both groups during 4 days of observation. Other pulmonary and systemic hemodynamic variables did not distinguish the two groups, and fat macroglobules in pulmonary capillary blood were comparably frequent. Oxygen delivery and consumption were similar in the actively treated and conservatively managed patients. All fractures united, but one patient had osteomyelitis following tibial rodding.

Intrapulmonary shunting was less evident in patients having immediate fracture fixation than in conservatively treated patients in this series. Operative stabilization of long-bone fractures reduces pulmonary dysfunction in multiply injured patients. Fat deposition within the pulmonary vascular bed may not be a proximate cause of pulmonary dysfunction in this setting.

▶ This is another study confirming the original observations of Border relative to the advantages of immediate fixation of long-bone fractures in preventing acute respiratory distress syndrome. Here, intrapulmonary shunting was less evident in patients having immediate fracture fixation compared to conservatively treated patients. Operative stabilization of long-bone fractures appeared to reduce pulmonary dysfunction in the multiply injured patient. As in other studies, the instance of fat macroglobules in blood aspirated from pulmonary capillaries was present but not significantly different between the immediate fixation and conservatively treated groups. This is just one more demonstration of the idea that fat embolism is probably rarely, if ever, a cause of pulmonary insufficiency following injury. Most of the ARDS following injury appears to be related to direct pulmonary injury or to sepsis.—G.T. Shires, M.D.

5 Wound Healing

Hidradenitis Suppurativa: Patient Satisfaction With Wound Healing by Secondary Intention

Bruce Silverberg, Clyde E. Smoot, Stuart J.F. Landa, and Robert W. Parsons (Univ. of Chicago and Michael Reese Med. Ctrs., Chicago)
Plast. Reconstr. Surg. 79:555–559, April 1987   5–1

In 1976 Ariyan and Krizek described three patients with perineal hidradenitis suppurativa who after excision achieved satisfactory closure that allowed spontaneous wound healing by secondary intention. This approach was used to treat 20 consecutive patients with hidradenitis suppurativa which involved the perineal, perianal, groin, and scrotal regions.

The group included 11 male and nine female patients aged 16 to 65 years. One was white and 19 were black. The involved skin and apocrine tissue were excised to a clean, unscarred level of subcutaneous tissue. To provide adequate drainage, adjacent fistula tracts were unroofed. Granulation tissue was excised. Postexcision wounds were too large for primary closure; average estimated excision was 300 sq cm. Dressings were changed four times a day and redressed with silver sulfadiazine after the patient took a sitz bath. One year after complete wound closure the surgical results and patient satisfaction were assessed.

All patients reported minimal inconvenience and interruption of daily activities from this treatment method. Analgesic requirements were minimal, and little reinforcement was needed to maintain vigorous wound care. Uncomplicated wound closure was achieved uniformly with unrestrictive, stable scars. Two patients were dissatisfied because of new onset of disease in previously uninvolved and unresected apocrine tissue.

This treatment approach was found to be satisfactory from the point of view of both the surgeon and the patient. Hospitalization time and costs were also reduced.

▶ There is no question that secondary healing, particularly in the perineum and buttocks, produces results superior to skin replacement. In the axillary area, however, it may be more practical to advance local skin flaps and obtain primary healing rather than nurse a secondary healing wound for a long period of time. Certainly, however, secondary healing is superior to free skin grafting following excision of hidradenitis suppurativa lesions.—E.E. Peacock, Jr., M.D.

Reaction to Injectable Collagen: Results in Animal Models and Clinical Use

Frank DeLustro, Susanne T. Smith, John Sundsmo, George Salem, Steven Kincaid, Larry Ellingsworth (Collagen Corp., Palo Alto, Calif.)
Plast. Reconstr. Surg. 79:581–594, April 1987   5–2

Zyderm collagen implant, a highly purified form of bovine dermal collagen, has been used to treat more than 200,000 patients in the United States for soft-tissue contour defects. Extensive clinical trials with Zyderm collagen and immunologic studies were reviewed.

In a multicenter study of 9,427 patients, 3% reported positive reactions to the intradermal test implant of Zyderm collagen. The predominant feature of this reaction was localized hypersensitivity at the skin test site. In a study population of 5,109, 1.1% had localized hypersensitivity reactions after Zyderm collagen treatment. Of the latter treatment responses reported since the end of clinical trials with Zyderm, 56% occurred after the first treatment, 28% after the second, 10% after the third, and 6% after subsequent exposures. These studies indicated that most patients receive a median of three treatments with Zyderm, but that most patients who are likely to develop sensitivity to it appear to respond immunologically to the test implant or first treatment. Forty-five percent of the patients with these treatment responses reported an onset of symptoms within 10 days, and 22% reported onset at more than 30 days after the last Zyderm collagen treatment. In 24% of the patients, erythema was the sole symptom; erythema and induration were seen in an additional 42%. Antibodies against Zyderm collagen were found in the sera of 88% of these subjects, but no reactivity against human collagen was observed. The sera from patients reporting only systemic symptoms did not have anticollagen antibodies.In animal models, Zyderm collagen was less immunogenic than other medical devices composed of bovine collagen. Sera from guinea pigs treated with collagen-derived hemostatic devices had significant levels of anti-implant antibodies (titers >640), whereas animals treated with Zyderm collagen had minimal responses (titers <40).

Data on the relative risk of a hypersensitivity reaction to Zyderm collagen in human beings suggest that this risk does not increase with multiple exposures; patients likely to develop an immune response to bovine collagen react most often to initial injections. The results of several animal models suggest that Zyderm collagen is less immunogenic than other commercial collagen devices when compared under similar conditions of administration.

▶ The editor has been opposed to widespread use of injectable animal collagen for two reasons: the material disappears rapidly, and the ultimate consequences of crossing a major histocompatibility locus are not fully identified in human beings. Regardless of how weak or how strong immunogenicity appears in a laboratory model, still too little is known about autoimmune disease and performed antibodies of the type that ruin transplantation to stimulate the immune system for cosmetic reasons.—E.E. Peacock, Jr., M.D.

The Influence of a Brief Preoperative Illness on Postoperative Healing
William H. Goodson III, J. Arthur Jensen, Luis Granja-Mena, Alberto

Lopez-Sarmiento, Judith West, and Jaime Chavez-Estrella (Univ. of Calif., San Francisco; and Univ. of Central Ecuador, Quito)
Ann. Surg. 205:250–255, March 1987

5–3

A study of wound healing at high altitudes was conducted with 26 patients who had appendectomies and 38 who had cholecystectomies. It was designed to evaluate the role of altitude-induced hypoxia in deposition of collagen, oxygen tension of subcutaneous tissue, and infection. Accumulation of hydroxyproline was used in response to an acute, standard wound stimulus as an index of wound healing capacity.

Hydroxyproline values were analyzed according to the type of operation and to whether or not supplemental oxygen had been administered. The supplemental oxygen did not have a significant effect on the accumulation in this study.

Patients who had appendectomies were younger and had shorter operations, but they were sicker in the immediate preoperative period. Postoperative fluid requirements were similar in the two groups. Among the patients who had cholecystectomies, 34% had been admitted to the hospital more than 24 hours before surgery for care until resolution of acute symptoms.

Appendectomy patients accumulated 20% less hydroxyproline than those who had cholecystectomy, and depression of the accumulation of hydroxyproline was related significantly to the length of preoperative illness. The authors believe this can explain the difference in accumulation of hydroxyproline in wounds, a unique situation because the brief illness did not produce lasting debility and the inflamed appendix, the source of illness, was not present during healing. It was also concluded that a postoperative decrease in perfusion was not the cause of the decreased accumulation of hydroxyproline in the wounds of appendectomy patients.

At least three explanations can be given for the fewer complications that were due to incisions in appendectomy patients: only minimal strength of repair is required, slower healing at 7 days probably does not mean healing is depressed permanently but reflects a slower start, and a 20% reduction in deposition of collagen may, by itself, not necessarily lead to complications.

Postoperative healing is influenced by the preoperative status of the patient in ways that are not included in the usual considerations of severe malnutrition (greater than 20% weight loss), continuing sepsis or drainage, or organ failure. That 34% of the cholecystectomy patients were admitted with acute illness but did not have a defect in formation of collagen at the wound suggests that controlling acute disease can ameliorate this defect.

▶ Although the numbers reported in this paper are clearly significant, the differences recorded in net collagen synthesis and deposition are not likely to be clinically significant for most patients. Nevertheless, the principle is presented well and may be the cause of clinically significant retardation of healing in some patients.—E.E. Peacock, Jr., M.D.

Local Heat Increases Blood Flow and Oxygen Tension in Wounds

John M. Rabkin and Thomas K. Hunt (Univ. of California, San Francisco)
Arch. Surg. 122:221–225, February 1987   5–4

Local heat is considered important in treating infections, but its mechanism of action is not well understood. In a recent survey of a group of surgeons about half believed that hot packs would not change perfusion, temperature, or oxygen tension in subcutaneous tissue, and about half thought they would. Opinion was also divided on whether oxygen tension in tissue would then rise or fall.

The effect of local hyperthermia on oxygen tension in subcutaneous tissue and perfusion was explored in 8 patients with the use of a subcutaneously implanted tonometer. The output of the oxygen electrode that was used is proportionate to the temperature (the temperature increment in oxygen tension being 2.5% per 1 C) (Fig 5–1). These patients were studied a total of 13 times with the hot pack.

Application of heat increased the temperature of subcutaneous tissue, as well as the oxygen tension. Mean oxygen tension in subcutaneous tissue rose by 39.5 mm Hg during oxygen breathing, an 80% increase over baseline measures. The corresponding mean subcutaneous temperature increased 4 C. A significant linear correlation was observed between the change in oxygen tension in subcutaneous tissue and subcutaneous temperature. By using the Fick principle, an average threefold increase in local perfusion was estimated.

These findings reaffirm the value of local hyperthermia in treating contaminated wounds and suggest a mechanism for its ability to alleviate infection. This mechanism implies that local hyperthermia may have prophylactic value as well.

▶ The use of hot, wet dressings occasionally is questioned by thoughtful surgeons. There probably is not a great deal of benefit from either heat or wet-

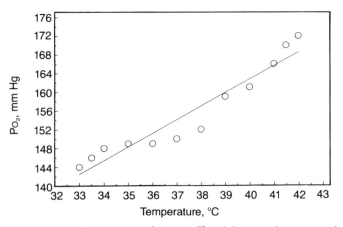

Fig 5–1.—Temperature calibration curve of oximeter. There is increment in oxygen tension (Po_2) of approximately 2.5% per 1 C. (Courtesy of Rabkin, J.M., and Hunt, T.K.: Arch. Surg. 122:221–225, February 1987.)

ness, but this study does show some benefit from heat and, of course, wet heat is more penetrating and therefore theoretically more useful than dry heat.—E.E. Peacock, Jr., M.D.

Dose and Time Effects of Nicotine Treatment on the Capillary Blood Flow and Viability of Random Pattern Skin Flaps in the Rat

C.R. Forrest, C.Y. Pang, and W.K. Lindsay (Univ. of Toronto, Canada)
Br. J. Plast. Surg. 40:295–299, May 1987   5–5

There is increasing evidence that cigarette smoking may increase the risk of skin flap necrosis. The apparent association between nicotine and cardiovascular disease prompted a study of the dose-related effects of nicotine on skin capillary blood flow and flap viability in rats with dorsal random-pattern skin flaps. Rats were given subcutaneous injections of doses of nicotine ranging up to 8 mg/kg of body weight twice daily over 5 weeks, starting 4 weeks before flap surgery.

Treatment with 2 mg/kg of body weight of nicotine or higher doses significantly reduced the length and area of skin flap survival compared with saline injections. Capillary blood flow decreased significantly, as did distal skin flap perfusion. If treatment began 2 weeks before flap surgery, no adverse effects were evident.

Nicotine apparently can lead to hypoperfusion and necrosis in acute random-pattern skin flaps. The effects of nicotine are time-dependent. Possible explanations for the effects of nicotine on skin flaps include direct endothelial cell damage; stimulation of norepinephrine release from sympathetic terminals or the adrenal glands; and altered local synthesis or release of prostaglandins and thromboxane.

▶ This good experimental study in an animal model shows that uncontrolled clinical observations suggesting loss of skin, particularly in rhytidectomy patients, is associated with use of nicotine. There are now basic as well as clinical data to support the recommendation that patients who are going to have skin flaps performed should reduce intake of nicotine to an absolute minimum.—E.E. Peacock, Jr., M.D.

Effects of Haemorrhage on Wound Strength and Fibroblast Function

D.E.M. Taylor, J.S. Whamond, and J.E. Penhallow (Royal College of Surgeons of England, London)
Br. J. Surg. 74:316–319, April 1987   5–6

Impaired wound healing can follow compensated oligemia, the loss of blood which is insufficient to result in clinical shock, if the blood is not replaced. Previous studies have indicated that a shift in the healing curve is caused by a defect in fibroblast function with respect to collagen. Two studies were conducted to further define this defect in fibroblast activity and the effects on skin and muscle layers of a laparotomy.

A midline laparotomy was performed in rats, with either 1 ml of blood/100 gm of body weight being removed from the proximal carotid artery (bled) or with the artery being tied (controls). The wound strength study included 11 control and nine bled animals that were killed after 22 days, and the anterior abdominal wall was removed for evaluation of width and strength of the skin and muscle layers.

The second part of the study involved 30 control and 31 bled animals that were killed 10 days after surgery. The wound was assessed histologically and autoradiographically using [$^{-3}$H]thymidine to measure cell replication, [^{3}H]leucine for general protein synthesis, and [^{3}H]proline for specific collagen metabolism.

The skin layer was 36.4% weaker in the bled animals compared to the controls, and the muscle layer was 22.2% weaker in the bled animals. These differences between groups were statistically significant. The density of fibroblasts, replication, and general protein synthesis were similar in the bled and control animals. However, collagen packing was 21% less dense in the bled animals and was associated with 32.8% more]^{3}H]proline uptake by fibroblasts. These differences were also statistically significant.

Although compensated oligemia affects the strength of both skin and muscle, the effect is greater on skin. The findings of this study suggest that a specific increase in collagen turnover with the rate of reabsorption being greater than that of synthesis may be the mechanism responsible for impaired wound healing.

These observations can be applied to surgical management so that in patients who have led replacement of blood loss an absorbable suture with a relatively long duration of strength loss or a bulk suture with a nonabsorbable monofilament is used for anastamoses and wound closure.

► Data continues to accrue showing that oligemia affects wound healing in ways that earlier measurements in anemic animals did not reveal. Longstanding chronic anemia does not have a significant effect upon wound healing, but sudden uncompensated hemorrhage obviously does.—E.E. Peacock, Jr., M.D.

Skin Closure Using Staples and Nylon Sutures: A Comparison of Results
Ian Stockley and Reginald A. Elson, (Northern Gen. Hosp., Sheffield, England)
Ann. R. Coll. Surg. Engl. 69:76–78, March 1987   5–7

The authors have compared skin closure with staples and sutures in clean orthopedic wounds in a study that was designed by using both methods in the same wound, with each wound affording its own control. There have been no previous reports of such a procedure in the literature. Over a 9-month period 129 patients who underwent elective or emergency hip and knee surgery and had incisions longer than 18 cm were studied.

All wounds were divided into thirds and closed with nylon-staples-

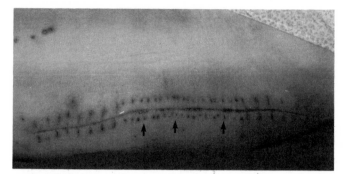

Fig 5–2.—Hip wound shows spreading of scar *(arrows)* after removal of staples following inversion of skin edges 16 days after operation. (Courtesy of Stockley, I., and Elson, R.A.: Ann. R. Coll. Surg. Engl. 69:76–78, March 1987.)

nylon or staples-nylon-staples, thus allowing a direct comparison between the two methods of closure in each wound and recognizing that in any one wound skin texture varies. A meaningful comparison was provided at the junction of sutures and staples.

The wounds were usually inspected on the 3d, 7th, and 14th postoperative days, and a final review was made 9 months to 1 year after operation. Of the hip wounds 48.5% healed without any complication or discomfort, and no difference could be seen between the segments at review. In 21.2% of cases staples were painful to remove, and in 6.1% of cases the nylon sutures were more painful.

Abnormal erythema developed in 8.1% of wounds around the staples, but not in the nylon segments. In 2% of wounds erythema developed around the nylon sutures but not around the staples. In 14.1% of wounds inversion had occurred after apparent satisfactory placement, and in all of them there was a variable tendency for the skin edges to gape when the staple from these parts was removed (Fig 5–2).

Of the knee wounds 60.0% healed without a problem. Clips were painful to remove in 18 wounds (33.3%) and in four of these marked erythema settled after removal. Only one patient said the nylon sutures were more painful to remove.

Overall, 51.2% of the wounds healed with no problem; staples tended to be more painful to remove than the sutures (24.0% versus 5.4%) and erythema was more common around them (7.8% versus 2.3%), especially in the knee wounds (13.3% versus 6.1%). Both types of closures exhibited a similar cosmetic appearance in uncomplicated wounds.

It would appear that the only advantage of stapling is the speed of execution, and this is difficult to balance against the higher cost and increased complication rate, which the authors state with some regret.

▶ It is uncanny that after 5,000 years we still have not found a way to close a wound any better than with sutures. Staples certainly are not a step forward.—E.E. Peacock, Jr., M.D.

Management of Hypertrophic Scars by Cross Hatching and Skin Grafting
S. Krupp and B. Deglise (Lausanne, Switzerland)
Eur. J. Plast. Surg. 10:18–20, July 1987   5–8

Burn injury promotes hypertrophic scar formation through exposing deeply burned areas to prolonged inflammation. Major functional and esthetic damage may result. Scar formation is especially likely to be a problem if burn management is delayed. The authors de-epithelialize the hypertropic scar, cross-hatch the scar tissue that is left in place, and repair the skin defect with a thin split-thickness graft. The scar tissue is incised along its junction with undamaged tissue before being cross-hatched down to intact underlying tissue. This allows the contracted tissues to expand and restore the size of the original skin defect. Either a single sheet of skin graft or a meshed graft then is applied and, if necessary, immobilized with a splint.

Six contracted scars were managed in this way in five burn-injured patients. Satisfactory results were obtained after follow-up periods of 1.5 to 3 years. Cross-hatching relieves the intrinsic tension of the hypertropic scar. Extrinsic tension is limited by incising the junction of the scar with the surrounding tissues. Grafting enhances collagenolytic activity within the maturing scar. This approach is relatively inexpensive and carries low morbidity, and the long-term results have been good.

► This is a trick the editor has used in treating pedunculated keloids for a number of years. The editor uses the surface of the keloid as a graft and excises the hypertrophic scar or keloid level with, but not into, uninvolved dermis rather than cross-hatching the scar.—E.E. Peacock, Jr., M.D.

Improvement of the Appearance of Full-Thickness Skin Grafts With Dermabrasion
June K. Robinson (Northwestern Univ.)
Arch. Dermatol. 123:1340–1345, October 1987   5–9

The cosmetic results of full-thickness skin grafting might be improved by dermabrading the rim of the junction of the graft with surrounding skin. Two hundred consecutive patients had basal-cell or squamous-cell carcinoma resected by Mohs histographic surgery, followed by the placement of full-thickness grafts 2–4 cm in diameter from the retroauricular or supraclavicular region. About half the patients had surgery on the nose. After 6–8 months, patients were randomized to either solar protection and topical lubricants, or dermabrasion.

Dermabrasion proved helpful in some cases for adjusting the level of the skin graft to the edge of the recipient site. Elevated grafts on the nose benefited most from dermabrasion. Depressed grafts remained depressed whether or not dermabrasion was carried out. Optimal improvement was reached 1 year after dermabrasion.

Dermabrasion appears to be most helpful where the grafted skin border is higher than the unoperated skin. The ideal plane for dermabrasion of normal surrounding skin is the papillary dermis. It is best to allow 6 months to pass after grafting before recommending dermabrasion to improve an elevated graft.

▶ A properly selected and performed full-thickness graft provides the best possible substitute for damaged or missing skin. The surrounding scar has been the only disadvantage. Dermabrasion has not been considered useful in reducing surrounding scar, and there has been some concern about the ability of a graft to withstand dermabrasion. This report suggests that plastic surgeons may have been too conservative trying to improve circumferential scar.—E.E. Peacock, Jr., M.D.

Mesh Grafts: An 18 Month Follow-Up
A.N. Herd, P.N. Hall, P. Widdowson, and N.S.B. Tanner (Queen Victoria Hosp., East Grinstead, England)
Burns 13:57–61, February 1987   5–10

The surgical value of meshed skin grafts in major burns is proven, but aesthetically, the use of 1:1.5 mesh has received mixed reviews. Long-term cosmetic results of sheet and meshed grafts have seldom been compared. The authors evaluated 34 patients who received either sheet or mesh grafts for cosmetic effects in an 18-month follow-up study.

Nine male and female panelists, ranging from plastic surgeons to lay observers, studied the patients. None was told the type of skin graft an individual patient had received. Nineteen patients received only sheet graft, 10 patients had predominately 1:4 mesh, and five patients received 1:1.5 mesh exclusively. Observers were asked to determine which type of graft the patient had received and whether the results were cosmetically acceptable.

Most observers identified sheet graft more readily than mesh. Experts identified nearly all 1:1.5 mesh but also usually incorrectly characterized sheet graft as mature mesh graft. All observers correctly identified 1:4 mesh, but inexperienced panelists tended to be unable to distinguish 1:1.6 mesh from sheet. Cosmetically, 1:4 mesh was considered unacceptable in nearly 50% of the cases, compared with 80% acceptance for 1:1.5 mesh. Sheet graft received a similarly favorable cosmetic rating.

It is concluded that, cosmetically, 1:1.5 mesh grafts are nearly indistinguishable from mesh grafts. Because of the enhanced survival rate of mesh grafts on wounds that are infected or have poor hemostasis, 1:1.5 mesh is recommended for wider use.

▶ Any observer who cannot tell the difference between a mesh graft of any dimension and a solid sheet graft has visual problems. A mesh graft should only be used when conservation of skin is necessary to save life. Expressed differently, the appearance of the graft is of no consequence when the proper indications for a mesh graft have been followed. Use of meshed skin grafts when conservation is not a factor is unthinkable in the judgment of the editor.—E.E. Peacock, Jr., M.D.

6 Infections

Infective Cutaneous Gangrene: Urgency in Diagnosis and Treatment

Fiona B. Bailie, I.P. Linehan, G.J. Hadfield, A.P. Gillett, and B.N. Bailey (Stoke Mandeville Hosp., Aylesbury, England)
Ann. Plast. Surg. 19:238–246, September 1987   6–1

Infective cutaneous gangrene is frequent in India and Africa, where it often presents as scrotal gangrene. Four cases were managed in a regional plastic surgery unit in an 18-month period.

CASE 1.—Girl, 16, was stepped on twice by a pony in a 6-week period. The foot became swollen and painful shortly after the second episode, and the patient became toxic. Cellulitis spread up the leg, and groin glands were enlarged. Examination revealed impending gangrene with blisters. On skin incision, pus exuded from the base of the little toe.

Beta hemolytic streptococcus group A was cultured; blood cultures were negative. Further surgical débridement was necessary before the area could be grafted. The wound took 3 months to heal, but finally the patient walked well with no major problems.

Infective cutaneous gangrene is classified as both necrotizing fasciitis and progressive bacterial gangrene. Usually some underlying pathology is present. Necrotizing fasciitis is caused by streptococcal infection of the fascia; subsequent dermal gangrene results from endarteritis obliterans. Progressive bacterial gangrene, caused by multiple organisms, represents a skin infection that gradually extends in area and depth.

Broad-spectrum antibiotics are given, and rapid exploration is carried out with decompression and débridement as indicated. Hyperbaric oxygen may be used in conjunction with surgical decompression and débridement, if anaerobes are present. Overwhelming sepsis is a life-threatening complication.

► When systemic signs of infection persist in spite of adequate antibiotic therapy but show no signs of cutaneous gangrene, acute necrotizing fasciitis should be suspected and deep fascia exposed and biopsied. Infective cutaneous gangrene usually is diagnosed early because of surface findings; acute necrotizing fasciitis often is not diagnosed early because of lack of such signs. The result of delaying the diagnosis of acute necrotizing fasciitis can be a mortality approaching 90%.—E.E. Peacock, Jr., M.D.

Fournier's Syndrome of Urogenital and Anorectal Origin: A Retrospective, Comparative Study

J.M. Enriquez, S. Moreno, M. Devesa, V. Morales, A. Platas, and E. Vicente (Hosp. Ramón y Cajal, Madrid)
Dis. Colon Rectum 30:33–37, January 1987   6–2

The authors describe experience with 24 male and 4 female patients from 1979 to 1986 with perianal and genital necrotizing infections and compared these cases with those that had a urologic primary focus and those which originated in the anorectal area. In 14 patients (group 1) the site was anorectal, in 10 (group 2) it was urogenital, and in 4 (group 3) the origin was unknown.

Overall mortality was 25%, with 28.5% mortality in patients in group 1 and 10% in those in group 2, not a statistical difference; two of the four patients in group 3 died a few hours after surgery.

Myonecrosis was found more often in group 1 patients, (50%) than in group 2 patients (10%). Although mortality was higher in patients with myonecrosis (50%) than in those without muscle involvement (16%), the difference was not statistically significant, and a definite correlation was not established in this study.

Six patients in group 1 had colostomies at the time of initial débridement, 1 had a delayed colostomy, and 1 had a suprapubic cystostomy; 4 patients in group 2 had a suprapubic cystostomy and 2 had perineal urethrostomies, but none required colostomy.

Because gangrenous infections from a colorectal source have a less clear form of presentation and can lead to delay in diagnosis, more incidence and a higher degree of myonecrosis, deeper extension, greater severity, and higher mortality, it is important to know the signs which should raise suspicion that an infection is not trivial. They include lack of

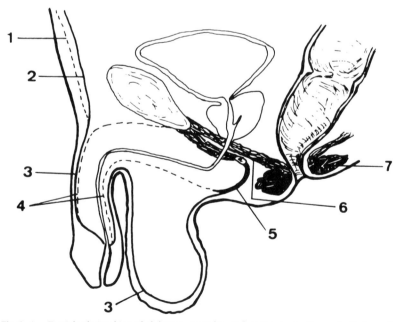

Fig 6–1.—Fascial relationships of abdomen, genitalia, and perineum: 1, Camper's; 2, Scarpa's; 3, Dartos; 4, Buck's; 5, Colles'; 6, levator; and 7, external anal sphincter. (Courtesy of Enriquez, J.M., et al.: Dis. Colon Rectum 30:33–37, January 1987.)

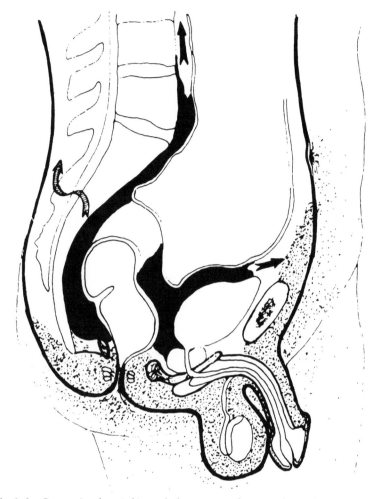

Fig 6–2.—Propagation from ischiorectal abscess *(spotted area)* and supralevator abscess *(black area)*. (Courtesy of Enriquez, J.M., et al.: Dis. Colon Rectum 30:33–37, January 1987.)

frank suppuration, progression of a painful erythema, skin necrosis or bullae around an abscess, crepitus or presence of gas in the plate, or absence of cicatrization of a perianal drain wound in a severely ill patient.

The fascial relationship among penis, scrotum, perineum, groin, and lower abdominal wall are shown in Figure 6–1. Different ways of extension after ischiorectal and pelvirectal abscess have been pointed out by Huber et al. (Fig 6–2).

Débridement must be radical and should be continued until the skin and subcutaneous tissue can no longer be separated from the deep fascia to avoid subsequent reconstructive problems. The precise limit of infection cannot be clarified until surgery is completed.

The authors recommend removal of any area of questionable viability because the most common error and cause of progression of the infection is inadequate aggressiveness in initial débridement and drainage. Antibiotics are only adjunctive to surgical therapy.

Of paramount importance in managing these patients is support therapy, adequate fluid replacement, hypernutrition, and wound reassessment. It may be necessary to do new débridements under anesthesia. Eight of these patients required skin grafting. Sphincteric function must be assessed before closure of the colostomy.

▶ One of the problems that has retarded progress in treatment of acute necrotizing fasciitis has been nomenclature. By definition, Fournier's gangrene is limited to the scrotum, but the principles of early diagnosis, early débridement, and repeated attempts to remove affected tissue are the same as when treating acute necrotizing fasciitis elsewhere. Early diagnosis and radical débridement are key. Antibiotics do not really seem to make a significant contribution unless extensive débridement is carried out earlier than commonly appreciated.—E.E. Peacock, Jr., M.D.

Effects of Wound Exudates on In Vitro Immune Parameters
McIntyre Bridges, Jr., Don Morris, John R. Hall, and Edwin A. Deitch (Louisiana State Univ., Shreveport)
J. Surg. Res. 43:133–138, August 1987   6–3

Local failure of host antibacterial defenses may contribute to surgical wound infection. The biologic activity of postsurgical wound exudates, or seroma fluids, on neutrophil and lymphocyte function was studied, and complement and fibronectin were quantified in the exudates. Samples were taken from 11 women in good general health who underwent mastectomy with axillary node dissection for breast cancer. A closed-system drainage device was placed at operation.

Wound exudates did not support opsonophagocytosis and killing of *Staphylococcus aureus* or *Pseudomonas aeruginosa* by control neutrophils, as did serum. They were less effective than serum as a neutrophil chemoattractant. The wound exudates also failed to support mitogen-induced lymphocyte blastogenesis as well as normal serum. A lack of normal humoral factors appeared to be responsible, for addition of normal serum to the wound exudates restored cellular activity to normal. Levels of plasma fibronectin and complement hemolytic activity in the wound exudates were reduced.

It appears that local collections of wound fluid may predispose to wound infection through impairing local host defenses. Seroma fluid within a surgical wound could impair host defenses by failing to supply cellular elements the humoral factors needed to optimize their function.

▶ Everything we know about wound healing cries out that wound exudate should not be allowed to remain on the surface of a wound. Change of dressings as often as necessary to prevent a collection of exudate may be all that is needed to start healing or prepare a wound for secondary closure. The conversion of wound exudate to wound transudate is key in knowing how long one should mechanically cleanse a wound to prevent immunologic and cellular complications, which prevent healing and encourage infection.—E.E. Peacock, Jr., M.D.

Reducing Wound Infections: Improved Gown and Drape Barrier Performance
Joseph A. Moylan, Kevin T. Fitzpatrick, and Kevan E. Davenport (Duke Univ.)
Arch. Surg. 122:152–157, February 1987   6–4

During a 21-month period 1,401 clean procedures and 780 clean-contaminated procedures were done to evaluate the use of a disposable gown and drape material that is made of spun-bonded fibers as a way to reduce wound infections, to define risk factors for developing infection when either the disposable material or a cotton gown and drape system is used, and to address the costs in using these systems.

The overall infection rate was 7.72% for the entire series, 2.78% for clean procedures, and 8.21% for clean-contaminated procedures. For the cotton system the infection rate was 6.51% and for the disposable system the rate was 2.83%. The rate of wound infections in both clean and clean-contaminated cases was significantly reduced by using the disposable system. Rates were 1.8% in clean and 4.8% in clean-contaminated procedures for the disposable system versus 3.8% in clean and 11.4% in clean-contaminated procedures when cotton was used. This effect was independent of all other factors.

Operations which lasted 90 minutes or more had an infection rate of 5.84%, and shorter procedures had a rate of 2.74%. Patients who did not receive preoperative antibiotics had an infection rate of 2.08% versus 7.23% for those who did, but there was no statistical difference in antibiotic use between the cotton or disposal groups. There was also no difference between the two materials by wound classification or sex.

Cost analysis was calculated for a community, university, and metropolitan hospital. For cotton the costs were $28.14, $48.56, and $18.63, respectively, per procedure; for disposable materials the cost was $25.78, $30.41, and $15.30, respectively, per procedure.

The risk of developing wound infection was 2½ times greater when cotton materials were used. As the length of operation increases, so does the risk of infection, which emphasizes the importance of barrier materials that must perform satisfactorily over lengthy surgical procedures.

Wound infections produced charges that exceeded significantly the diagnosis-related groups (DRG) payments in almost every case, and the disposable system was significant in reducing infections and affecting cost savings, which can be accrued by conversion to disposables as well as by preventing overrun on DRG payments.

▶ This report is bad news to legions of surgeons who despise paper drapes. The "feel" of drapes is not as important, perhaps, as the "feel" of a suture, but the rustle of paper and the difficulty of keeping things in place make older surgeons yearn for cloth around the field. If infections have been reduced and overall costs lowered, however, such yearning will have to be forgotten.—E.E. Peacock, Jr., M.D.

Incisional Infection After Colorectal Surgery in Obese Patients
Per-Olof Nyström, Anders Jonstam, Henning Höjer, and Lennart Ling (Univ. Hosp., Linköping, and Regional Hosp., Helsingborg, Sweden)
Acta Chir. Scand. 153:225–227, March 1987   6–5

Obese persons may have lowered tolerance to bacterial contamination of incisional wounds and therefore be at an increased risk of infection. A prospective study of colorectal surgery was carried out in which the subcutaneous fat layer in the incisional wound was measured and correlated with the occurrence of infection. All 189 patients in the study received systemic antibiotic prophylaxis. The patients were operated on electively at two hospitals.

Twenty wound infections occurred, for a prevalence of 10.6%. The overall average thickness of subcutaneous fat in the wounds was 3 cm, and the average wound length was 19 cm. Fat thickness was 1.2 cm greater on average in infected wounds. No such difference in wound length was observed. When the fat layer was 3.5 cm or more in thickness,

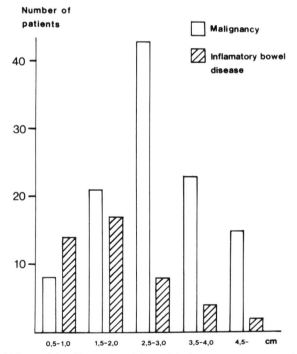

Fig 6–3.—Thickness of the subcutaneous abdominal fat layer in 110 patients with colonic cancer and 45 with inflammatory bowel disease. (Courtesy of Nyström, P.-O., et al.: Acta. Chir. Scand. 153:225–227, March 1987.)

one fifth of wounds were infected. Among patients with cancer, infection occurred in 24% of those with a thick fat layer and in 8% of the others (Fig 6–3).

A significantly increased abdominal wound infection rate was associated with a subcutaneous fat layer 3.5 cm or more in thickness in this study. This degree of obesity apparently carries an increased risk of wound infection after colorectal surgery. An increased wound area may be more important than the inferior resistance of fat to bacteria.

▶ These are interesting data to support what every experienced abdominal surgeon almost intuitively has known. Unfortunately, the same data apply to an intestinal anastomosis. Experienced surgeons have known for years that obesity, diabetes, and obstruction are all serious factors when contemplating intestinal anastomosis.—E.E. Peacock, Jr., M.D.

Ketoconazole Prevents *Candida* Sepsis in Critically Ill Surgical Patients
Gus J. Slotman, and Kenneth W. Burchard (Brown Univ.; Rhode Island Hosp.; and VA Med. Ctr., Providence)
Arch. Surg. 122:147–151, February 1987   6–6

To determine whether or not ketoconazole can prevent colonization of yeast or invasion in critically ill adult surgical patients a prospective, randomized, double-blind placebo-controlled study was conducted of 57 patients in a surgical intensive care unit (ICU) who had three or more clinical risk factors for *Candida* infection. Twenty-seven patients received 200 mg of ketoconazole via the gastrointestinal tract daily, and 30 patients received placebo.

In ketoconazole-treated patients the incidence of colonization with yeast species was significantly lower than in the placebo-treated group: 8 of 27 versus 18 of 30. With ketoconazole therapy disseminated *Candida* invasion did not occur, but it developed in five of the 30 patients who had placebo, a significant difference. Positive *Candida* cultures first developed in the colonized ketoconazole-treated patients on study day 4.5 (median), compared with a median of 10 days for the placebo-treated group. The yeast species that was cultured and the incidence of concomitant nonfungal bacteremia were similar for both groups.

Overall mortality was 32% for this study, 26% for the ketoconazole-treated group, and 37% for the placebo-treated group, which was not significantly different; mortality was also similar for colonized and non-colonized patients. However, in colonized placebo-treated patients who were older than age 55 years there was a significantly increased mortality, compared with that of younger patients: 50% versus 0%. There were no other clinical factors associated with increased mortality in any subgroup. Patients with yeast invasion had a mortality of 60%. Median stay in the surgical ICU for the ketoconazole-treated group was significantly lower than that of the placebo-treated group: 6.0 versus 12.5 days.

The results indicate that ketoconazole significantly reduces colonization of critically ill surgical patients by yeast. Invasive *Candida* sepsis was prevented in these patients; none developed it, although 30% became colonized with yeast, a significant finding. The effect on mortality of ketoconazole was not clearly defined in this study because the rate was similar for both groups, as well as for the colonized patients in each treatment group. That 60% of patients with disseminated *Candida* sepsis in this study died suggests an increased risk of mortality with yeast invasion. Although ketoconazole does not affect overall survival, it may reduce mortality in selective subgroups and it is recommended that it be administered to patients at risk for *Candida* colonization and dissemination.

▶ This is an important contribution. Even though amphotericin B is not as dangerous as previously thought and taught, it is still a very dangerous drug. Another agent is a timely contribution.—E.E. Peacock, Jr., M.D.

Effect of Topical and Systemic Antibiotics on Bacterial Growth Kinesis in Generalized Peritonitis in Man
Z.H. Krukowski, H.M. Al-Sayer, T.M.S. Reid, and N.A. Matheson (Aberdeen Univ. and City Hosp., Aberdeen, Scotland)
Br. J. Surg 74:303–306, April 1987   6–7

Antibiotic peritoneal lavage is still frowned upon or largely discredited worldwide, and the lack of a prospective controlled trial in patients with severe generalized peritonitis possibly underlies this scepticism on the value of tetracycline lavage, especially outside the United Kingdom. The bacterial counts of 28 patients with peritonitis of small intestinal, appendicular, or colonic origin and of less than 48 hours' duration were studied.

A wide variation in the concentration of viable organisms in the peritoneal fluid was found, but there was a significant difference between the effect of preoperative and no preoperative systemic antibiotics.

In the first sample of 14 patients who had preoperative antibiotics the growth rate was slower, and the difference was significant throughout the incubation period. The rate of growth detection in lavage patients was significantly reduced throughout the incubation period, regardless of whether antibiotics had been given before operation, except after 8-hour incubation in the group which did not receive antibiotics.

After tetracycline lavage in 14 patients, 5 of whom had received antibiotics before operation, there was complete inhibition of bacterial growth in the residual peritoneal fluid, regardless of whether preoperative antibiotics had been given, an effect which was still present in a fluid sample that was taken 1 hour after tetracycline lavage in 6 cases.

Patients who received antibiotics before operation were not selected randomly; rather, antibiotics were given to those for whom there was clinical concern about any delay in initiating treatment. Furthermore, the lack of randomization is irrelevant with respect to the conclusions of the authors regarding the effect of tetracycline lavage. There was a variation of between 2 and 8 hours in the timing of operation and taking of bacteriologic samples in relation to the administration of the preoperative systemic antibiotics, but the authors do not believe this detracts from the validity of their observations.

Bacterial growth in the peritoneal fluid still occurred after preoperative systemic antibiotics, although it was impaired. The effect of systemic antibiotics on bacterial growth was augmented temporarily by the dilutional effect of saline lavage on the concentration of organisms in the peritoneal fluid.

In contrast, lavage with tetracycline abolished bacterial growth, and the dilutional effect of saline lavage is clearly enhanced by addition of a high concentration of a nontoxic broad-spectrum antibiotic; complete inhibition of the bacterial growth occurred despite the relatively limited spectrum of tetracycline. Its effect is attributable to a high topical concentration of antibiotic.

On the basis of the present observations it is believed that systemic antibiotics should be given as soon as a diagnosis of peritonitis is made.

▶ So many reports have been presented indicating that peritoneal lavage with an antibiotic is not important in the treatment of generalized peritonitis that this study should be recorded. The data presented are suggestive of tetracycline lavage being helpful, but the measurements are only indirect and do not answer definitively the question of whether the problems caused by peritoneal lavage outweigh any theoretical or experimentally derived advantages.—E.E. Peacock, Jr., M.D.

Effect of Blood Transfusions on Immune Function: III. Alterations in Macrophage Arachidonic Acid Metabolism
J. Paul Waymack, Lois Gallon, Uno Barcelli, Orrawin Trocki, and J. Wesley Alexander (Univ. of Cincinnati)
Arch. Surg. 122:56–60, January 1987   6–8

Surgical patients often require blood transfusions during and after surgery, but the effect of transfusions on immune function and resistance to infection remains uncertain. Allogeneic blood transfusions have reduced cell-mediated immunity in rats. The effects of transfusion on production of prostaglandin metabolites by cultured macrophages were examined in a rat model in which 1-ml transfusions were administered.

Allogeneic blood transfusions decreased macrophage migration in response to inflammatory stimulation and increased the production of prostaglandin E, a strongly immunosuppressive arachidonic acid metabolite. Syngeneic transfusions did not alter either macrophage migration or arachidonic acid metabolism. Leukotriene B production did not differ significantly in the various animal groups.

Immunosuppression associated with blood transfusion appears to be related to increased prostaglandin E synthesis. Prostaglandin E probably is the most immunosuppressive of all arachidonic acid metabolites. It significantly impairs T lymphocyte blastogenesis and also interferes with macrophage differentiation and phagocytosis. The failure of allogeneic transfusions to increase macrophage production of leukotrienes indicates that the net effect of transfusion is strongly toward immunosuppression.

▶ Still another excellent reason to reduce to an absolute minimum the number of transfusions patients receive.—E.E. Peacock, Jr., M.D.

Surgery in Patients With Acquired Immunodeficiency Syndrome
Gene Robinson, Samuel E. Wilson, and Russell A. Williams (Harbor-Univ. of California Med. Ctr., Torrance; and Univ. of California, Los Angeles)
Arch. Surg. 122:170–175, February 1987   6–9

The authors studied the clinical courses of operations which were performed on 21 patients with acquired immunodeficiency syndrome (AIDS), between 1982 and 1985. Average age of the 20 men and 1 woman was 36 years at time of surgery.

Procedures included seven emergency and 24 elective operations. Seven patients underwent multiple procedures, with one patient having four. There were 4 thoracostomies, 2 celiotomies, and 1 craniotomy emergency operation. The elective operations were done for diagnostic and therapeutic indications, including thoracotomy with open lung biopsy on four occasions and abdominal operations in five patients. Long-term central venous access catheters were placed because of malnutrition in 4 patients, 1 patient had a tracheostomy, and 4 had neurologic procedures.

After emergency procedures, the 30-day operative mortality was 57%; for elective surgery the rate was 43%. By January 1986 mortality for all patients was 76%. The time from diagnosis of AIDS to death ranged from 2 to 45 weeks (mean duration, 31 weeks).

The most common infective agent was cytomegalovirus (CMV), and the next most common operative finding was Kaposi's sarcoma (KS). In one patient *Candida* pseudohyphae and ulcerations with acute and chronic cholecystitis were found; although reports of *Candida* cholecystitis exist, none were seen in association with AIDS. Toxoplasmosis and an unusual ameba were protozoan infectious agents in this group.

As seen in two patients brain biopsy specimens may be nondiagnostic, and evidence of toxoplasmosis emerged only later on repeated biopsy or at autopsy. In one patient ventriculostomy and medical treatment reduced intracerebral pressure and swelling from toxoplasmosis in the basal ganglia.

The most common opportunistic infection in AIDS patients is *Pneumocystis carinii* pneumonia; 24% of these patients had it, and it was found in half of the thoracostomies that were done for pneumothorax after bronchoscopy.

▶ There really isn't anything surprising about this study. One of the reasons AIDS was recognized is that physicians, in general, and surgeons, in particular, have more often evaluated during the last few decades the immunologic status of patients rather than just having tried to eliminate bacteria. It is not acceptable in 1988 to operate electively upon a patient whose immune response appears depressed following skin tests.—E.E. Peacock, Jr., M.D.

Immunity Against Tetanus and Response to Revaccination in Surgical Patients More Than 50 Years of Age
Ole Simonsen, Arne V. Block, Anette Klærke, Michael Klærke, Keld Kjeldsen, and Iver Heron (State Serum Inst., Copenhagen, Denmark, and Ålborg Hosp., Denmark)
Surg. Gynecol. Obstet. 164:329–334, April 1987   6–10

Tetanus has occurred after a wide range of surgical procedures. Most cases are thought to be of exogenous origin. Older patients are at an increased risk, for immunocompetence declines with advancing age. A questionnaire dealing with vaccination history was given to 178 surgical patients older than 50 years. Sixty-eight patients found to be inadequately vaccinated were offered revaccination, and 44 underwent revaccination and blood sampling 4 weeks later. Thirty-one of these patients subsequently had surgery. Sera were analyzed by the ELISA technique.

Forty-seven percent of 127 evaluable patients had never been vaccinated against tetanus. Two thirds had serum antitoxin concentrations below the protective level. A study of vaccinated patients showed a continuous decline in immunity following vaccination. Patients given a complete three-dose primary vaccination during the previous 5 years or who were revaccinated within the previous 10 years were well protected. Revaccination consistently provided adequate antibody concentrations. Revaccination some days before operation appeared to be optimal.

It appears that surgical patients should be revaccinated, if necessary, at least some days before operation to assure adequate serum antitoxin levels. Elderly patients apparently have no special requirements.

▶ Most surgeons do not think of tetanus infection as a postoperative complication. It should be remembered that tetanus spores can live in the body for many years without producing clinical tetanus. Repeated trauma such as that caused by surgery can release tetanus organisms and produce typical clinical tetany. Medical and legal repercussions can be enormous.—E.E. Peacock, Jr., M.D.

7 Burns

Hypomagnesemia: A Multifactorial Complication of Treatment of Patients With Severe Burn Trauma
John J. Cunningham, Ran D. Anbar, and John D. Crawford (Shriners Burn Inst., Boston; Massachusetts Gen. Hosp., Boston; and Harvard Univ.)
JPEN 11:364–367, July–August 1987   7–1

Magnesium deficiency may be associated with burn injury. Because hypomagnesemia impairs renal potassium reabsorption, burn patients are at risk of hypokalemia. Magnesium and potassium status were assessed in six severely burn-injured adolescents. The average burn covered 82% of the total body surface. All patients required IV potassium in the early phase to maintain a serum potassium greater than 3.5 mEq/L. The parenteral nutrition solution used contributed 1 mEq/kg of potassium and 0.4 mEq/kg of magnesium daily. Enteral nutrition with Traumacal provided 20 mEq/L of potassium and 17 mEq/L of magnesium.

All patients with hypomagnesemic. Two of five patients were hypomagnesemic during gentamicin therapy, and all five were hypomagnesemic during subsequent treatment with tobramycin. Five patients had further episodes of hypomagnesemia in the absence of aminoglycoside therapy. Detailed studies of one patient showed that hypomagnesemia occurring during tobramycin therapy was associated with refractoriness to potassium repletion. Magnesium supplementation prevented recurrent hypokalemia during a subsequent phase of hypomagnesemia induced by diuresis.

The need for magnesium replacement increases in patients recovering from severe burn injury. Commercially available enteral products may not contain adequate amounts of magnesium for these patients; early restoration of enteral nutrition in postburn patients therefore will require magnesium supplementation of available commercial formulations.

▶ Although magnesium deficiency is primarily seen in malabsorption syndromes, the problem can occur in burned patients and often is overlooked. This paper serves as a timely reminder.—E.E. Peacock, Jr., M.D.

Regulation of Lipolysis in Severely Burned Children
Robert R. Wolfe, David N. Herndon, Edward J. Peters, Farook Jahoor, Manu H. Desai, and O. Bryan Holland (Univ. of Texas and Shriners Burns Inst., Galveston, Tex.)
Ann. Surg. 206:214–221, August 1987   7–2

Basal free fatty acid (FFA) flux is elevated after burn injury. Since catecholamines stimulate lipolysis and are chronically increased in severely burned patients, they may be important in stimulating lipolysis in this setting. Lipolytic responsiveness to infused epinephrine was studied in 12 severely burn-injured children. Aggressive excisional treatment was carried out after fluid resuscitation. The response of lipolysis to β-blockade with propranolol also was studied.

Infusion of epinephrine at a rate of 0.015 μg/kg/minute stimulated lipolysis in four of seven patients, as evidenced by the rate of appearance of glycerol. Resting energy expenditure, nitrogen excretion, and substrate oxidation did not change significantly. No lipolytic response was seen in three patients who underwent greater fascial excisions than the others. β-Blockade led to a prompt reduction in the glycerol appearance rate in all patients. The potential energy available as plasma FFA was reduced much more than the overall rate of energy expenditure.

The rate of appearance of FFA after severe burn injury may be limited by a reduced amount of endogenous fat following excisional treatment. The deficiency may adversely affect energy metabolism. In the long term, fat removal may influence the ability to perform exercise. The present findings do not support the use of adrenergic blocking agents to lower the metabolic rate in this setting.

▶ Burned patients exhibit alterations in triglyceride, cholesterol, carnitine, fatty acid, lipoprotein, and prostaglandin metabolism. Although glucose is more effective than fat as a ready source of energy, conservative administration of fat, particularly linoleic acid provides nutritional support evenly rather than sporadically, as when infrequent meals are the only source of energy.—E.E. Peacock, Jr., M.D.

The Effect of Burn Wound Excision on Measured Energy Expenditure and Urinary Nitrogen Excretion
Carol S. Ireton-Jones, William W. Turner, Jr., and Charles R. Baxter (Univ. of Texas and Parkland Mem. Hosp. Burn Ctr., Dallas)
J. Trauma 27:217–220, February 1987   7–3

After major thermal injury, energy expenditures increase. The Curreri formula is often used to predict caloric needs, and modifications that take into account changes in burn wound size have been suggested. The effect of wound closure on metabolic needs in 20 patients (15–59 years old; mean ± SD, 27 ± 10 years) with burns over more than 30% of their body surface was assessed by measured energy expenditure (MEE) as evaluated by calorimeter, by the Curreri formula (CEE), by a modified Curreri formula (MCEE) that took into account the percentage of open wound remaining, and by urine urea nitrogen (UUN) excretion.

Three patients died during this study. Nine patients showed net decreases in MEE over 17–77 days postburn, while 11 patients had net increases in MEE from 8 to 99 days postburn. The MEE and percentage of open wounds were not correlated. The MCEE and MEE were not correlated. Caloric intake and MEE were only weakly correlated. The UUN excretion was not correlated with percentage of open wounds.

Curreri formula estimates of energy requirements of burned patients, even when adjusted for percentage of open wound remaining, appear to be of limited usefulness. Serial measurement of energy expenditure provides a more accurate assessment. Protein catabolism correlates poorly with energy expenditure, and protein needs should be evaluated by UUN excretion.

▶ The mystery of how to account for all of the expenditure of energy, even to the extent of death from a negative nitrogen balance, continues. One of the oldest theories—that burned tissue produces toxins that drive metabolism off scale, therefore necessitating excision of damaged tissue to prevent energy depletion—does not appear now to be a complete explanation or answer to the problem. It is certainly a major component, however, and other benefits can be derived from getting a closed wound besides correction of accelerated metabolism.—E.E. Peacock, Jr., M.D.

Fever as a Predictor of Infection in Burned Children
Ruth Ann Parish, Alvin H. Novack, David M. Heimbach, and Loren R. Engrav (Univ. of Washington and Harborview Med. Ctr., Seattle, Wash.)
J. Trauma 27:69–71, January 1987   7–4

Children with burns often develop fever, but the course and duration of these fevers have not been evaluated. The records of 223 children admitted to a regional burn center from 1979 to 1982 were reviewed to determine the predictive value of fever as an indicator of infection in burned children. The highest rectal temperature during each 8-hour period was recorded. A fever was defined as a rectal temperature of 38.2°C or higher.

The highest mean temperature occurred 38 to 96 hours after burn injury and appeared at the same time whether or not the child had infection. Each of the 23 children with infections and 145 of 200 noninfected children had one episode of fever during the first 2 weaks postburn, indicating that fever was not specific for the presence of infection. Similarly, fever was not a significant predictor of infection in children younger than 4 years or those with burns over more than 20% of the total body surface area. The presence of infection was readily determined by physical examination alone in all but 2 children with infection.

The presence of fever is not a specific indicator of infection in all burned children. The physical examination is a reliable source of information about wound infection, sepsis, or other childhood infections, and it should be the primary tool used in making the diagnosis of infection in burned children.

▶ This simple presentation of a clinical observation that people who do not take care of children routinely or for a variety of conditions often overlook has been responsible for overtreatment of many burned children. The paper also points out that accurate direct observations, such as those gained in a good physical examination, can be more valuable in assessing the condition of a sick child than merely looking at the temperature chart.—E.E. Peacock, Jr., M.D.

A Ten-Year Review of *Candida* Sepsis and Mortality in Burn Patients
Jai K. Prasad, Irving Feller, and Philip D. Thomson (Univ. of Michigan)
Surgery 101:213–216, February 1987   7–5

The records of 233 burn patients who since 1975 were found to have had *Candida* at any time during their hospital course were reviewed. Average age of the 233 patients was 36 years, and the average burn covered 46.5% of total body surface. Those with candidemia had a mean age of 38 years and a larger average burn area: 57.2% of total body surface. Those who died had a mean age of 54 years, and their burns covered a mean of 67.2% of body surface.

Candida-positive cultures were obtained from wounds in 199 patients and from urine in 46, sputum in 46, and blood in 70. Of 70 patients with candidemia, 38 died: 23 from gram-negative bacterial sepsis, 6 with mixed bacterial and *Candida* sepsis, 5 with generalized candidiasis, 2 from hemorrhagic shock, 1 from heart failure, and 1 from respiratory failure. All 23 patients who died of bacterial sepsis had been treated with amphotericin B, as had six who died of mixed bacterial and *Candida* sepsis and who had also received aminoglycoside antibiotic. Despite treatment with amphotericin B, five patients died of proved candidiasis.

The incidence of *Candida* was shown to be 13.5%, which was lower than that in the study of Spebar and Pruitt, which showed 30%, and the 63.5% incidence that was reported in a pediatric study by MacMillan et al.

The incidence in the present study may be explained by a comprehensive program of prevention and early detection. As soon as *Candida* sepsis was detected, treatment with amphotericin B was begun, and if there was no clinical response within 24 hours the dose was increased. If after 2 weeks of initial therapy there was unacceptable clinical response or if a breakthrough of *Candida* had occurred, the dose of amphotericin B was increased for another 2 weeks, and this regimen proved efficacious. The infection was controlled with few side effects.

The incidence of candidemia of 4.0% in this series agrees with that noted by Spebar and Pruitt of 3.4%, but mortality in the present study was 54% versus 76.9% in their study. These differences cannot be explained by age or extent of the body surface that was burned, but they may be explained by the early and aggressive use of amphotericin B.

Twenty-three patients died with gram-negative septicemia. The six who died from mixed bacterial and *Candida* sepsis may be said to have died of mixed infection, but they have to be placed in the *Candida* group. A third group of five patients died despite amphotericin B therapy. It appears there are actually three types of patients in this group, although the numbers are small: eleven patients with candidemia died of *Candida* sepsis, and the death rate was only 15.7% (11 of 70). The other four died of organ system failure that was unrelated to *Candida* sepsis.

The authors believe aggressive prevention and a diagnostic program for *Candida* sepsis should be carried out in all burn patients and that treatment for *Candida* wound sepsis and candidemia should be initiated early.

▶ Two facts are worthy of emphasis. The first is that *Candida* sepsis becomes more common as other infections are controlled, and second, amphotericin B is not as dangerous as previously believed and should be instituted earlier than most surgeons have thought.—E.E. Peacock, Jr., M.D.

Leukopenia Secondary to Silver Sulfadiazine: Frequency, Characteristics and Clinical Consequences
Patricia Smith Choban and Wendy J. Marshall (Eastern Virginia Med. School, Norfolk, Va.)
Am. Surg. 53:515–517, September 1987   7–6

Leukopenia, found in about 5% of burn-injured patients treated with silver sulfadiazine (SSD), may be a risk factor for infectious complications in this setting. Seventy-seven patients with thermal injuries seen within 24 hours of injury were reviewed. The patients, with a mean age of 29 years, had an average body surface burn of 23%.

Thirty-four patients were treated with SSD and had serial white blood cell (WBC) counts. Seventeen others received silver nitrate, and five received other topical treatment. Fifty-six percent of the patients treated with SSD had a WBC count less than 5,000, as did 12% of those treated with silver nitrate. Leukopenia was most evident in SSD-treated patients with burn injuries exceeding 15% of the body surface. Leukopenia generally occurred on the second postburn day and resolved when treatment was discontinued. A reduction in mature neutrophils was chiefly responsible for the neutropenia. No increase in septic complications or opportunistic infections was associated with leukopenia, and there was no difference in the final outcome.

More than half the burn-injured patients in this study who received SSD treatment had leukopenia. Patients with larger burns were most at risk. This leukopenia appeared to be self-limited and was not related to an increased occurrence of infectious complications.

▶ Although, as this paper correctly points out, leukopenia that develops secondary to administration of silver sulfadiazine is not a significant complication as far as final outcome is concerned, it should be noted that other silver salts are probably more effective now in controlling local infection than silver sulfadiazine. Silver pipemidate is one such compound.—E.E. Peacock, Jr., M.D.

Management of Burned Long Bones

Daniel S. Sellers, Philip F. Parshley, David W. Waldram, Stephen H. Miller, and Robert J. Demuth (Oregon Health Sci. Univ. and Emanuel Hosp., Portland)
J. Trauma 27:322–325, March 1987   7–7

Proper management of burns involving osseous tissues is controversial. The authors describe two such patients, managed by standard soft-tissue coverage techniques, who both sustained fractures of the burned bone several months later.

Man, 50, received an electrical burn. The anterior compartment of the lower leg was débrided until one half the circumference of the tibia was exposed. Autografts were placed 24 days later with 80% take overall, except over the exposed tibia. The nonviable bone was removed and covered. On postburn day 106, the patient was dancing at home and developed a stress fracture of the previously burned bone.

Man, 24, had been burned to the bone by a space heater. The area was débrided and covered with xenograft and later with autograft. The patient was at home walking on postburn day 136, when the previously burned femur fractured.

Both of these patients had stress fractures in bones that had been burned and débrided. The following guidelines are proposed in light of this experience. Minimize débridement and decortication. Early vascularized muscle coverage should prevent desiccation and infection. Prophylactic fixation should be used to protect the bone during healing. Activity should be restricted until healing is complete.

▶ The key to successful therapy, of course, is rapid coverage before osteomyelitis occurs. The problem is compounded when there is a fracture. Splitting the unique tibialis anterior muscle so that a portion can be rotated over the bone does not interfer with muscle function and usually provides immediate successful coverage.—E.E. Peacock, Jr., M.D.

Face Burn Reconstruction: Does Early Excision and Autografting Improve Aesthetic Appearance?

J.L. Hunt, G.F. Purdue, T. Spicer, G. Bennett, and S. Range (Univ. of Texas., Dallas; and Parkland Mem. Hosp., Dallas)
Burns 13:39–44, February 1987   7–8

Recently attention has been directed toward improving the ultimate cosmetic and functional deformities of the burned face by means of early excision and grafting. The authors have evaluated both the technique and esthetic result of early excision and split-thickness autografting (STAG) of full-skin-thickness face burns.

Twenty-five patients with full-skin-thickness face burns underwent surgery 4 to 14 days after the burn. Thirteen had excision and STAG in one stage; seven of them had excision of eschar that covered the entire face.

Twelve patients had a two-stage procedure. Eschar was excised at the

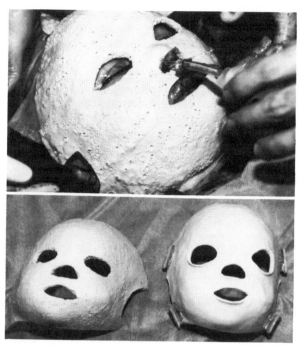

Fig 7–1 (top).—Porous silicone mask is fitted over face after autografting.
Fig 7–2 (bottom).—Hard Polyflex II plastic mask *(right)* fits over silicone mask *(left)*. Both act as pressure dressing.
(Courtesy of Hunt, J.L., Burns 13:39–44, February 1987.)

first operation, and the wound was covered with a biologic dressing. The wound was then autografted 24 to 72 hours later. In nine of these patients the full-thickness burn involved the entire face. The last seven patients had a pressure dressing in the form of a silicone face mask that was applied over the autograft in the second stage (Figs 7–1 and 7–2). Follow-up ranged from 3 months to 5.5 years.

Results showed that postoperative autograft loss secondary to subgraft hematoma was much less, but it was not completely eliminated with the two-stage procedure. Once it was realized that metal staples were as good as sutures to secure skin, their more liberal use resulted in less graft slippage and decreased operating time in both treatment groups.

Three patients who had the one-stage procedure and one who had the two-stage procedure required an additional operation to skin graft open areas that had been inadequately excised. Two patients in the two-stage group needed repair of severe bilateral upper and lower eyelid ectropion within 4 weeks of primary excision. No patient needed a second operation to reautograft an area because of local wound sepsis.

Twenty-four percent of all patients were readmitted for release of contracture or revision of scar. Common indications were eyelid ectropion, medial canthal contracture, microstomia, lip ectropion, and hypertrophic scar. The number of operations ranged from one to six.

These preliminary results are encouraging and warrant assessment by surgeons at other hospitals. When early excision of full-skin-thickness face burns is used, cautious optimism about the ultimate esthetic result by both the surgeon and the patient is advised.

▶ Mercifully, uniform third degree burns over a wide area of the face are rare. Knowing this, a thoughtful surgeon will be very conservative and débride only obviously dead tissue that already is separating by normal enzymatic digestion. The principle of wide early excision of all questionably viable tissue does not apply to facial burns. Scarred skin following deep second degree burn frequently is more acceptable cosmetically than a split-thickness or even a full-thickness graft.—E.E. Peacock, Jr., M.D.

Composite Autologous-Allogeneic Skin Replacement: Development and Clinical Application
Charles B. Cuono, Robert Langdon, Nicholas Birchall, Scott Barttelbort, and Joseph McGuire (Yale Univ.)
Plast. Reconstr. Surg. 80:626–635, October 1987   7–9

Grafting of autologous keratinocyte cultures directly to a burn wound has been effective but does not replace lost dermis. Viable allogeneic dermis is not immunologically inert, but removal of the epidermal component might eliminate most cells that express class II major histocompatibility complex (MHC) product. The residual dermis might be the best natural recipient site for autologous keratinocytes. A composite grafting method was developed in which excised burn wounds are resurfaced with unmatched allograft. Keratinocyte cultures are initiated from the patient. After removing allogeneic epidermis, the dermal bed is resurfaced with keratinocyte cultures. Cryopreserved skin grafts 0.015–0.017 inch thick are utilized. Two cases are described.

CASE 1.—Man, 47, with hypertension and pulmonary disease, sustained 55% total body surface area (TSBA) burns, circumferential from nipples to ankles. Eighty percent of burn area was full-thickness, but there was no inhalation injury. Z-index was 5.3, with mortality probability at 90%. Hypertonic resuscitation was uneventful. Bilateral lower-extremity escharotomies were performed on day of admission. On postburn day 3 excised areas were resurfaced and keratinocyte cultures were initiated. On day 15, lower extremity allografts were excised, and wounds were resurfaced with standard autografts expanded 3:1. On day 32, allograft between the xiphoid and umbilicus was dermabraded and resurfaced with keratinocyte. The procedure was repeated on infraumbilical on day 42. On day 71, the patient (fully ambulatory) was discharged; Jobst compression garments were worn 6 months thereafter. At 11 months postgraft, all areas remained well healed.

CASE 2.—Man, 32, sustained 65% TSBA burns, 70% full-thickness, including upper extremities, anterior and posterior trunk, and lower extremities to knees. Z-index was 5.9, with mortality probability at 95%. Patient was intubated for respiratory failure and resuscitated with Parkland regimen. Half the burn wounds were excised on day 4, including upper extremity. Hands and fingers were resurfaced with autografts, and viable allograft was used elsewhere. Keratinocyte cultures were begun on day 4. Escharectomy with allograft was completed on day 11. Adult respiratory distress syndrome (ARDS) and tubular necrosis improved. On day 27, allograft skin was abraded from upper extremities and resurfaced with keratinocyte, which became coalescent. Candidiasis developed. On day 48, allograft was excised from posterior and anterior trunk, and wound was resurfaced with keratinocyte. The patient improved but developed panlobar pneumonia on day 53 and died of respiratory failure. Biopsy revealed successful engraftment of keratinocyte.

It appears that allogeneic dermis can function as dermis and support engraftment and the integration of cultured autologous keratinocyte sheets. The combined procedure provides permanent skin replacement. The long-term fate of allogeneic dermis and its fibroblasts requires further study.

▶ This paper is reminiscent of the collagenous "ghosts" originally described by Thomas Gibson in his first report on the use of allografts in treating burned patients. The collagenous portion of dermis can make a contribution to wound healing, and the combination of autologous and allogeneic skin, therefore, may be even better than the artificial dermis described by Burke et al.—E.E. Peacock, Jr., M.D.

The Influence of Inhalation Injury and Pneumonia on Burn Mortality
Khan Z. Shirani, Basil A. Pruitt, and Arthur D. Mason (U.S. Army Inst. of Surgical Research, Fort Sam Houston, Tex.)
Ann. Surg. 205:82–87, January 1987   7–10

Pulmonary complications resulting from inhalation of toxic gases and products of incomplete combustion adversely affect the prognosis of burn patients. Cutaneous burns activate the complement cascade, inducing intrapulmonary leukocyte aggregation, release of oxygen-free radicals, and pulmonary damage. Because global immunosuppression is proportional to burn area, respiratory tract infections are the most common complication of burns. This article reviews a retrospective study conducted to determine how inhalation injury and pneumonia reduce burn patient survival.

The records of 1,058 consecutive burn patients were analyzed for status of inhalation injury on admission, development of pneumonia during hospitalization, and survival. The 487 patients at risk for inhalation injury had been examined by bronchoscopy or Xenon 133 lung scan, or both. Chest roentgenograms and smears of sputum or endotracheal secretions were studied if pneumonia was suspected. Of the group of 1,058 patients, pneumonia occurred in 141 of 373 (38%) with inhalation injuries and in 60 of 685 (8.8%) without inhalation injury. Individually, inhalation injury and pneumonia increased mortality by a maximum of 20% and 40%, respectively; together, they increased mortality by a maximum of 60%. The increase in mortality from inhalation injury and pneumonia was greatest among patients with moderate burns.

These data suggest that inhalation injury and pneumonia have significant, independent, and additive effects on mortality among burn patients. When considered along with age and total burn size, inhalation injury and pneumonia can be used to predict the survival rate.

▶ There is not much new in this paper, but it is worthy of presentation and review because thinking about pulmonary injury early and treating it early is still key to preventing fatal termination after inhalation injury.—E.E. Peacock, Jr., M.D.

8 Transplantation

A Perspective on Long-Term Outcome in Organ Transplantation
R.D. Guttmann (Royal Victoria Hosp. and McGill Univ., Montreal, Quebec, Canada)
Transplant. Proc. 19:67–73, February 1987   8–1

A long-range perspective in organ transplantation can be obtained by examining (1) whether long-term data are available and adequate to provide an accurate picture, especially in renal transplantation; (2) some of the specific medical problems occurring in long-term transplant patients; and (3) the status of patients with successful allografts who continue to take chemical immunosuppressive drugs with no obvious medical problems, and why they might have potential susceptibility to long-term complications such as malignancy and infection.

From a survey of leading transplant centers, 32%, 22%, and 19% of grafts were surviving at 5–9, 10–14, and 15–19 years, respectively, in nonliving donor renal transplantation; and the graft survival rates for similar time periods for cardiac allograft recipients were 14%, 11%, and 2%. The major problems in renal allograft patients are a variety of viral and bacterial infections, hepatitis, occlusive vascular disease, bone disease, and cancer, aside from chronic graft rejection, according to the present survey. From published reports of renal transplant recipients, after 5 years it is clear there is continued graft, patient loss, and significant medical complications in the survivors. Attention has been centered on hepatitis B as a major medical problem where it is clear that the chronic carrier state leads to long-term chronic liver disease, including cirrhosis and hepatoma. For unclear reasons, the incidence of bone disease has been markedly reduced during the past 15 years in patients who received transplants, but malignancy remains a significant long-term problem.

In assessing the immune response in terms of in vivo delayed-type hypersensitivity skin tests, it was observed that as a function of posttransplant time an increasing proportion of patients develop delayed cutaneous anergy, associated in the short term with an increase in surgical complications and serious bacterial infections and in the long-term with chronic viral infections and fatal malignancy. Studies have allowed the author's group to develop a picture of the immune system environment in the long-term patient (table) where the true T lymphocyte population is reduced markedly and the Leu-7^+ cell populations coexpressing T lymphocyte markers are expanded. From further studies addressing the question of whether or not abnormally expanded Leu-7^+/Leu-4^+/Leu-11^- populations of cells have T cell function, the author's group studies have now revealed that they lack T cell function, do not possess interleukin 2 (IL-2) receptors, and cannot be induced to express IL-2 receptors using

119

THE DISTORTED LYMPHOCYTE SUBPOPULATIONS IN PERIPHERAL BLOOD IN THE HEALTHY
LONG-TERM RENAL ALLOGRAFT RECIPIENT RECEIVING CHRONIC
CHEMICAL IMMUNOSUPPRESSION*

Lymphocyte Subset	Defined by Monoclonal Antibodies†	Normal Activity	PBL Pool Size in Long-term Recipients
Total T cells	LEU-4+/LEU-7⁻/LEU-11⁻	T function	Decreased
T helper	LEU-3+/LEU-7⁻/LEU-11⁻	Helper function	Decreased
T cytotoxic/suppressor	LEU-2+/Leu-7⁻/LEU-11⁻	Cytotoxic/suppressor function	Decreased
LGL	LEU-4+/LEU-7+/LEU-11⁻	No NK function No T function	Markedly expanded
LGL	LEU-4 /LEU-7+/LEU-11+	Moderate NK function	No change
LGL	LEU-4 /LEU-7⁻/LEU-11+	Potent NK function	Markedly decrease

*Abbreviations: **PBL**, peripheral blood lymphocytes; **LGL**, large granular lymphocytes.
†Becton Dickinson Monoclonal Antibody Center, Mountain View, Calif.
(Courtesy of Guttmann, R.D.: Transplant. Proc. 19:67–73, February 1987.)

IL-2. There seems to be a markedly and abnormally expanded subpopulation of non-NK large granular lymphocytes with phenotype Leu−7⁺/Leu−4⁺/Leu−11⁻ in long-term stable renal allograft recipients who are at increased risk of developing cancers and chronic viral infections.

A significant number of very young children will in the future have heart, liver, and kidney transplants; consequently, a thorough analysis of risks and benefits must be undertaken to determine the appropriateness of this therapy.

▶ In this careful and very well done survey of the long-term perspective in organ transplantation presented by Dr. Guttmann to the Transplantation Society in its 1986 meeting, the harsh realities of long-term effects of chronic disease and chronic immunosuppression are portrayed. Continued attrition due to rejection-related phenomena; infection, especially viral; and tumor development continue to claim grafts and lives throughout several decades of follow-up. It is important, especially with the dramatic short-term improvements recently noted with the use of cyclosporine and other new immunosuppressive regimens, to be reminded that organ transplantation is meant to provide long-term benefits of both quantity and quality of life, and reports of this sort must encourage further efforts to solve these long-term problems. This is one of the several very potent reasons to continue to emphasize clinical and bench research in transplantation immunobiology, and to de-emphasize dissemination of organ transplantation into the community. Centers of research and excellence in organ transplantation must be provided with the patients and the resources necessary to continue investigation in order to fulfill the enormous expectations widely held for organ transplantation.—O. Jonasson, M.D.

Regulation of Alloantigen Expression in Different Tissues

J.W. Fabre, A.D. Milton, S. Spencer, A. Settaf, and D. Houssin (Queen Victoria Hosp., East Grinstead, England; and Hôpital Paul Brousse and Hôpital Cochin, Paris)
Transplant. Proc. 19:45–49, February 1987
8–2

The class I and class II antigens of the major histocompatibility complex (MHC) are known to function as immunoregulatory molecules for T lymphocyte reactions. Both delayed-type hypersensitivity and cytotoxic and antibody responses are likely to play a role in allograft rejection. The bulk of the cytotoxic T cell response is directed at class I antigens, whereas the bulk of the inflammatory delayed-type hypersensitivity response is stimulated by class II antigens.

Transplanted organs differ widely in their expression of class I antigens at the time of grafting. Species differences in class I expression also exist, and there are interindividual differences within species. The parenchymal cells of many grafts initially have little or no class I expression and therefore are not vulnerable to cytotoxic T cells. Class II antigens are stronger transplantation antigens than are those of class I.

All grafts except those of CNS tissue carry strongly class II—positive interstitial dendritic cells in their connective tissues. Most than merely class II expression is required for stimulating T cells. The kidney is the only commonly transplanted organ that has class II—positive parenchymal cells at the time of grafting.

If induction of the MHC is important in the rejection process, prevention of induction may effectively suppress rejection. Preliminary studies suggest that treatment in vivo with E prostaglandins can prevent induction of the MHC in allografts.

▶ In these studies, antigen expression on the allograft is examined. Immunogenicity of the grafted tissue is certainly a major stimulus of the immune response. Other studies with dispersed cells or tissues have had encouraging results, with absent or more easily controlled rejection reactions when antigen presentation is inhibited or suppressed.—O. Jonasson, M.D.

The Relation Between Major Histocompatibility Complex (MHC) Restriction and the Capacity of Ia to Bind Immunogenic Peptides

Soren Buus, Alessandro Sette, Sonia M. Colon, Craig Miles, and Howard M. Grey (Natl. Jewish Ctr. for Immunology and Respiratory Medicine, Denver)
Science 235:1353–1358, March 13, 1987   8–3

Protein antigens must be processed by accessory cells in order to be recognized by T cells. T cells of the helper subset only recognize protein antigens in the context of Ia molecules on accessory cells. The function of Ia may be to specifically bind only certain peptides, thus selecting the determinants to be presented. Ia and antigen then interact specifically prior to T cell recognition.

In each of the 12 experiments that examined binding of labeled proteins to Ia, Ia—antigen interaction was demonstrated. Every Ia molecule was capable of binding some but not all peptides.

All peptides bound to more than one Ia molecule. In 11 of 12 cases, the peptide bound most strongly to the restriction element. The data indicate a determinant selection process of MHC restriction in which Ia molecules select peptides created during antigen processing and subsequently present them to T cells. A single Ia molecule is capable of binding many different unrelated peptides, clearly distinguished from the antigen-antibody reaction.

Major Histocompatibility Complex (MHC) Restriction of Foreign Transplantation Antigens in Rats Rendered Tolerant at Birth
Hiromitsu Kimura, Lise Desquenne-Clark, Megumu Miyamoto, and Willys K. Silvers (Univ. of Pennsylvania; and Hamamatsu Univ., Hamamatsu, Japan)
J. Exp. Med. 164:2031–2037, December 1986   8–4

If mice and rats are inoculated with MHC-incompatible bone marrow cells (BMC) at birth, they become tolerant of the transplantation antigens that are present on the donor cells. Earlier the authors proposed that MHC restriction accompanies the induction of tolerance. To test this hypothesis, rats which had been inoculated with foreign BMC at birth were challenged with third-party skin grafts that were compatible with either the foreign inoculum or with the host.

Eleven of 12 mice accepted third-party skin grafts when foreign transplantation antigens were compatible with the BMC inoculum. Only three of 14 grafts were accepted when the graft was MHC-compatible with the host.

Lewis.1N rats were made tolerant at birth with BMC that were prepared from Wag donors. After 7 weeks these rats received grafts of Wag skin, BN.B2 skin, or BN skin.

It was found that Bn.B2 grafts are MHC-compatible with Wag, whereas BN grafts have the same minor histocompatibility antigens of BN.B2 but the MHC of Lewis.1N. All the Wag grafts were accepted, thus confirming induction of tolerance. Four of nine BN.B2 skin grafts were accepted, but all six BN grafts were rejected.

These results support the hypothesis that MHC restriction of foreign transplantation antigens occurs when tolerance is induced.

▶ The phenomenon of MHC restriction has been complex and difficult to comprehend. In the clear and sophisticated studies reported by Buus and colleagues (Abstract 8–3), the Ia molecules of marrow cells were found to pick and choose among peptide antigens for presentation to T cells. They showed that a single Ia molecule is capable of binding many peptides, and only in combination with the Ia (MHC) do these peptides then become satisfactory antigens.

This concept was applied in the studies reported by Silver's group (Abstract 8–4) in which clever use of histocompatibility differences in rodents was made to demonstrate that it was also MHC restriction of foreign transplantation antigens that was significant in the induction of tolerance.

Basic studies such as these are contributing to our more complete understanding of the donor-host compatibility relationships.—O. Jonasson, M.D.

Antagonistic Effects of γ Interferon and Steroids on Tissue Antigenicity

Dariusz Leszczynski, Bernadette Ferry, Huub Schellekens, Peter H.v.d. Meide, Pekka Häyry (Univ. of Helsinki, Finland, and the Primate Ctr., Rijswijk, The Netherlands)

J. Exp. Med. 164:1470–1477, November 1986   8–5

Very few kidney vascular endothelial cells express class II antigens, and in those that do, the level of expression is low. Human and rat heart and liver have a low level of class II expression on endothelial cells; the major class II antigen-expressing cells are the dendritic cells (DC). The authors investigated the stability of the level of class II antigen expression in rat organs.

Male rats weighing about 200 gm were used. Gamma interferon (rIFN-γ) was obtained from cultures of a transformed Chinese hamster ovary cell line carrying the gene encoding rat IFN-γ. Double indirect immunofluorescence was performed. Three days after a single intraperitoneal injection of rIFN-γ, the number of Ia^+ rabbit antiserum to factor VIII-related antigen (FVIII-RAg$^-$DC) increased in heart tissue 3.6-fold, from 23.5 cells/sq mm to 85.1 cells/sq mm. The number of Ia^+ FVIII-RAg$^+$ capillary endothelial cells increased 6.5-fold. The response of liver endothelial cells to IFN-γ, particularly in the central vein area, was much more marked than in the heart or kidney. After injection, the number of liver Ia^- phagocytic cells, most of which were in the central vein area, decreased, whereas the number of Ia^+ phagocytic cells increased, which indicates an in situ activation of Kupffer cells. Administration of a single bolus of 300 mg/kg methylprednisolone with 10^5 U/kg of IFN-γ completely abolished the effects of IFN-γ on endothelial cells and DC in all three organs. A single bolus of methylprednisolone by itself was inefficient, although repeated small doses were highly efficient. The baseline expression of class II on the capillary endothelial cells and the density of tissue DC were decreased in rat heart and kidney to a dose range of 1–3 mg/kg/day. In the liver, baseline class II expression of capillary endothelial cells was almost abolished at a dose of 1 mg/kg/day.

These results indicate that the level of class II antigen expression in rat organs are unstable. It may be modulated by exogenous administration of drugs. Steroids and rIFN-γ had antagonistic effects on class II antigen presentation.

▶ Häyry's group in Helsinki has undertaken systematic studies of antigen expression in various cells in organ allografts and on the regulation of this expression. These studies reaffirm the potent role of gamma interferon in the enhancement of the expression of class II antigen by endothelial cells and make the important observation that steroids, in doses well within the therapeutic range for humans, completely abolish the stimulus to increased expression and actually lower baseline expression of class II antigens in organ allografts. These are important and necessary basic studies as further explorations of the graft and possible modification of its antigenicity are explored.—O. Jonasson, M.D.

Ultraviolet Irradiation of Canine Dendritic Cells Prevents Mitogen-Induced Cluster Formation and Lymphocyte Proliferation

Joseph Aprile and H. Joachim Deeg (Fred Hutchinson Cancer Research Ctr. and Univ. of Washington)

Transplantation 42:653–660, December 1986   8–6

Work in rodents has implicated dendritic cells (DC) in the process of antigen presentation and T cell activation. In this study dendritic cells in peripheral blood were identified in the dog on the basis of properties that were originally described in rodents. The authors have assessed these properties in canine DC.

Cells of low-buoyant density that were rosette negative, plastic nonadherent, Ia positive, nonspecific esterase negative and nonphagocytic were obtained. These cells had large irregular nuclei, multiple spherical mitochondria, and elongated cytoplasmic projections, and did not contain phagosomes. They had the characteristics of rodent DC. The dendritic cells reconstituted the proliferative response to lectin (Con-A) and $NaIO_4$ of accessory cell-depleted lymphocytes. The proliferative response consisted of a clustering of lymphocytes around DC, followed at 48 to 72 hours by lymphocyte blastogenesis and at 72 to 96 hours by lymphocyte proliferation. Ultraviolet (UV) irradiation of the DC prevented this response.

A direct interaction of DC and lymphocytes is involved in T cell activation and proliferation. This process is sensitive to UV irradiation of the DC.

▶ Reduction of antigenicity of the grafted tissue by removing or inactivating antigen presenting cells in the graft is also an attractive means of ensuring specific acceptance of grafted tissue. Especially in combination with minimal immunosuppression, this technique has been successfully applied in a number of experiments. In this study, antigen-presenting dendritic cells have been identified and studied in the dog and have been shown to be necessary for activation and lymphocyte blastogenesis in the recipient. Ultraviolet irradiation inhibited this effect.

Further work in modification of the graft, especially the grafts of cells and tissues rather than whole vascularized organs, seems worthwhile.—O. Jonasson, M.D.

Assessment of Multi-Organ System Engraftment by Genotypic Typing Using Restriction Fragment-Length Polymorphisms and by Phenotypic Typing Using a Microcytotoxicity Assay

Bruce R. Blazar, Christine C.B. Soderling, and Daniel A. Vallera (Univ. of Minnesota and Inst. of Human Genetics, Minneapolis)

J. Immunol. 137:3338–3346, Nov. 15, 1986   8–7

In this study Southern blotting was used to assess the engraftment status of recipients of murine marrow grafts. A probe that distinguishes the two strains (pMK 1440) was used to probe restriction digests of DNA from cells of the recipient.

Recipients were treated with lethal doses of radiation and infused with bone marrow cells. Two weeks after transplantation, the animals were killed, and DNA was extracted from spleen, bone marrow, and thymocytes. No host cells were detected in spleen or bone marrow cells, indicating that irradiation was complete.

Southern blotting provides useful information during this early period when H-2 typing is often uninformative. Southern blotting was compared to H-2 typing at later postengraftment stages. There was good agreement between the two methods. Southern blotting could also be used to detect sex mismatching between donor and recipient.

Although Southern blotting is more time-consuming and expensive than H-2 typing, it can be used to obtain information in the early postengraftment period. It is more sensitive than H-2 typing in a microcytotoxicity assay. These results indicate the superiority of the Southern blotting technique for the quantitation of donor cell engraftment.

▶ Using highly sophisticated techniques of molecular genetics, these authors were able to document the proportion of host and donor cells in a bone marrow transplant model in mice. The alternate technique, that of serologic typing for the histocompatibility markers on cells, is often difficult due to technical and antigen density problems. These problems are also often present in histocompatibility testing in human subjects. The development and application of more sophisticated but more reliable methodology for assessment of donor and recipient compatibility would be a valuable contribution.—O. Jonasson, M.D.

Kidney Function in Heart-Lung Transplant Recipients: The Effect of Low-Dosage Cyclosporine Therapy
Elaine M. Imoto, Allan R. Glanville, John C. Baldwin, and James Theodore (Stanford Univ.)
J. Heart Transplant. 6:204–213, July–August 1987   8–8

Cyclosporine nephrotoxicity has become a major complication of heart-lung transplantation. Recent recipients have been converted from prednisone/cyclosporine immunosuppression to a triple-drug regimen consisting of steroid, azathioprine, and a lower dose of cyclosporine. Nineteen heart-lung transplant recipients who survived the operation received high doses of cyclosporine to maintain postoperative trough serum levels of 150–300 ng/ml, and later levels of 100–150 ng/ml. Eleven of these patients later converted to lower doses of cyclosporine, maintaining trough serum levels of 75–100 ng/ml. The dose of azathioprine was 1– 1.5 mg/kg of body weight, maintaining the white blood cell count at $5 \times 10^3/\mu l$ or greater.

Low-dose cyclosporine recipients had lower creatinine levels and higher creatinine clearance values in the early postoperative period (table). Renal function also was improved in the outpatient period, in

Comparison of the Early Postoperative and Outpatient Creatinine Levels, Creatinine Clearance, and Cyclosporine Levels in Long-Term Heart-Lung Transplant Survivors Treated With High- or Low-Dosage Cyclosporine

	High-dosage cyclosporine			Low-dosage cyclosporine			
	Mean	SE	N	Mean	SE	N	p^*
After operation							
Creatinine levels†	1.84	0.14	19	0.96	0.82	8	<0.001
Creatinine clearance‡	46.33	3.79	19	62.47	4.64	8	<0.026
Cyclosporine levels§	337.96	25.08	19	204.30	13.27	8	<0.001
Outpatient							
Creatinine levels†	1.88	0.13	19	1.05	0.10	8	<0.001
Creatinine clearance‡	52.64	6.56	18	67.05	7.53	5	0.052
Cyclosporine levels§	221.92	25.29	19	106.60	9.80	8	<0.001

*P Value for the Mann-Whitney U statistic.
†Serum creatinine in milligrams per deciliter.
‡Twenty-four-hour creatinine clearance in milliliters per minute.
§Trough serum cyclosporine level in nanograms per milliliter, measured by radioimmunoassay.
(Courtesy of Imoto, E.M., et al.: J. Heart Transplant. 6:204–213, July–August 1987.)

contrast to the high-dose recipients. Two low-dose recipients had significant improvement in creatinine clearance.

Low-dose cyclosporine eliminates wide fluctuations in renal function following heart-lung transplantation. Irreversible interstitial fibrosis may be avoided in this way. Triple-drug immunosuppression can be adequate at trough serum cyclosporine levels below 100 ng/ml. Low-dose treatment should start early in the course. Patients with chronic azotemia from long-term cyclosporine therapy also may benefit from a reduction in dosage.

Modification of Experimental Nephrotoxicity With Fish Oil as the Vehicle for Cyclosporine

Lawrence Elzinga, Vicki E. Kelley, Donald C. Houghton, and William M. Bennett (Oregon Health Sci. Univ., Portland, and Brigham and Women's Hosp., Boston)
Transplantation 43:271–273, February 1987   8–9

Cyclosporine is an effective immunosuppressive drug, but acute renal dysfunction is a common complication. Increased renal eicosanoids could mediate the toxic effect of cyclosporine. Therefore, fish oil rich in eicosapentaenoic acid (EPA), an inhibitor of renal eicosanoid synthesis, was substituted for the conventional olive oil cyclosporine vehicle in male rats.

Male rats were pretreated with 1 cc of fish or olive oil for 2 weeks. Then cyclosporine, 12.5 mg/cc, was added to the vehicle, and the animals received 50 mg/kg for 2 weeks. Control animals continued to receive vehicle alone. Glomerular filtration rate was significantly reduced in the cyclosporine-in-olive-oil group, $0.28 \pm .05$ ml/minute per 100 gm, as compared to the olive oil controls, $0.70 \pm .04$. While the rate was reduced in the cyclosporine-in-fish-oil group, $0.47 \pm .07$, as compared to the fish oil controls, $0.74 \pm .04$, it was significantly higher than in the cyclosporine-in-olive-oil group. Renal cortical levels of the vasoconstrictor, thromboxane B_2, were elevated only in the cyclosporine-in-olive-oil group. There were fewer proximal tubular vacuolar changes in the cyclosporine-in-fish-oil group than in the cyclosporine-in-olive-oil group.

Use of an EPA-rich medium for the delivery of cyclosporine ameliorates cyclosporine nephrotoxicity. This is associated with lower renal cortical levels of thromboxane B_2. The mechanism of EPA activity, the optimal protocol, and its effects on immunosuppression are not yet known.

Evidence That Renal Prostaglandin and Thromboxane Production Is Stimulated in Chronic Cyclosporine Nephrotoxicity
Thomas M. Coffman, David R. Carr, William E. Yarger, and Paul E. Klotman (Duke Univ. and Durham VA Med. Ctr.)
Transplantation 43:282–285, February 1987   8–10

Cyclosporin A (CsA) is a potent immunosuppressive agent, but its use is associated with nephrotoxicity. It has been suggested that CsA has direct effects on the metabolism of arachidonic acid (AA). The authors have examined the effects of CsA toxicity on the production of AA metabolites by the kidney.

Male ACI rats were anesthetized, and their right kidney was removed. The left kidney was denervated and the renal artery was clamped for 30 minutes to simulate ischemia. These rats were then given CsA, 50 mg/kg/day, for 12 to 14 days.

Pretreatment of these postischemic, denervated rats with CsA resulted in significant nephrotoxicity with marked decreases in both glomerular filtration rate and renal blood flow, as compared to rats that did not receive CsA. Rats that were treated with CsA had increased renal production of thromboxane B_2 (TXB_2), prostaglandin E_2 and 6-keto prostaglandin $F_{1\alpha}$ (6-keto $PGF_{1\alpha}$).

Arachidonic acid stimulated greater production of renal eicosanoid in the animals that were treated with CsA. Increased urinary excretion of TXB_2, 2,3-dinorTXB_2 and 6-keto-$PGF_{1\alpha}$ occurred in rats with CsA nephrotoxicity, compared to control rats.

Thus CsA nephrotoxicity is associated with alterations in AA metabolism in the kidney. These data suggest that inhibition of vasoconstrictor products of metabolism of AA may alleviate the toxic effects of CsA.

Who Should Be Converted From Cyclosporine to Conventional Immunosuppression in Kidney Transplantation, and Why
D.J. Versluis, G.J. Wenting, F.H.M. Derkx, M.A.D.H. Schalekamp, J. Jeekel, and W. Weimar (Univ. of Rotterdam, the Netherlands)
Transplantation 44:387–389, September 1987   8–11

Cyclosporine may cause reversible and, with longer exposure, persistent nephropathy; but early conversion to conventional immunosuppres-

128 / Surgery

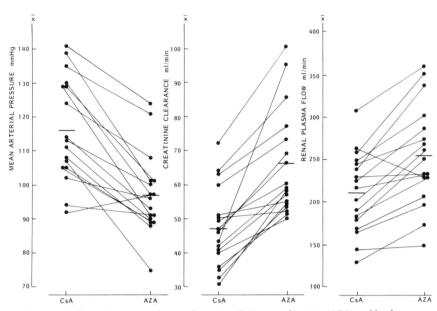

Fig 8–1.—Effect of conversion from cyclosporine *(CsA)* to azathioprine *(AZA)* on blood pressure, creatinine clearance, and effective renal plasma flow at 3 months after conversion. (Courtesy of Versluis, D.J., et al.: Transplantation 44:387–389, September 1987.)

sion may lead to irreversible rejection of a renal allograft. Twenty-three cadaver kidney recipients participated in a conversion study. Cyclosporine and prednisone were given from the day of transplantation, the former to produce trough plasma levels of 50–150 ng/ml. The patients were electively converted to azathioprine a year after transplantation, when renal function was stable. No rejection had occurred in the previous 6 months. The dose of azathioprine was 2 mg/kg.

Five patients had biopsy-proved rejection within 6 weeks of conversion; four were recipients of a second allograft. Two patients lost their grafts from rejection. Four of seven patients given a second allograft rejected it at the time of conversion. Creatinine clearance increased after conversion, as did the renal plasma flow (Fig 8–1). Blood pressure (BP) declined; and plasma renin activity increased significantly.

Recipients of a second renal allograft are especially at risk of graft rejection when converted from cyclosporine to azathioprine. Maintenance of cyclosporine for a year does not provide for safer overall engraftment. Renal dysfunction and hypertension are reversible even after late conversion.

▶ Although it has been the availability of cyclosporine that has made heart and heart-lung transplantation a successful form of therapy, the nephrotoxicity of cyclosporine has proven to be of serious consequence in these extrarenal transplant recipients. Studies in the past from Stanford have shown clear-cut evidence of progressive and long lasting renal dysfunction, with documented progression to renal failure in a number of patients and with hypertension in nearly all. Imoto's report (Abstract 8–8) attempts to achieve the best immuno-suppressive results available with cyclosporine and also to avoid the nephrotox-icity, by reducing the dose and supplementing the immunosuppression with conventional (azathioprine-prednisone) types of drugs. The long-term follow-up in these heart-lung transplant recipients does seem to clearly indicate perma-nent and irreversible structural changes due to cyclosporine in long-term recip-ients, and the recommendations of this paper for dose reduction are worthy of serious consideration.

The mechanism of cyclosporine nephrotoxicity is as yet unknown. However, it appears to be related to renal vasoconstriction and decreased renal perfusion. In Elzinga's article (Abstract 8–9), this concept is further investigated, compar-ing a standard olive oil medium for dissolving the lipid soluble cyclosporine with a fish oil medium that is known to inhibit cyclooxygenase metabolites. When the levels of the vasoconstrictor thromboxane B_2 can be depressed with the use of this fish oil vehicle, renal plasma flow is maintained and glomerular filtra-tion rate is less severely depressed than in rats receiving cyclosporine in olive oil.

In the paper by Coffman (Abstract 8–10), further investigation of renal pros-taglandin and thromboxane production is reported. Again in a rat model, in-creased renal production of thromboxane B_2 and other renal eicosanoids was documented, suggesting that cyclosporine nephrotoxicity might be attacked through inhibiting the production of these vasoconstrictor prostaglandins.

In a final paper in this series on renal nephrotoxicity of cyclosporine (Abstract 8–11), a group from the University of Rotterdam in the Netherlands has con-verted renal transplant recipients from cyclosporine to azathioprine immuno-suppression 12 or more months after transplantation and has documented that renal function improved dramatically almost immediately after conversion. While a substantial number (22%) of the patients who were converted did have a rejection, the improvement in renal physiology in the remainder was quite dramatic. However, the implication that this functional improvement is equated with absence of anatomical or permanent pathologic change in the kidney after 12 months of cyclosporine is unsubstantiated, since no histologic evidence of this was sought. In the heart and heart-lung transplant recipients reported in the previous papers, renal biopsies clearly showed structural damage, even though functional abnormalities often reverted toward normal, at least over the short term.—O. Jonasson, M.D.

Cancers Following Cyclosporine Therapy
Israel Penn (Univ. of Cincinnati and Cincinnati VA Med Ctr.)
Transplantation 43:32–35, January 1987   8–12

Any immunosuppression will lead to cancer if it is intense and long enough. Cyclosporine-related cancer was studied in a series of 2,563 or-gan transplant recipients who developed 2,740 cancers de novo following transplantation. There were 142 tumors in 141 cyclosporine-treated pa-tients.

COMPARISON OF COMMON NEOPLASMS FOLLOWING CYCLOSPORINE
AND CONVENTIONAL IMMUNOSUPPRESSION

	Conventional (2598 Tumors)*	%	Cyclosporine (142 Tumors)	%
Skin cancers	1032	40	22	15
Lymphomas	319	12	58	41
Carcinomas of cervix	151	6	3	2
Kaposi's sarcoma	85	3	11	8
CA vulva/perineum	75	3	0	0

*Occurred in 2,422 patients.
(Courtesy of Penn, I.: Transplantation 43:32–35, January 1987.)

Malignancy appeared 5 years after the start of conventional immuno-suppression, and, in contrast, 20 months after the start of cyclosporine therapy. Only eight of the latter patients were treated with cyclosporine alone. Recipients of extrarenal organs, particularly the heart, were especially at risk of cyclosporine-related tumor. Only 2% of conventionally immunosuppressed patients received extrarenal organs compared with one fourth of the cyclosporine group. Lymphoma was much more frequent in cyclosporine-treated patients than in those given conventional immunosuppression (table). Kaposi's sarcomas also were more frequent in the cyclosporine group, while conventionally treated patients more often developed skin cancers. The lymphomas occurred a relatively short time after transplantation in cyclosporine recipients. Extranodal lymphoma and CNS involvement both were more frequent in this group.

Cyclosporine may, by inhibiting signals from T cells in response to antigens, permit excessive B cell responses leading to lymphoproliferative disorders. Epstein-Barr virus is suspected of causing lymphomas in renal transplant recipients. The risk of excessive immunosuppression must be kept in mind, particularly in cyclosporine recipients, who are at particular risk of developing life-threatening tumors of internal organs.

▶ In his usual careful and concise fashion Dr. Penn has now analyzed the malignancies occurring in patients treated with cyclosporine as their major immunosuppressive drug. He has found a substantial incidence of lymphomas and Kaposi's sarcoma and a much lesser incidence of skin cancer than is found in patients given "conventional" immunosuppression with azathioprine, prednisone, and antilymphocyte serum. The lymphomas appear rapidly in cyclosporine treated patients and appear to be partly a consequence of dose. Early experience with cyclosporine was with much higher doses than are currently employed, and the incidence, as more experience is gained with proper use of this powerful immunosuppressive drug, may be less frightening. However, we have only a short experience with the use of cyclosporine, and longer periods of observation will be required before the pattern of malignancy is better understood.—O. Jonasson, M.D.

Long-Term Survival of Skin Allografts in Rats Treated With Topical Cyclosporine

Chung-Sheng Lai, Terrence A. Wesseler, J. Wesley Alexander, and George F. Babcock (Univ. of Cincinnati and Shriners Burns Inst., Cincinnati)
Transplantation 44:83–87, July 1987   8–13

Topical use of the immunosuppressive drug cyclosporine (CsA) could prove convenient and less toxic than systemic administration. Topically applied CsA was evaluated in differing regimens in a skin allograft model involving Buffalo and Lewis rats. Cyclosporine prepared in olive oil and dimethyl sulfoxide was administered topically in conjunction with the placement of 3 × 3-cm allografts. Applications of CsA, 5 or 10 mg, were made for 10, 20, or 28 days.

Allograft survival increased with the duration of topical CsA treatment when a dose of 10 mg per day was used. Rejection usually began 5–8 days after withdrawal of topically applied CsA. Long-term allograft survival was observed in rats given CsA continuously for 100 or 120 days. Even application of CsA at a site distal to the allograft prolonged graft survival. Animals given high doses had mild anemia, lymphocytopenia, and neutrophilia. Cellular infiltration of allografts was less evident in treated animals.

A short course of topically applied CsA significantly prolongs the survival of skin allografts in rats. A high local concentration of topically applied CsA may be important in prolonging graft survival. This approach is a convenient and effective one with minimal side effects. It may prove especially useful in burn-injected patients who require extensive skin grafting.

▶ This nice little experiment shows that topical cyclosporine, when applied in modest doses directly to a skin allograft, will prolong survival of that graft essentially indefinitely. Of course, the cyclosporine is readily absorbed through the skin and into the circulation and can accumulate to toxic levels, but the effect appears to be largely related to localized concentrations of the drug. Implications for treating burned patients requiring major skin allografting are immediately evident.—O. Jonasson, M.D.

A Multifactorial System for Equitable Selection of Cadaver Kidney Recipients

Thomas E. Starzl, Thomas R. Hakala, Andreas Tzakis, Robert Gordon, Andrei Stieber, Leonard Makowka, Joeta Klimoski, and Henry T. Bahnson (Univ. of Pittsburgh, and VA Med. Ctr., Pittsburgh)
JAMA 257:3073–3075, June 12, 1987   8–14

The authors developed an objective system for allocating cadaver kidneys and applied it to 270 renal transplant procedures done in 1986. Recipients were given points for waiting time, antigen matching, antibody analysis, medical urgency, and logistic practicality. Points were assigned for each antigen matched at the A, B, and DR histocompatibility loci. Preformed cytotoxic antibodies were measured.

Kidneys were given to patients with the highest point totals in 98% of cases. Sixty operations were retransplantations. A majority of kidneys were from other procurement agencies. Seven patients also received livers or hearts, six of them at the same time as the renal transplant. All patients who were passed over by the system received a kidney within a few days or weeks.

This is the first report of using a computerized point system to allocate cadaver kidneys. Whether similar selection methods can be applied to liver and heart transplantation remains to be determined. Preliminary candidate stratification for these procedures is much more restrictive than for renal transplantation.

▶ This system for kidney allocation, which has been proposed and adopted by Starzl's group in Pittsburgh, attempts to codify an objective system of recipient selection in order that organ allocation be as fair as possible.

Unfortunately, the system as prescribed by Dr. Starzl, while objective, de-emphasizes certain priorities that are likely to improve outcome of organ transplantation and therefore cannot be ignored. These include relevant HLA antigen matching and prior immunologic history. Emphasis of length of time on the waiting list should be dismissed from these criteria, in my opinion, because of the frequent manipulation of this statistic in the pretransplant period and the failure to correlate length of time on the waiting list with outcome.

Nonetheless, Dr. Starzl's system is a major improvement over the usual non-structured methods of choosing the recipients, especially for kidney transplants, and his group is to be congratulated on the development and implementation of a system that works for them.—O. Jonasson, M.D.

Kidney Transplantation From Anencephalic Donors
Wolfgang Holzgreve, Fritz K. Beller, Bernd Buchholz, Manfred Hansmann, and Kurt Köhler (Westf. Wilhelms Univ., Münster, and Univ. of Bonn, West Germany)
N. Engl. J. Med. 316:1069–1070, April 23, 1987   8–15

The authors have successfully carried out three kidney transplantations from two anencephalic fetuses, with follow-up exceeding 1½ and 2½ years, respectively. Both kidneys of an anencephalic fetus of 38 weeks' gestation were used, each in a child undergoing long-term hemodialysis. Both transplants functioned without complication. The second case involved a twin pregnancy with one healthy and one anencephalic fetus delivered at 36 weeks' gestation. The kidneys of the anencephalic fetus were transplanted to an adult patient, who remained well with standard immunosuppression therapy.

Brain development is absent in the anencephalic fetus, allowing termination of gestation at any time. The affected fetus cannot survive for longer than a few weeks. The parents may well feel relieved at the prospect of kidney donation. The use of organs from an anencephalic child requires respect for the fetal donor and a concern for the parents' psychologic situation.

▶ The anencephalic infant as an organ donor has recently become a controversial issue. The question that is debated has to do with the definition of brain death, a diagnosis difficult to make in infancy in any case, and a concept difficult to apply to this severe congenital anomaly. These infants are "brain-absent," neither "brain-alive" nor "brain-dead." Since these infants have been considered potential sources of heart donors for neonatal cardiac transplant now being performed for the hypoplastic left heart syndrome, it is important to educate the professional and the lay public to the acceptability of the diagnosis of "brain-absent" in these unfortunate infants with only a brief life expectancy on life support systems.—O. Jonasson, M.D.

▶ ↓ The following three papers (Abstracts 8–16 to 8–18) address histocompatibility testing and donor recipient matching in cadaver renal transplantation.—O. Jonasson, M.D.

The Effect of First Cadaver Renal Transplant HLA-A, B Match on Sensitization Levels and Retransplant Rates Following Graft Failure
Fred Sanfilippo, Nancy Goeken, Gary Niblack, Juan Scornik, and William K. Vaughn (Duke Univ., Univ. of Iowa, and Iowa City VA Med. Ctrs., Vanderbilt Univ. and Nashville VA Med. Ctrs., and Univ. of Florida)
Transplantation 43:240–244, February 1987   8–16

Patients with renal graft failure tend to be more sensitized by exposure to an allogeneic graft and consequently have to wait longer for a cadaver kidney. Data were reviewed on 449 first cadaver renal allograft recipients, who underwent transplantation at four centers in 1978–1982 and developed graft failure by 1985. Of 383 evaluable patients, 182 were placed on an active waiting list for retransplantation.

Poorly HLA-matched patients had shorter first-transplant survival times and a greater rise in panel-reactive antibody levels after graft failure compared with better-matched patients. Patients with lower peak

INFLUENCE OF 1 DEGREE CADAVER RENAL TRANSPLANT HLA-A,
-B MATCH ON REGRAFT RATES

HLA-A, B match	Regraft rate	
	All patients (n=182)	White patients (n=121)
0, 1	36/72 (50.0%)*	22/39 (56.4%)†
2–4	77/110 (70.0%)*	61/82 (74.4%)†

*Significance of difference, P < .01.
†Significance of difference, P = .05.
(Courtesy of Sanfilippo, F., et al.: Transplantation 43:240–244, February 1987.)

antibody levels tended to receive regrafts more frequently. Patients with a good first-transplant HLA-A, -B match were retransplanted significantly more often than those with a poor match (table). The relative risk of not being regrafted for patients with a poor initial HLA match was 1.69.

Poor HLA matching at primary cadaver kidney transplantation relates to increased sensitization following graft failure. Among patients placed on a waiting list for regrafting, those previously well matched are regrafted more often than those with poor initial matching. The effect of cyclosporine on the degree of sensitization after graft failure in relation to HLA match remains to be determined.

Substantial Benefits of Tissue Matching in Renal Transplantation
Walter R. Gilks, Benjamin A. Bradley, Sheila M. Gore, and Peter T. Klouda for the Users of the UK Transplant Service (Cambridge and Bristol, England)
Transplantation 43:669–674, May 1987   8–17

Many reports have claimed benefits from tissue matching in renal transplantation, but there is little solid statistical support for such benefit. The authors analyzed 2,282 first cadaver kidney transplants to determine the influence of tissue matching on graft survival. Data were analyzed by the stratified piecewise proportional hazards regression method.

Substantially improved graft survival was associated with DR compatibility and, at most, one A or B mismatch. Lesser degrees of tissue matching, however, conferred little apparent advantage. Few graft recipients have benefited substantially from tissue matching as yet, partly because of unsolved technical problems in DR typing.

Tissue matching improves the outcome of renal transplantation, whether or not cyclosporine is used for immunosuppression. Comparable benefit has been demonstrated in North America and Europe.

It is estimated that, with a pool of 3,000 patients awaiting transplantation, considerable improvement in graft survival can be expected in more than half the recipients. Exchange of kidneys on a regional, rather than a national, basis in the United Kingdom would unduly limit the opportunity to obtain beneficial matching.

The Effect of Zero HLA Class I and II Mismatching in Cyclosporine-Treated Kidney Transplant Patients
James Cicciarelli, Paul I. Terasaki, and M. Ray Mickey (Univ. of California, Los Angeles)
Transplantation 43:636–640, May 1987   8–18

Tissue matching appears to enhance the results of cadaver kidney transplantation, even in cyclosporine-treated patients. The value of tissue matching was assessed by estimating graft survival in more than 15,000 renal graft recipients, more than 3,500 of whom received cyclosporine.

PERCENTAGE OF PROBABILITY OF OBTAINING ZERO-MISMATCH RECIPIENTS
FOR A RANDOM DONOR*

HLA system	Recipient pool size							
	100	200	400	800	1500	3000	6000	10,000
A, B, DR	1.5	2.5	3.9	6.0	8.5	12	16	19
B, DR	6.2	10	15	22	29	38	48	54
DR†	60	76	89	95	98	99	99.7	99.9

*Effective pool size (ABO matching, patient availability, etc.) was assumed to be 30% of nominal pool size.
†Calculation based on gene frequency estimates for white populations.
(Courtesy of Cicciarelli, J., et al.: Transplantation 43:636–640, May 1987.)

Mismatching had a definite effect if HLA-A, -B, or -DR loci alone were taken into account. When the DR locus was combined with the A or B locus, markedly improved results were obtained by matching. The difference between the best and worst matches for A, B, and DR matching was 17%. If only one antigen was mismatched, graft survival declined markedly compared with zero mismatching for class I and class II antigens. When zero mismatching was combined with cyclosporine, 88% graft survival was achieved. Cyclosporine improved graft survival except in zero A, B, DR mismatch cases. Cyclosporine improved graft survival 10%–14% for all categories of mismatched patients; DR matching is possible with relatively small recipient pool sizes (table).

In renal transplantation, HLA matching remains very important, even with the use of cyclosporine for immunosuppression. The good graft survival rates obtained with zero mismatching of class I and class II antigens suggest that kidney sharing and large recipient pool sizes are a reasonable approach to transplantation.

▶ There has been a widespread feeling among clinicians involved in renal transplantation that cyclosporine is sufficiently powerful as an immunosuppressive drug to overcome the effects of HLA mismatching, and therefore attempting to match donor and recipient is not only unnecessary but might compromise the excellent 1-year graft survival of approximately 75%, because of increase in cold ischemia time while transporting the kidneys to matched recipients. Because of this widespread attitude, there has been an increasing tendency toward local and regional use of kidneys procured from cadaver donors and a reluctance to participate in organ sharing programs.

Sanfilippo and his colleagues (Abstract 8–16) have studied the effect of HLA matching or lack thereof on subsequent course of patients following rejection of a first cadaver renal allograft. Although this study encompassed patients treated prior to the use of cyclosporine, their information is of considerable interest. They have shown that mismatch for each HLA-A and -B, presumed targets of the immune response, yields patients with higher levels of preformed antibody and with a significantly reduced chance for retransplantation compared to patients who have lost their first kidneys even though matched for HLA-A and -B. Poor HLA matching appeared to be correlated with increased sensitization following graft failure.

The UK Transplant Service (Abstract 8–17) analyzed over 2,000 first cadaver kidney transplantation procedures by a sophisticated statistical approach and have demonstrated a marked benefit of providing a zero mismatched A, B, and DR organ. They showed a slight benefit if one antigen was mismatched but no subsequent benefits in that poorly matched recipients were at high risk for graft loss. In their calculations, a recipient pool size of 5,000 would provide a zero antigen mismatched donor for approximately 30% of the recipients and convey a highly significant survival advantage.

Terasaki's group (Abstract 8–18) analyzed 15,000 transplants with 3,500 patients receiving cyclosporine. These investigators emphasized that a zero mismatch provided highly significant and large survival advantages but that any mismatch was deleterious. In their calculations of pool size, a recipient pool size of 10,000 people would match 19% of recipients with a zero antigen mismatched donor and 99.9% with a DR compatible donor.

Taken together, these careful statistical studies make a powerful case for national organ sharing and the development of a large recipient pool size.—O. Jonasson, M.D.

Phenotypic Composition and In Vitro Functional Capacities of Unmodified Fresh Cells Infiltrating Acutely Rejected Human Kidney Allografts
Bernard M. Charpentier, Marie-Anne Bach, Philippe Lang, Bernadette Martin, and Daniel Fries (Univ. Paris-Sud; Hôpital Paul Brousse, and Inst. Pasteur, Paris)
Transplantation 44:38–43, July 1987   8–19

The cells of the immune system that destroy foreign tissues remain uncertain, although it is known that contact of alloantigen and immune cells triggers interactions among several cell populations and soluble mediators. The authors examined renal graft-infiltrating cells (GIC) in the setting of graft rupture secondary to intense acute cellular rejection. Eight patients given cadaver kidney grafts participated in the study. Cell surface markers of isolated GIC were examined, and functional in vitro assays were carried out.

The mononuclear cells infiltrating the grafts were 80%–90% lymphocytes and 15%–20% monocytes, with very few polymorphs present. No stimulatory hyporesponsive state was evident, in contrast to patients having good graft tolerance. Three of five patients had lymphocytotoxins in their renal eluates. Some of the patients with lymphocytotoxins had unexpectedly high serum antibody levels. Studies of unmodified GIC indicated that OKT8[+] cells predominated.

T cells, especially OKT8[+] cells, are important in this type of acute irreversible renal allograft rejection. However, anti-HLA antibodies can be eluted from these grafts, despite histologic evidence of acute cellular rejection, indicating that other potential effector mechanisms of cell destruction also are present. The findings underline the complexity of transplant rejection.

▶ This group has studied the effect and mechanisms in situ in severely rejecting renal allografts. Although the model is a severe one, that is, rupture of the allograft due to acute rejection, some useful information is obtained because of the large numbers of cells present in the graft that can be retrieved for study without further enzymatic or stimulating treatment. As expected, the cells infiltrating the graft were activated T cells with cytotoxic capabilities. Also, as expected in severe acute rejection, antibody and inflammatory mediators could be detected and were probably participants.—O. Jonasson, M.D.

Prolongation of Renal Allograft Survival in Antilymphocyte-Serum– Treated Dogs by Postoperative Injection of Density-Gradient–Fractionated Donor Bone Marrow

William C. Hartner, Sally R. De Fazio, Takahashi Maki, Thomas G. Markees, Anthony P. Monaco, and James J. Gozzo (Northeastern Univ. and Deaconess Hosp., Boston)
Transplantation 42:593–597, December 1986   8–20

Previous work in mice had shown that injected fractionated donor bone marrow cells allowed prolonged survival of skin allografts; to extend this work, fractionated bone marrow injections were used in canine renal transplants. Outbred dogs were treated with rabbit or horse antilymphocyte serum (ALS) for 6 days prior to and 7 days following kidney transplantation. Two weeks after transplantation, fresh or frozen unfractionated donor bone marrow or a Percoll gradient bone marrow fraction (BM Fr3) was infused into the dogs.

Infusion of bone marrow and BM Fr3 significantly prolonged the time during which the allograft functioned (Fig 8–2). The BM Fr3 was significantly more effective than whole bone marrow. Frozen bone marrow

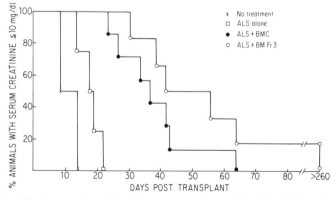

Fig 8–2.—The duration of survival with a serum creatinine ≤ 10 mg/dl in kidney allografted dogs. Daily ALS treatment was from day −6 through day +7 relative to kidney allografting on day 0. Unfractionated bone marrow *(BMC)* at $3–10\times10^{7}$ viable cells/kg, or fraction 3 bone marrow *(BM Fr3)* at $2–4\cdot10^{7}$ viable cells/kg was administered at days +13 or +14. The number of dogs was: 2 with no treatment, 4 with ALS and BMC, and 5 with ALS and BM Fr3. (Courtesy of Hartner, W.C., et al.: Transplantation 42:593–597, December 1986.)

was as effective as fresh bone marrow. Reduced lymphocyte responses to donor cells, third party cells, Con A, PHA, and pokeweed mitogens suggested that the animals were immunosuppressed. By 60 days after the transplant, normal responsiveness had returned to the mitogens and the third-party cells, but not to donor cells.

Therefore, treatment of recipient dogs with ALS and fresh or frozen fractionated bone marrow prolongs the function of kidney allografts by inducing specific long-lasting immunosuppression. This may have useful applications in human transplantation.

▶ Monaco's group have extended their exciting observations of "tolerance" induction in mice with antilymphocyte serum and donor bone marrow pretreatment into a large animal species, the dog. In these outbred animals, kidney allografts were accepted with what appeared to be reconstitution in all other respects. Further work in large animal species must precede clinical trials of this treatment modality, but the promise of inducing specific tolerance is most encouraging.—O. Jonasson, M.D.

Renal Transplant Patients Treated With Total Lymphoid Irradiation Show Specific Unresponsiveness to Donor Antigens in the Mixed Leukocyte Reaction (MLR)

Danny Chow, Vivian Saper, and Samuel Strober (Stanford Univ.)
J. Immunol. 138:3746–3750, June 1, 1987   8–21

Total lymphoid irradiation (TLI) reduces peripheral blood mononuclear cell proliferation in renal transplant recipients, but the mixed leukocyte reaction (MLR) subsequently recovers. Nine transplant recipients prepared with TLI were followed up after transplantation with stable graft function for at least 18 months. The MLR to normal allogeneic stimulator cells recovered substantially in all patients. Fresh posttransplant blood mononuclear cells were used as responder cells in the MLR against frozen donor or third-party stimulator cells to identify specific unresponsiveness to donor antigens. The only immunosuppressive agents were rabbit antithymocyte globulin and low dose prednisone. There was no more than one rejection episode.

Seven of the nine patients failed to respond significantly above background levels to donor cells but did respond adequately to third-party cells. Preliminary efforts to identify antigen-specific suppressor cells were unsuccessful. The background response of posttransplant responder cells was about half that of pre-TLI cells.

Specific immune tolerance of allogeneic organ grafts is associated with specific unresponsiveness to donor cells in the MLR. The present patients who were unresponsive to donor cells continued to undergo limited immunosuppressive therapy, so that it is not clear whether they are truly tolerant of their grafts.

▶ Strober's group at Stanford has continued to evaluate the utility of total lymphoid irradiation (TLI) as a means of inducing specific immunologic tolerance of an organ allograft in humans. In this study of nine patients more than 18 months posttransplant with stable good renal function on low dose prednisone maintenance immunosuppression, immune competency toward other third-party cells had become reestablished as measured in the MLR. Seven of these nine, however, demonstrated no reactions to donor cells in culture, indicating a degree of specific donor tolerance.

Although TLI is an expensive and cumbersome method of pretreatment and causes considerable morbidity in the proposed recipients, an outcome of specific immunologic tolerance to an organ allograft with no need of immunosuppressive maintenance drug therapy would be highly desirable and worth the initial investment.—O. Jonasson, M.D.

Use of Cytomegalovirus Immune Globulin to Prevent Cytomegalovirus Disease in Renal-Transplant Recipients

David R. Snydman, Barbara G. Werner, Beverly Heinze-Lacey, Victor P. Berardi, Nicholas L. Tilney, Robert L. Kirkman, Edgar L. Milford, Sang I. Cho, Harry L. Bush, Jr., Andrew S. Levey, Terry B. Strom, Charles B. Carpenter, Raphael H. Levey, William E. Harmon, Clarence E. Zimmerman II, Michael E. Shapiro, Theodore Steinman, Frank LoGerfo, Beldon Idelson, Gerhard P.J. Schröter, Myron J. Levin, James McIver, Jeanne Leszczynski, and George F. Grady (New England Med. Ctr., Brigham and Women's Hosp., Children's Hosp., Beth Israel Hosp., University Hosp., and VA Hosp., Boston; University Hosp., Denver, and other participating institutions)

N. Engl. J. Med. 317:1049–1054, Oct. 22, 1987   8–22

Cytomegalovirus (CMV) is the main viral pathogen in renal transplant recipients. Cytomegalovirus-seronegative recipients of transplants from CMV-seropositive donors are at high risk for serious CMV disease. The authors carried out a multi-institutional, randomized, controlled trial to investigate the use of a CMV hyperimmune globulin modified for intravenous administration to prevent primary CMV disease.

Fifty-nine CMV-seronegative recipients of kidneys from donors with antibodies against CMV were assigned to receive intravenously CMV immune globulin or no treatment. The immune globulin was given in doses of 150 mg/kg of body weight within 72 hours of transplantation, then 100 mg/kg 2 and 4 weeks after transplantation, followed by 50 mg/kg given at 6, 8, 12, and 16 weeks postoperatively. The incidence of virologically confirmed CMV-associated syndromes was 60% in control subjects and 21% in immune globulin recipients (table). Fungal or parasitic superinfections occurred in 20% of control subjects and in none of the immune globulin recipients. Rates of graft loss and mortality did not significantly differ between the two groups. One globulin recipient died of CMV pneumonia complicated by pseudomonas sepsis. Immune globulin had no effect on overall viral isolation or seroconversion rates. In patients who received therapy for graft rejection, immune globulin reduced the attack rate of serious CMV disease from 54% to 15%. Of the 205 immune globulin infusions, 6% were associated with possible side effects. Therapy did not need to be stopped for any of the reactions noted.

OUTCOMES IN 24 PATIENTS RECEIVING CYTOMEGALOVIRUS
(CMV) IMMUNE GLOBULIN AND 35 CONTROL PATIENTS

OUTCOME	GLOBULIN	CONTROLS
	no. (%)	
Clinical		
Virologically confirmed CMV syndrome	5 (21)	21 (60)*
Fungal or parasitic opportunistic infection	0	7 (20)†
Death	1 (4)	5 (14)
Graft loss	4 (17)	10 (29)
Virologic		
CMV viremia	6 (25)	15 (43)
Viral isolation (any site)	13 (54)	20 (57)
Seroconversion	17 (71)	27 (77)

*$X^2 = 8.86; P < .01.$
†Fisher's exact test, $P = .05.$
(Courtesy of Snydman, D.R., et al.: N. Engl. J. Med. 317:1049–1054, Oct. 22, 1987.)

These data indicate that prophylactic use of CMV immune globulin provides substantial protection for the renal transplant recipient at risk for primary CMV disease. Cytomegalovirus-seronegative candidates receiving kidneys from CMV-seropositive donors should be considered for globulin prophylaxis.

▶ In these studies high titer antibody to cytomegalovirus was used to confer passive immunity to CMV infection in the immunosuppressed renal transplant recipient. This strategy implies that donors as well as recipients are tested for CMV antibody as an indicator of latent CMV infection. The results were striking in that morbidity was substantially reduced in the patients receiving the antibody treatment. Although plasma infusions carry some risk of disease transmission, most notably HIV infection, the price paid for a primary CMV infection in a transplant recipient is very high, and this therapy seems justified. In fact, it seems to be a major advance.—O. Jonasson, M.D.

Opportunistic Strongyloidiasis in Renal Transplant Recipients
James S. Morgan, William Schaffner, and William J. Stone (Vanderbilt Univ. and VA Med. Ctr., Nashville)
Transplantation 42:518–524, November 1986   8–23

Strongyloides stercoralis is an intestinal nematode of man distributed worldwide. It may persist for decades in the normal host as a chronic subclinical infection (Fig 8–3) but become life-threatening in the immunocompromised state. Hyperinfection is an augmentation of the normal life cycle seen in heavily infected or compromised hosts.

Of a total of 41 episodes of documented infection with *S. stercoralis* reported in 29 renal transplant recipients, in more than half the cases its evidence was present prior to transplantation. In 11 patients, eosino-

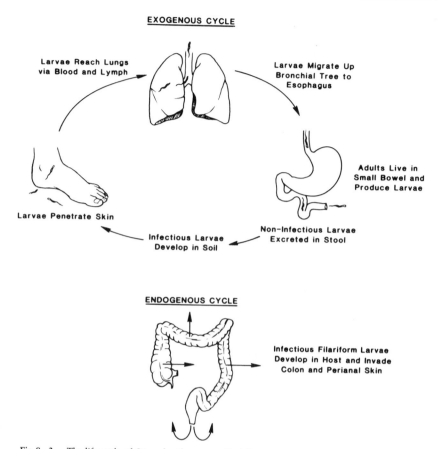

EXOGENOUS CYCLE

Larvae Reach Lungs via Blood and Lymph

Larvae Migrate Up Bronchial Tree to Esophagus

Larvae Penetrate Skin

Adults Live in Small Bowel and Produce Larvae

Infectious Larvae Develop in Soil

Non-Infectious Larvae Excreted in Stool

ENDOGENOUS CYCLE

Infectious Filariform Larvae Develop in Host and Invade Colon and Perianal Skin

Fig 8–3.—The life cycle of *Stronglyoides stercoralis*. The exogenous cycle is characterized by rhabditiform larvae from human stool being transformed into invasive filariform larvae through an external phase. Man is then infected through cutaneous contact with soil. The endogenous cycle results from filariform larvae forming within or on the human host and invading the intestine or skin immediately *(autoinfection)*. (Courtesy of Morgan, J.S., et al.: Transplantation 42:518–524, November 1986.)

philia, 5%–53%, was noted in the peripheral blood. Three had strongyloidiasis documented prior to transplantation. Clinical symptoms were often misleading. Fever was the initial symptom complex in 17 patients. Among other initial presentations were GI complaints, pulmonary symptoms, and bacteremia.

In all cases primary treatment was thiabendazole. When thiabendazole was ineffective other antihelminthic agents were usually also unable to eradicate worm burdens. Of the 29 patients, 15 died.

In renal transplant recipients, opportunistic infection with *S. stercoralis* is a potentially preventable cause of disease and death. In diagnosing the pulmonary phase of strongyloidiasis, the value of sputum cytology may have a broader application than currently recognized.

It is recommended that all renal transplant candidates submit at least four stools for ova and parasite examination. Until larvae have been absent from screening specimens for 6 months, monthly treatment of 25 mg/kg thiabendazole, twice daily for 2 days, is recommended.

▶ This is a good review of an infrequently recognized complication of immunosuppression following organ transplantation. The recommendations for screening and for treatment of high risk populations are very useful.—O. Jonasson, M.D.

Effect of Antiidiotypic Antibodies to HLA on Graft Survival in Renal Allograft Recipients
Elaine Reed, Mark Hardy, Alan Benvenisty, Conrad Lattes, Jeffrey Brensilver, Robert McCabe, Keith Reemstma, Donald W. King, and Nicole Suciu-Foca (Columbia Univ., St. Luke's Roosevelt Hosp. Med. Ctr., New York, and Univ. of Chicago)
N. Engl. J. Med. 316:1450–1455, June 4, 1987   8–24

Survival of renal transplants in presensitized patients may be explained by acquisition of an antiantibody, or anti-idiotypic antibody (Ab2), which reacts with determinants in the binding site of anti-HLA antibody (Ab1), thereby suppressing the proliferation of Ab1-producing B cells. The possible influence of anti-idiotypic antibody was studied in 20 recipients with a history of presensitization to donor HLA antigens.

Sera taken at the time of transplantation contained no antibodies against donor class I or class II antigens. Sera from nine patients blocked donor-specific anti-HLA antibody in historic positive samples. Samples from nine other patients potentiated cytotoxic activity. Potentiating antibody was strongly associated with irreversible rejection, and blocking antibody with graft survival (table).

Presensitized patients with Ab1-potentiating antibody are likely to have early renal allograft rejection, while those with Ab2 can be expected to tolerate the graft. Anti-idiotypic antibody to HLA also may explain the beneficial effect of transfusions, as well as maternal tolerance of an allogeneic conceptus. Studies of anti-idiotypic autoimmunity may provide

ALLOGRAFT SURVIVAL IN PATIENTS WITH ANTIBODIES THAT
BLOCK OR THAT POTENTIATE THE CYTOTOXIC ACTIVITY OF
ANTIDONOR HLA ANTIBODIES

ALLOGRAFT SURVIVAL	BLOCKING ANTIBODIES		POTENTIATING ANTIBODIES	
	PRESENT	ABSENT	PRESENT	ABSENT
Less than 1 mo	0	10	9	1
More than 1 yr	9	1	0	10
Total	9*	11*	9†	11†

*$P < .001$ by Fisher's exact method.
†$P < .001$ by Fisher's exact method.
(Courtesy of Reed, E., et al.: N. Engl. J. Med. 316:1450–1455, June 4, 1987.)

a basis for deciding whether a patient can receive a second graft that shares HLA antigens with a previous transplant.

Antiidiotypic Antibodies to Human Major Histocompatibility Complex Class I and II Antibodies in Hepatic Transplantation and Their Role in Allograft Survival
T. Mohanakumar, C. Rhodes, G. Mendez-Picon, M. Wayne Flye, and H.M. Lee (Med. College of Virginia, Richmond, and Washington Univ., St. Louis)
Transplantation 44:54–58, July 1987   8–25

The immune response to HLA antigens is subject to idiotype network regulation, and the final state of responsiveness may reflect a balance of idiotypic and anti-idiotypic components. Antibodies to anti-HLA class I and II antigens now have been found in liver allograft recipients with functioning grafts. The role of anti-idiotypic antibodies to anti-MHC was studied in ten liver-graft recipients, for whom serial serum samples were obtained before and after transplantation.

Seven patients developed strong specific anti-anti-HLA activity, and all of them have maintained well-functioning allografts. The inhibitory activities of posttransplant sera were cyclical. Neither pretransplant sera nor normal human AB sera exhibited inhibitory activity. The inhibitory antibodies were monospecific, but some recipients with inhibitory antibodies appeared to cross-react with major cross-reactive groups.

Active removal of antibodies followed by suppression of the immune response to major histocompatibility (MHC) antigens may have a role in tolerance of liver allografts. The present experience suggests that development of anti-MHC blocking activity is critical for the continued tolerance of such allografts. Anti-idiotypic antibodies to anti-MHC may alter some T cell functions in the recipient, therefore benefiting the graft.

▶ These two articles (Abstracts 8–24 and 8–25) describe the development of antibodies to preformed antibody, or "anti-idiotypic antibodies," in presensitized patients. Such antibodies are believed to be major components of the network theory of regulation of the immune response. These anti-idiotypic antibodies block the action of the cytotoxic antibodies and perhaps suppress the proliferation of cytotoxic antibody producing B cells. In the paper from Suciu-Foca's group (Abstract 8–24), patients with a previously positive cytotoxic antibody toward donor cells who were found to have a negative cross-match at the time of transplantation received a cadaver renal allograft. Half of these patients had a successful graft, and half failed. Of those failing, no anti-idiotypic antibody was found, whereas those with successful grafts had this blocking antibody. Similarly in the paper by Mohanakumar's group (Abstract 8–25), anti-idiotypic antibodies were found and were associated with long-term success in liver allografts.

Tolerance of the allografts even in the presence of sensitization is a very interesting observation and worthy of further investigation. Why grafts succeed, in contrast to the question of why grafts fail, may eventually prove to the most interesting aspect of investigation.—O. Jonasson, M.D.

Evidence for an Immune Response to HLA Class I Antigens in the Vanishing-Bileduct Syndrome After Liver Transplantation
P.T. Donaldson, J. O'Grady, B. Portmann, H. Davis, G.J.M. Alexander, J. Neuberger, M. Thick, R.Y. Calne, and Roger Williams (King's College, London, and Addenbrooke's Hosp., Cambridge, England)
Lancet 1:945–948, April 25, 1987   8–26

The relation between HLA class I and II antigen matching and rejection with particular reference to the vanishing bile duct (VBD) syndrome, a type of chronic rejection accurately definable on both histologic and clinical criteria, was investigated in 62 patients who had survived liver transplantation from 3 to 109 months. Sera were also treated for the presence of lymphocytotoxic antibodies to donor HLA antigens developing subsequent to liver transplantation. The patients were classified into three groups: (1) those with normal graft function, 42 patients; (2) those with chronic graft rejection (VBD syndrome), 14 patients, with clinical and biochemical evidence of severe progressive cholestasis; and (3) those with chronic graft malfunction unrelated to VBD syndrome, 6 patients.

Complete mismatch for class I antigens was present more often in patients with VBD than in other groups ($P < .025$), and complete mismatch for class II antigens was significantly less frequent ($P < .02$). The combination of a complete mismatch for class I antigens with a partial/complete match for class II antigens was significantly associated with the VBD syndrome. Of 7 patients with this pattern, 6 had progressed to the

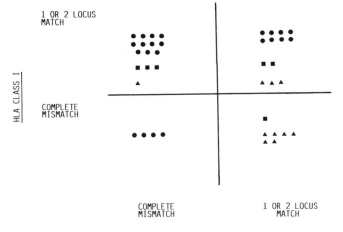

Fig 8–4.—Relation of graft matching to development of VBD syndrome. ●, normal graft function; ■, chronic graft malfunction unrelated to VBD syndrome; ▲, VBD syndrome. (Courtesy of Donaldson, P.T., et al.: Lancet 1:945–948, April 25, 1987.)

VBD syndrome in comparison with only 4 of the remaining 32 ($P <$ .0005) or to 1 of 15 with the opposite combination, i.e., a complete mismatch for class II antigens and a partial or complete match for class I antigens ($P < .005$; Fig 8–4).

Lymphocytotoxic antibodies were detected in 22 (35%) of all patients: in 8 of 14 (57%) of those with VBD syndrome; and in 14 of 48 (29%) of those without the syndrome. The antibodies proved reactive with either class I determinants or non-HLA determinants except for one case, where an antibody reacting with donor-specific HLA class II antigen was identified.

The findings of this study contrast with early clinical studies where neither HLA status nor lymphocytotoxic antibodies were found to relate to rejection, most likely because chronic rejection has now been more clearly defined. Finding a correlation between the occurrence of VBD syndrome and a complete donor-recipient mismatch for HLA class I antigens supports the hypothesis that these antigens are the target of a host immune response consistent with the known pathology of this syndrome, where the predominant damage is to bile duct epithelium. The finding of a close correlation between a partial or complete donor–recipient class II match and the development of the VBD syndrome was unexpected.

▶ It is interesting that the manifestation of chronic rejection in liver allografts is often the vanishing bile duct syndrome. The bile duct epithelium is apparently the target of the rejection response in these chronic patients, and Calne's group shows in this series that incompatibility for HLA class I antigens or pre-existing cytotoxic antibodies against HLA class I were significantly associated with the late occurrence of this bile duct lesion.—O. Jonasson, M.D.

Allogeneic Hepatocyte Transplantation in the Rat Spleen Under Cyclosporine Immunosuppression

Leonard Makowka, George Lee, Christopher S. Cobourn, Emmanuel Farber, Judith A. Falk, and Rudolf E. Falk (Univ. of Toronto)
Transplantation 42:537–541, November 1986   8–27

The spleen is a favorable site for the survival and growth of single-cell suspensions of hepatocytes. Allogeneic hepatocytes were transplanted to the spleens of recipient rats and were maintained in these allogeneic hosts.

Single-cell suspensions of hepatocytes from normal male ACI-strain rats were injected into the spleen of allogeneic male Fischer rats that had had a 70% hepatectomy and had been treated with 2-acetylaminofluorene to prevent regeneration of the residual host liver. The recipients received cyclosporine (CsA), 3 mg/kg/day, after transplantation.

Histologic examination of the spleen 2 days after transplantation demonstrated an area of replacement by hepatocytes. The area of replacement had expanded by 7 days. If CsA was not administered, no hepatocytes could be detected at 7 days. If CsA was withdrawn, the hepatocytes were rejected.

Allogeneic hepatocytes can colonize the spleen of recipient rats if the hosts are immunosuppressed with CsA. The transplanted cells can be maintained for at least 2 weeks if treatment with CsA is continued. Further study may allow this technique to be applied to the problem of replacement of hepatic function or for acute hepatic failure in human beings.

▶ In ongoing studies of liver cell transplantation in rats with acute hepatic failure, Makowka's group has demonstrated excellent hepatic cell survival and proliferation in the splenic tissue of immunosuppressed allogeneic recipients. These are very encouraging findings and deserve further trials in large animals.—O. Jonasson, M.D.

Segmental Small Intestinal Allografts: II. Inadequate Function With Cyclosporine Immunosuppression: Evidence of a Protein-Losing Enteropathy

Jack Collin, Ashley R. Dennison, Roger M. Watkins, Peter R. Millard, and Peter J. Morris (Univ. of Oxford, Oxford, England)
Transplantation 44:479–483, October 1987   8–28

Long-term survival of intestinal allografts is reported with cyclosporine (CsA) immunosuppression, but its effects of intestinal function are uncertain. The authors performed terminal ileal autografts or allografts, using Thiry-Vella segments in dogs, and administered CsA to dogs with allografts in a dose of 20 mg/kg of body weight daily. Continuity of the nontransplanted gut was restored after 5–6 weeks, and all nontransplanted small bowel was excised 3 months after autografting.

In autografted animals, body weight was maintained at 88% of baseline by absorption from the autografted intestine. Cyclosporine produced reversible impairment of intestinal absorption. Allografted animals survived a mean of 63 days; deaths within 9 weeks of transplantation were due to peritonitis from graft rejection. Later deaths were secondary to inadequate intestinal absorption. Absorption and motility were comparable to those of autografts in the first month, but large volumes of high protein-content fluid were lost from the allografted Thiry-Vella segments. The dogs with allografts became hypoalbuminemic. Allografts often were viable at autopsy but exhibited mucosal atrophy, medial fibrosis, and vascular changes of rejection.

Cyclosporine substantially prolongs the survival of intestinal allografts. Early absorptive function is adequate, but a protein-losing enteropathy promotes weight loss, and eventually death, from malnutrition. Improved immunosuppression is needed to ensure adequate function of the transplanted small bowel before the procedure is used clinically.

▶ In these studies the classic model of the short segment Thiry-Vella loop was either allotransplanted or autografted in dogs, and absorption and motility studies were carried out before and after restoration of intestinal continuity. The immunosuppressive regimen of cyclosporine only, in large doses, was clearly inadequate to prevent acute and chronic rejection, and the dogs with allografted loops were unable to sustain their nutrition due to a severe protein-losing enteropathy. The authors conclude that clinical trials of small bowel allografting are quite premature until the major issue of adequate immunosuppression has been solved.—O. Jonasson, M.D.

Fatal Gastrointestinal Hemorrhage Caused by Cytomegalovirus Duodenitis and Ulceration After Heart Transplantation

Nigel H. Bramwell, Ross A. Davies, Arvind Koshal, G.N.W. Tse, Wilbert J. Keon, and Virginia M. Walley (Univ. of Ottawa, Univ. of Ottawa Heart Inst., and Ottawa Civic Hosp., Ottawa, Canada)
J. Heart Transplant. 6:303–306, September–October 1987   8–29

The compromised immune status of organ transplant recipients makes them susceptible to a variety of viral infections. Recently, a cytomegalovirus (CMV)-associated enterocolitis and colonic ulceration were in patients with acquired immunodeficiency syndrome (AIDS) and in kidney transplant recipients. A man who suffered a fatal gastrointestinal hemorrhage from duodenal ulcers 50 days after heart transplantation is described.

Man, 61, had severe atherosclerotic coronary artery disease. He had been a heavy smoker with a history of non-insulin-dependent diabetes mellitus. Heart transplantation was performed. Immunosuppression therapy included orally ad-

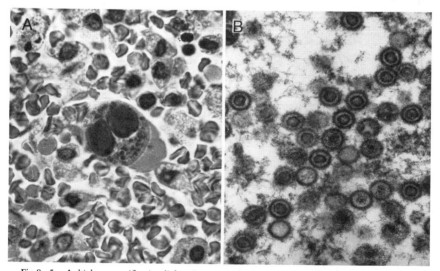

Fig 8–5.—**A,** higher magnification light microscopy showing cell with characteristic cytomegalovirus (CMV) intranuclear and intracytoplasmic inclusions are particularly characteristic of CMV cytopathology. (Hematoxylin, phloxine, and saffron stain; original magnification, ×512.) **B,** electron micrograph showing multiple CMV viral particles with characteristic dense core and surrounding envelope in nucleus of infected cell. (Original magnification, ×114,000.) (Courtesy of Bramwell, N.H., et al.: J. Heart Transplant. 6:303–306. September–October, 1987.)

ministered cyclosporine, methylprednisolone, acetylsalicylic acid, and dipyridamole. Endomyocardial biopsy specimens obtained on days 14, 21, 29, and 44 after surgery showed no evidence of rejection. The patient never received pulsed
prednisone or other acute rejection therapy. On postoperative day 50, the patient
passed a great quantity of frank blood rectally. Fiberoptic esophagogastroduode-
noscopy showed esophagitis with ulceration at the gastroesophageal junction,
prepyloric erosions, and duodenitis. A bleeding vessel was found in the third part
of the duodenum, as well as a 1-mm, shallow ulcer with arterial bleeding. The
ulcer was oversewn along with another small, shallow linear ulcer. The patient
died of rebleeding at multiple sites of mucosal ulceration into the bowel 52 days
after heart transplantation. Microscopic examination showed rare scattered foci
of cells with CMV viral effects. Virus-associated tissue necrosis and inflammation
were restricted to the gastrointestinal tract and lung. Large clusters of
CMV-infected cells associated with mucosal ulceration, inflammatory infiltrates,
and vasculitis were noted in the duodenum. The nature of the CMV infection
was confirmed by numerous giant cells with the typical intranuclear, intracytoplasmic inclusions on light microscopy and viral particles on electron microscopy
(Fig 8–5).

This unusual case is the first report of a fatal CMV-associated gastrointestinal hemorrhage after heart transplantation. Microscopically,
clusters of CMV-infected cells were localized in the ulcerative lesions of
the gastrointestinal muscosa. A vasculitic picture in such cases is a frequent accompaniment.

▶ The causative role of CMV in GI tract mucosal ulcerations in the immunosuppressed patient has recently been recognized. Although CMV apparently is localized in areas previously diseased, the association of CMV infection and vasculitis in the mucosa of the colon and duodenum in patients who bleed and
perforate appears to be that of cause and effect. Care to avoid exposing the
recipient to a primary CMV infection by transplantation of a CMV-positive donor
organ should be carefully avoided. Consideration should be given in these patients to administration of the CMV immune globulin.—O. Jonasson, M.D.

**Temporary Use of the Jarvik-7 Total Artificial Heart Before
Transplantation**
Bartley P. Griffith, Robert L. Hardesty, Robert L. Kormos, Alfredo Trento,
Harvey S. Borovetz, Mark E. Thompson, and Henry T. Bahnson (Univ. of
Pittsburgh)
N. Engl. J. Med. 316:130–134, Jan. 15, 1987   8–30

The Jarvik-7 artificial heart was implanted in six patients who were
not expected to live for more than a few hours and for whom a heart
transplant was not available. Only the contraindication of overt infection
was to prevent each patient from receiving a heart transplant as soon as
possible.

There was a total of 52 days (range 1 to 18) of device support for these
six patients. Four were extubated and three could get from their bed to a

chair with assistance. Five had successful transplantation, but the sixth died of candidal sepsis and multiorgan failure on the 18th day while still on the artificial heart. Except for the latter patient the preoperative function of the noncardiac organs was stabilized or improved in every patient.

Removing the artificial heart and the associated prosthetic material did not complicate unduly orthotopic cardiac transplantation. Four of the five with successful transplants are alive and well at 12, 8, 4, and 2 months after transplantation; one died of rejection 60 days afterward.

Two patients had serious infection which was related to their death. At autopsy the artificial heart and multiple organs of one patient showed macroscopic *Candida albicans.* In another patient mediastinitis developed on the 20th day after transplantation, and there was irreversible rejection on the 60th day.

Although no patient had a stroke, all explanted devices showed some deposition of small white thrombi in the inner and outer crevices that formed between the polished valve rings and their polycarbonate housings and between the housings and the Dacron vascular conduits.

The smaller 70-ml Jarvik-7 heart was used in the last three patients, and it performed well. During two procedures in which the 100-ml device was used, red thrombi were found, which are more threatening than the irregular aggregates of platelets that are common along the creases formed by the valves and their housings.

That an embolic complication did not occur was due to good fortune, aggressive anticoagulation, and the short duration of support, and underscores the need to use the Jarvik-7 device only if necessary and for as short a period as possible.

Patients with a high level of incompatibility against a panel of HLA antigens have been excluded because the authors do not intend to use the currently available total artificial heart for long-term support. In these patients, compatibility with a randomly available donor is not likely.

Use of the Jarvik-7 artificial heart provided a bridge from almost certain death to satisfactory cardiac transplantation in four of the six patients in this study.

▶ This is yet another exciting report from the cardiac transplant group at the University of Pittsburgh, who have been actively extending the boundaries of heart transplantation to a wider group of potential recipients. In this study, patients with a predicted life expectancy measured in hours were treated with excision of the native heart and implantation of the Jarvik-7 artificial heart as a bridge to transplantation. In four of six patients this was a successful bridge, and the authors recommend its use in selected patients who are preterminal and for whom a heart donor can reasonably be expected to be found within a few days of artificial heart support. Of course, this raises other issues of priority for the scarce organ donor resource, but if organ distribution is maintained fairly and equitably, the approach outlined by Griffith and his colleagues seems reasonable.—O. Jonasson, M.D.

9 Oncology and Tumor Immunology

The Autoimmune Nature of Cancer

Richmond T. Prehn and Liisa M. Prehn (Inst. for Med. Research, San Jose, Calif.)

Cancer Res. 47:927–932, Feb. 15, 1987

9–1

It appears that tumor-specific immunity in the murine MCA-induced sarcoma system usually facilitates oncogenesis, rather than inhibiting it. An intermediate level of antitumor immune reactivity is most conducive to oncogenesis. Immune spleen cells show dose dependent facilitation or inhibition of tumor cells, and the same molecular species of antibody can facilitate or inhibit tumor growth, depending on its concentration.

The immune reaction most conducive to oncogenesis is a significantly positive reaction, not a minimal one. Tumors of low antigenicity develop best in an environment with a highly responsive immune system, but those of high antigenicity grow better in a less immune-responsive environment.

The inverse relation between the strength of the oncogenic stimulus and the optimal level of host immune response may reflect the immunogenicity of the tumor, which varies with the dose of oncogene. In human beings immunodepression appears to potentiate cutaneous oncogenesis. The finding that patients with acquired immunodeficiency syndrome (AIDS) who present with Kaposi's sarcoma live longer than those without this neoplasm suggests that residual immune capacity is not only beneficial but it also may actively facilitate growth of the sarcoma. It is likely that the specific antitumor immune response serves vital functions under normal conditions, thus outweighing its detrimental effects in relation to cancer. Many supposedly nonimmunogenic tumors may actually be facilitated by the immune reaction. The means of preventing autoimmune disorders may be applicable to the prevention of some cancers.

▶ In this brief article on perspectives in cancer research, the authors present an argument, based on four general sets of observations, supporting the hypothesis that the immune response to tumor development includes an autoimmune component which frequently facilitates tumor development as well as normal host defense mechanisms. The conflicting observation of suppression and antitumor activity of host immune response continues to provide rich areas for basic investigations into mechanisms and control of malignancy.—O. Jonasson, M.D.

Augmentation of the Antimetastatic Effect of Anticoagulant Drugs by Immunostimulation in Mice

Elieser Gorelik (Natl. Cancer Inst., Frederick, Md.)
Cancer Res. 47:809–815, Feb. 1, 1987   9–2

Intravascular observation of tumor cells has shown them in close association with platelets or surrounded by fibrin. Anticoagulant drugs, which can prevent this association, have an antimetastatic effect. This effect was studied in mice with stimulated or depressed natural killer (NK) cell activity following injection with BL6 melanoma or Lewis lung carcinoma (3LL) cells.

Treatment with the anticoagulant warfarin or the NK cell stimulator polyinosinic-polycytidylic acid (poly I:C) prevented metastasis formation in 22%–38% of the mice. Combined treatment prevented metastases in 78%–90% of the mice. When mice were treated with anti-asialo G_{M1} serum or cyclophosphamide (CY), both of which suppress NK cell activity, tumor colonization of the lungs increased. The antimetastatic effect of poly I:C was associated with NK cell stimulation. Warfarin did not stimulate NK cell activity, but it did have an effect on the elimination of tumor cells (Fig 9–1). Three-week-old C57BL/6 and beige C57BL/6 mice have low NK reactivity. These mice received the same treatments as above to determine whether their low level of NK activity would be sufficient to demonstrate the same responses. More metastases

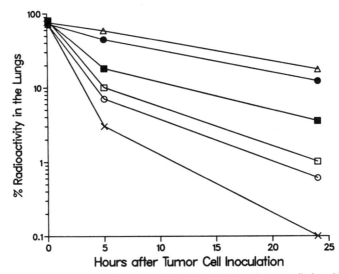

Fig 9–1.—Effect of warfarin on elimination of radiolabeled BL6 melanoma cells from lungs of NK-depressed or -stimulated mice. C57BL/6 mice were treated with poly I:C (100 μg) or anti-asialo G_{M1} serum (0.25 ml, dilution 1:40). Mice received warfarin (8 mg/L drinking water) 2 days before IV injection of 2.5 × 10^5 ^{111}In oxide-labeled BL6 melanoma cells (radioactivity, 2 cpm/cell). The level of radioactivity remaining in the lungs was determined 10 min and 6 and 24 hr after tumor cell administration. ■, controls; □, poly I:C; ○, warfarin; ×, poly I:C plus warfarin; △, anti-asialo G_{M1} serum; ●, anti-asialo G_{M1} serum plus warfarin. (Courtesy of Gorelik, E.: Cancer Res. 47:809–815, Feb. 1, 1987.)

were seen in young mice than in older mice. Nevertheless, heparin and poly I:C did have antimetastatic effects. Even the reduced level of NK activity found in these animals appeared sufficient to potentiate the antimetastatic effects of anticoagulants.

These data indicate that prevention of fibrin deposition on tumor cells increased the antitumor activity of NK cells. The interaction of the tumor cells with fibrinogen and NK cells occurred in the blood. Administration of anticoagulants or fibrinolytic agents might have an antimetastatic or antitumor effect when combined with other therapies.

▶ In these interesting experiments, the author explores the mechanism of intravascular tumor cell elimination by normal host surveillance mechanisms, the natural killer, or NK, cells. The import of cancer cells in the circulating blood has been hotly debated for many decades. A number of investigators have found correlations of the presence of cancer cells in the blood stream with the development of metastatic disease and developed means of adjuvant systemic chemotherapy to control this phase of the disease. Undoubtedly this remains the major basis for the use of such adjuvant chemotherapy today. Others have felt that the mere documentation of the presence of cancer cells in the blood stream has little practical significance, in that the majority of these cells are eliminated.

From the results of the experiments reported by Gorelik, it appears that cancer cells actually in the circulating blood are vulnerable to destruction by NK cells. Stimulation of NK cell activity accelerates tumor cell clearance. Anticoagulant drugs, such as the warfarin used in Dr. Gorelik's studies, prevent fibrin coagulation and produce a substantial antimetastatic effect. The combination of these two treatments greatly potentiates antimetastatic treatment.—O. Jonasson, M.D.

▶ ↓ The next five papers (Abstracts 9–3 to 9–7) deal with the treatment of metastatic cancer by lymphokine-activated tumor cells and interleukin-2, one of the principal lymphokines.—O. Jonasson, M.D.

A Progress Report on the Treatment of 157 Patients With Advanced Cancer Using Lymphokine-Activated Killer Cells and Interleukin-2 or High-Dose Interleukin-2 Alone
Steven A. Rosenberg, Michael T. Lotze, Linda M. Muul, Alfred E. Chang, Fred P. Avis, Susan Leitman, W. Marston Linehan, Cary N. Robertson, Roberta E. Lee, Joshua T. Rubin, Claudia A. Seipp, Colleen G. Simpson, and Donald E. White (Natl. Insts. of Health, Bethesda, Md.)
N. Engl. J. Med. 316:889–897, April 9, 1987   9–3

A previous study of 25 patients with advanced cancer treated with a single course of lymphokine-activated killer (LAK) cells and interleukin-2 reported some objective regressions of metastatic cancer. The effects of this therapy, called adoptive immunotherapy, were studied in 157 patients with metastatic cancer for whom standard therapy had failed or was not available.

One hundred eight patients received 127 courses of therapy with LAK cells and high dose interleukin-2, and 49 patients received 53 courses of high dose interleukin-2 alone. Prior therapy had been given to 103 patients in the first group and to 45 in the second group; many had also undergone chemotherapy, radiotherapy, hormonal therapies, or other experimental immunotherapies. Of 106 evaluable patients receiving LAK cells and interleukin-2, eight had complete responses. Fifteen had partial responses, and ten had slight responses. Among those with complete responses, the median duration of response was 10 months; among those with partial responses, it was 6 months. The patients with the longest complete response were still in remission 22 months after the completion of therapy. Of 46 patients evaluable treated with high dose interleukin-2 alone, one had a complete response and remained in remission for more than 4 months, five had partial responses and remained in remission for 2 to more than 11 months, and one had a minor response. Common side effects observed were hypotension, weight gain, oliguria, and elevation of bilirubin and creatinine levels; they resolved promptly after interleukin-2 therapy was stopped. Four of the 157 patients died from treatment-related causes.

These findings demonstrate that this immunotherapeutic approach can produce marked tumor regression in some patients for whom no other effective therapy is currently available. Further attempts to increase therapeutic efficacy and decrease toxicity and complexity are needed.

Constant-Infusion Recombinant Interleukin-2 in Adoptive Immunotherapy of Advanced Cancer

William H. West, Kurt W. Tauer, John R. Yannelli, Gailen D. Marshall, Douglas W. Orr, Gary B. Thurman, and Robert K. Oldham (Biological Therapy Inst. and Biotherapeutics, Inc., Memphis and Franklin, Tenn.)
N. Engl. J. Med. 316:898–905, April 9, 1987   9–4

Adoptive immunotherapy with recombinant interleukin-2 (IL-2) has induced regression of some cancers, but it may produce marked fluid retention and cardiopulmonary compromise. A study was made of constant infusion of IL-2 rather than bolus dosing. A dose-escalation schedule was tried in an attempt to obtain optimal biologic effects. Forty-eight patients with advanced cancer resistant to standard treatment participated in the study. A 24-hour infusion was given in 5-day cycles with 5-day rest intervals. Leukapheresis was interposed between IL-2 infusions.

Thirteen of 40 evaluable patients had partial responses, and two others had minor responses. Many toxic effects were evident (Table 1). Some, such as weight gain and resting dyspnea, occurred only in patients with poorer baseline performance. Three of six renal cancers and five of ten melanomas responded partially to IL-2 infusion therapy (Table 2). Responses were associated with good performance status; a baseline lymphocyte count of more than 1,400/cu mm; and an induced lymphocyte count of 6,000 or higher. The best lymphocytosis resulted from a priming dose of 3×10^6 U/sq m daily.

TABLE 1.—Toxic Effects in 40 Patients
Receiving Constant Infusions of rIL-2

Toxic Effect	No. of Patients
Fever	40
Fatigue	40
Anemia	40
Hypoalbuminemia	40
Eosinophilia	40
Rash	40
Nausea	12
Diarrhea	14
Stomatitis	10
Bilirubin >3 mg/dl	5
Creatinine >3 mg/dl	12
Sodium <125 mmol/liter	2
Confusion	4
Weight gain >10 percent	5
Dyspnea	6
Hypotension	14
Tachyarrhythmia	1
Congestive heart failure	1
Myocardial infarction	0
Admission to ICU*	6
Treatment-associated death (sepsis)	1

*ICU, intensive care unit.
(Courtesy of West, W.H., et al.: N. Engl. J. Med. 316:898–905, April 9, 1987.)

TABLE 2.—Analysis of Responses
According to Tumor Type

Type	Responses/Total
Melanoma	5/10*
Renal cancer	3/6
Lung cancer	1/5
Parotid cancer	1/2
Ovarian cancer	1/1
Breast cancer	0/1
Hodgkin's disease	1/1
Nodular mixed lymphoma	1/1
Colon cancer	0/13

*Two additional patients of these 10 with melanoma had minor responses.
(Courtesy of West, W.H., et al.: N. Engl. J. Med. 316:898–905, April 9, 1987.)

Infused recombinant IL-2 may lead to marked regression of refractory cancer with relatively acceptable toxicity. Such treatment might be examined in patients with a smaller tumor burden and apparently intact immune function.

The Requirements for Successful Immunotherapy of Intraperitoneal Cancer Using Interleukin-2 and Lymphokine-Activated Killer Cells

Reyer T. Ottow, Alexander M.M. Eggermont, E. Philip Steller, and Paul H. Sugarbaker (Natl. Insts. of Health, Bethesda, Md.)
Cancer 60:1465–1473, Oct. 1, 1987   9–5

Adjuvant treatment of the peritoneal cavity might prove useful in some patients with gastrointestinal (GI) or ovarian malignancies. An evaluation was made of adoptively transferred cells, along with their biologic response modifier interleukin-2 (IL-2), in a murine model of intraperitoneal tumor. A weakly immunogenic 3-methylcholanthrene-induced sarcoma, MCA-105, was utilized.

Intraperitoneal tumor mass decreased significantly when both lymphokine-activated killer (LAK) cells and exogenous IL-2 were given. Prolonged survival also was evident with this treatment (Fig 9–2). Allogeneic and syngeneic LAK cells were equally effective. Cells generated from normal donors were as reactive as those obtained from tumor-bearing donors. Treatment was effective in immunocompromised hosts. Both IL-2 derived from a subline of EL-4 thymoma and recombinant IL-2 proved effective in controlling intraperitoneal tumor. Peritoneal exudate cells had high levels of LAK cytotoxicity.

Intraperitoneal tumor in mice is effectively treated by high dose IL-2, and a greater effect is obtained when LAK cells are given intraperitoneally at the same time. Such treatment may be helpful in the immunocompromised host. Clinical trials should evaluate intraperitoneal IL-2 administration, with and without adoptive transfer of LAK cells to the same body site.

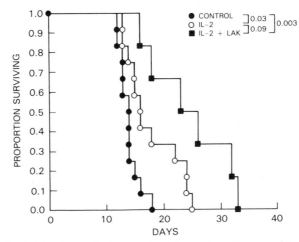

Fig 9–2.—Survival benefits in mice inoculated with intraperitoneal tumor and treated with 25,000 units of IL-2 intraperitoneally twice a day, or IL-2 days 3 through 7 and 1×10^8 LAK cells intraperitoneally on day 3. (Courtesy of Ottow, R.T., et al.: Cancer 60:1465–1473, Oct. 1, 1987.)

Intraperitoneal Administration of Interleukin-2 in Patients With Cancer

Michael T. Lotze, Mary C. Custer, and Steven A. Rosenberg (Natl. Cancer Inst., Bethesda, Md.)

Arch. Surg. 121:1373–1379, December 1986   9–6

Reports have showed that interleukin-2 (IL-2) serves as the second signal in mitogenesis of lymphocytes and stimulates directly the generation of lymphokine-activated killer cells that lyse fresh human tumor cells.

Seven patients with intraperitoneal metastases of melanoma, ovarian carcinoma, or colorectal carcinoma were treated three times daily with intraperitoneal (IP) administration of recombinant IL-2 as a bolus infusion through an indwelling Tenckhoff catheter to determine the toxicity, efficacy in peritoneal and nonperitoneal sites, and immunologic effects.

Toxic effects that were seen with this treatment were felt to be comparable with those in patients who were receiving IL-2 intravenously. All

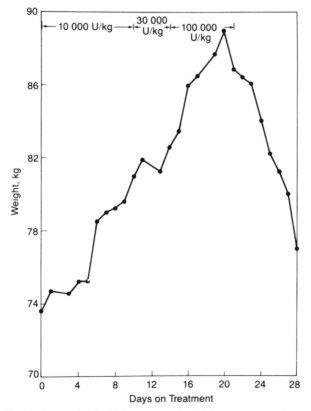

Fig 9–3.—Weight gain associated with intraperitoneal administration of recombinant interleukin-2. Increase in weight is secondary to increased intravenous and oral fluids that were required to maintain blood pressure and treat oliguria. Presumed leaky capillary syndrome that was due to interleukin-2 or indirectly secondary to release of other mediators is postulated. Marked ascites was noted. (Courtesy of Lotze, M.T., et al.: Arch. Surg. 121:1373–1379, December 1986.)

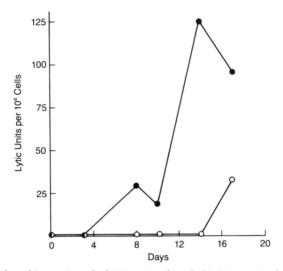

Fig 9–4.—Prolonged intraperitoneal administration of interleukin-2 is associated with development of natural killer and lymphokine-activated killer cells in vivo. In addition to 100-fold expansion of recoverable cells from peritoneal cavity, marked augmentation in natural killer activity *(solid circles)* during end of 2-week therapy with ability to lyse fresh tumor in 4-hour release assay (sodium chromate Cr51) was found. No lymphokine-activated killer cell activity *(open circles)* could be detected in peripheral blood. Similar results were obtained in second patient. Assay was run at effector-to-target ratios of between 1:1 and 40:1. (Courtesy of Lotze, M.T., et al.: Arch. Surg. 121:1373–1379, December 1986.)

patients developed fever, chills, and ascites, and all gained weight (Fig 9–3). The edema and congestion that developed within the extremities, torso, and individual organs was thought to represent a capillary leak syndrome.

Four patients required pressor support with infusions of dopamine hydrochloride or phenylephrine hydrochloride. One patient with extensive IP tumor could not be successfully treated because of dense adhesions and tumor.

One of the seven patients had a dramatic decrease in the size and number of multiple pulmonary, hepatic, and splenic metastases from melanoma with progressive shrinkage for several months. Seven months later a single brain metastasis was noted and treated with craniotomy, excision, and brain irradiation; the patient was alive with continued shrinkage of pulmonary lesions after 14 months.

Intraperitoneal administration is associated with sustained high levels of IL-2 in the peritoneal cavity and low levels in the serum (Fig 9–4). However, intraperitoneal IL-2, administered at maximal tolerated doses to achieve a therapeutic effect, also caused prohibitive toxicity, especially edema and ascites; therefore, use of intraperitoneal IL-2 alone for the treatment of intraperitoneal tumors, has been abandoned.

The marked increase in total IP cells noted during IP IL-2 therapy suggests the interesting possibility of use of this regimen to expand the population of activated lytic cells for use in treatment.

Interleukin 2-Activated Human Lymphocytes Exhibit Enhanced Adhesion to Normal Vascular Endothelial Cells and Cause Their Lysis

Nitin K. Damle, Laura V. Doyle, Jeffrey R. Bender, and Edward C. Bradley (Stanford Univ.)

J. Immunol. 138:1779–1785, March 15, 1987   9–7

Interleukin-2 (IL-2) stimulates human lymphoid cells to proliferate and differentiate to cytotoxic effector cells, the IL-2-activated killer (IAK) cells. Adoptive immunotherapy with IAK cells induces tumor regression in vivo but also produces significant toxicity, including vascular leakage, with resultant edema and weight gain. The IAK cells were demonstrated to adhere strongly to endothelial cells and lyse them, which might contribute to systemic toxicity from high infused doses of IL-2.

Lymphocytes activated by IL-2 exhibited increased adherence to vascular endothelial-cell monolayers. The effect was dose-dependent. No such effect was observed with tumor cells, fibroblasts, or epithelial cells. A strong cytolytic effect on endothelial-cell targets was noted. Human and bovine endothelial cells, corneal cells, and NK-resistant Daudi cells all were lysed. Lysis was mediated by both IL-2-activated large granular lymphocytes and small agranular lymphocytes.

Destruction of endothelial cells by adhering IAK cells may help explain the systemic toxicity resulting from infusion of high doses of IL-2. It is not clear why IAK activity is seldom noted within circulating lymphocytes from IL-2-treated patients, but most IAK cells might be sequestered about the vascular endothelium.

▶ Mononuclear cells in the peripheral blood, the peritoneal cavity, and the lymphocyte aggregates infiltrating tumors have been stimulated in a nonspecific fashion by various lymphokines, especially interleukin-2 (IL-2), and have responded by proliferating and attaining cytotoxic activity for tumor cells. Cells expanded in in vitro cultures by IL-2 have been used in passive transfer experiments either intravenously or into the peritoneal cavity, and a few remarkable tumor regressions have been achieved in both experimental and clinical models. The toxicity of IL-2 treatment is profound, however, especially due to a vascular leakage syndrome with massive edema, pulmonary insufficiency, and renal failure. The first paper in this series is by Rosenberg's group at the National Cancer Institute (Abstract 9–3); these investigators continue to report marked tumor regression in some patients for whom no other effective therapy was available. These reports, although accompanied by notations of severe toxicity, have continued to drive this field forward.

The second paper, by West's group (Abstract 9–4), attempts to ameliorate some of the vascular leakage syndrome toxic effects with a carefully controlled constant infusion of courses of high dose IL-2. Careful analysis of the factors associated with successful treatment indicated that patients in the last stages of their illnesses were poor candidates for this rigorous treatment, but in the good risk patient, especially one with melanoma, substantial tumor regression is achievable. Vascular leakage syndrome did appear considerably less with their methods of administration.

The third paper (Abstract 9–5) discusses adoptively transferred LAK cells and IL-2 used intraperitoneally in a mouse model. This approach is particularly appealing for application to tumors implanted onto peritoneal surfaces, such as ovarian cancer.

The next report (Abstract 9–6), again from the National Cancer Institute, addressed the clinical application of interperitoneal IL-2. Again, severe toxicity from the vascular leakage syndrome severely compromised any benefits.

The final report in this series specifically addresses the vascular leakage syndrome (Abstract 9–7) and suggests that this syndrome is caused by an inappropriate cytolytic effect of LAK cells on normal vascular endothelial cells. In these careful studies, the investigators have challenged the concept that LAK cells routinely spare normal tissues by demonstrating that activated mononuclear cells exhibit strong adhesion to endothelial cells and then lyse them. The investigators suggest that binding of lymphoid cells to endothelial cells is the first stage in passage from the circulation into lymphoid or nonlymphoid tissue and is required for access of the LAK cells to the tumor cells. In the presence of high doses of IL-2 and many LAK cells, the authors imply that cytotoxicity and the vascular leakage syndrome occur at a rate in direct proportion to the dose of IL-2 given to the patient.—O. Jonasson, M.D.

Recombinant Interferon Enhances Monoclonal Antibody-Targeting of Carcinoma Lesions In Vivo
John W. Greiner, Fiorella Guadagni, Philip Noguchi, Sidney Pestka, David Colcher, Paul B. Fisher, and Jeffrey Schlom (Natl. Cancer Inst., Bethesda, Md.; FDA, Bethesda; Rutgers Med. School, Piscataway, N.J.; and Columbia Univ.)
Science 235:895–898, Feb. 20, 1987   9–8

A characteristic that is common to most, if not all, populations of human carcinoma cells is the heterogeneity in the expression of tumor-associated antigens. Within the population antigen-negative cells can escape detection and therapy. Rendering a population of human tumor cells more homogeneous for the expression of an antigen could result in augmentation of the binding of monoclonal antibodies (mAbs) and thus provide more efficient diagnostic or therapeutic results.

Of eight different recombinant species of human leukocyte interferon α (Hu-IFN-α) that were previously described, Hu-IFN-αA was the most potent in augmenting the binding of mAbs to defined cell surface human tumor antigens. The increased expression of surface antigen was a result of an increase in the amount of surface tumor antigen per cell and a higher percentage of antigen-positive cells, which provided a more homogeneous population of antigen-expressing tumor cells.

It can now be reported that Hu-IFN-αA can augment the binding of a mAb to human carcinoma cells in vivo. The authors investigated the possibility that the use of Hu-IFN-αA in treating athymic mice that bear human colon carcinoma xenografts could enhance the level of expression of the 90-kD tumor antigen and augment the localization of labeled mAb B6.2 to the colon tumor.

The findings indicated that in addition to an overall increase in expression of tumor antigen within the cell population, the interferon treatment results in an increase in the percentage of antigen-positive cells within that population from approximately 50% to more than 90%. The results suggest enhanced synthesis of the surface antigen as a possible mechanism.

In the athymic mice WiDr cells were grown as subcutaneous tumors. When the mice were treated with 50,000 or 250,000 units of the interferon for 5 days and had their human colon tumors measured for the binding of ^{125}I-labeled B6.2, there was a significant increase in the amount of B6.2-reactive 90-kD tumor antigen in the tumor extracts.

Thus, treatment with Hu-IFN-αA appears to alter the biology of a human tumor cell population. Previous in vitro studies revealed that this was due to the increased amount of antigen that is expressed per cell as well as an increase in the percentage of antigen-expressing cells within the population. Different laboratories are evaluating numerous mAbs by using both experimental models and clinical protocols to determine their usefulness in managing human carcinomas.

The ability to increase expression of antigen on tumor cells by pretreatment with human recombinant interferon could result in a more accurate discrimination between tumor and nontumor tissue in an immunodiagnostic procedure, and mAbs can be used to deliver therapeutic doses of radionuclides, toxins, or effector cells to the tumor site.

▶ In this logical extension of the labeling studies reported in the previous paper, a potent lymphokine, recombinant human leukocyte interferon alpha, has been used to enhance the expression of the tumor-associated antigens in a line of cultured human colon cancer cells. Under the influence of interferon, the tumor cells show substantial increase in labeling with antibody, due not only to increased label per cell but to increases in the proportion of cells in the tumor expressing the antigen. The author suggests that enhancement of tumor antigen expression might substantially increase the antibody labeling for therapeutic as well as diagnostic purposes. These are imaginative studies and are found to be productive areas of investigation.—O. Jonasson, M.D.

Tumor Necrosis Factor Enhances HLA-A,B,C, and HLA-DR Gene Expression in Human Tumor Cells
Klaus Pfizenmaier, Peter Scheurich, Carsten Schlüter, and Martin Krönke (Max Planck Society, Göttingen, West Germany)
J. Immunol. 138:975–980, Feb. 1, 1987   9–9

Tumor necrosis factor-α (TNF-α) has direct tumoricidal activity, stimulates metabolic activities, and serves the expression of cell surface antigens on nonmalignant cells. Tumor necrosis factor-α has been found to upregulate constitutively expressed HLA genes in various human tumor cells.

Tumor necrosis factor-α enhances both constitutive and interferon-γ (IFN-γ)-induced HLA class I and II antigen expression by upregulating HLA gene transcription. In addition, a posttranscriptional level of gene expression is influenced in some tumor cells. The factor reversibly promoted IFN-γ-induced HLA gene expression at the level of mRNA transcription. However, HLA class I membrane expression was enhanced in Colo 205 cells without apparent change in steady-state mRNA levels.

It is possible that TNF-α, like IFN-γ, may produce tumor rejection by a direct tumoricidal action and also by enhancing HLA antigens and inducing tumor-specific immune responses. Enhancement of HLA expression by combined treatment with IFN-γ and TNF-α might potentiate the immunogenicity of tumors, particularly those with cells expressing few or no HLA antigens.

▶ The immune response to human tumors is predicted on the expression of antigens on tumor cell surfaces and host recognition of these antigens. This investigation was concerned with a lymphokine tumor-necrosis-factor-α, which is known to exert direct lytic effects on tumor cells under certain conditions. Yet these studies showed that TNF-α supplemented the effect of immune interferon-γ and enhanced HLA class I and II antigen expressions by upregulating HLA gene transcription as well as increasing a posttranscriptional level of gene expression. The authors point out that the expression of a critical density of antigens on tumor cells is a prerequisite for tumor rejection, and the observation that TNF potentiates antigenicity may be useful in planning strategies for therapy.—O. Jonasson, M.D.

Identification of Specific Cytolytic Immune Responses Against Autologous Tumor in Humans Bearing Malignant Melanoma

Linda Mesler Muul, Paul J. Spiess, Elaine P. Director, and Steven A. Rosenberg (Natl. Cancer Inst., Bethesda, Md.)
J. Immunol. 138:989–995, Feb. 1, 1987   9–10

There is evidence that lymphocyte infiltration of tumors reflects an immune response against the tumor. Human tumor may induce suppressor cells or factors that inhibit the function of infiltrating lymphocytes. Expanded tumor-infiltrating lymphocytes (TIL) from six patients having malignant melanoma proved to be cytotoxic in a chromium-release assay for their own autologous fresh melanoma tumor cells but not for normal autologous cells.

The TIL from freshly excised melanomas proliferated in the presence of viable tumor cells. Repeated passages led to a very high proportion of Leu-2⁻, Leu-3⁺4⁺ lymphocytes. Expanded TIL from three patients were specifically cytotoxic only for autologous melanoma cells but not for allogeneic melanoma cells. The other three preparations had limited capacity to kill allogeneic fresh tumor targets. A majority of expanded TIL were Leu-3$^+$ in five of six instances.

Patients with melanoma raise an immune response against autologous tumor. The mechanism of killing is not clear, but the Leu-3$^+$ T cells may recognize and kill tumor in conjunction with class II histocompatibility antigens. Human lymphocytes with antitumor reactivity might be useful in the adoptive immunotherapy of tumors. The isolation of lymphocytes that are selectively reactive with autologous tumor indicates the existence of tumor-specific antigens on human tumors.

▶ The peripheral blood is a poor place to monitor the immunobiologic activity occurring in a localized area such as a rejecting organ transplant or a tumor. The mononuclear cell infiltrate found associated with many tumors may provide a much more relevant population of cells to study. Some have argued that the infiltrating mononuclear cells are actually suppressor cells, inhibiting an immune response; others have felt that these cells enhance the expansion of tumors by providing growth factors. In this study, Dr. Rosenberg's group has identified a population of lymphoid cells in the infiltrate around a tumor that, when stimulated to proliferate by IL-2, demonstrates cytolytic activities specifically directed against the autologous tumor or, in some instances, similar allogeneic tumors. Demonstration of this specific antitumor cytotoxicity by tumor-infiltrating lymphocytes was a major achievement. Although the series is small and the results are highly variable (maximum expansion with IL-2 varies from three times to 95,000 times), these cells appear to be highly effective in tumor cell lysis and provide evidence for the existence of tumor-specific antigens on human tumors.—O. Jonasson, M.D.

Suppressor Cell Activity in Melanoma-Draining Lymph Nodes
D.S.B. Hoon, R.J. Bowker, and A.J. Cochran (Univ. of California, Los Angeles)
Cancer Res. 47:1529–1533, March 15, 1987   9–11

In previous reports the authors have used histology and immunohistology to show significantly reduced paracortical (T zone) activity in nodes which are located near primary or metastatic melanoma. In the present study suppressor cell activity in melanoma-draining lymph nodes that were located at different distances from a tumor were examined by using a reliable Con A suppressor induction cell assay. All the nodes that were examined were obtained from axillary and groin dissections and were identified histologically to be tumor free.

In most patients the nodes proximal to the tumor, A nodes, had more suppressor cell activity than those distal to the tumor, C nodes. The high levels of Con A-induced suppressor cell activity in pooled melanoma-draining lymph node lymphocytes (LNL) supported previous observations that immune suppression does exist in such nodes. Average overall Con A suppressor cell activity among the patients was 73%. Substantial node-to-node variation in suppressor cell activity was indicated on examination of LNL from single tumor-oriented nodes. The nodes that were closest to the tumor were significantly more suppressive than those that were located farther away.

The cause of increased suppressor cell activity in proximal tumor-draining lymph nodes has yet to be determined. Possible factors may be melanoma-derived products that pass from tumor cells to the proximal nodes; migration of suppressor cells from the tumor area to the regional nodes, with possible additional recruitment or activation of presuppressor cells in the node, or both; and melanoma cells that seed in the nodes and induce suppression. Suppressor cell activity may also reflect normal immunoregulatory activity toward high T cell activity that is induced by antigenic stimulation. The major inducers of suppression in nodes near a tumor are most likely the first two possibilities.

This study confirmed results of immunohistologic studies which showed that lymph nodes proximal to melanoma have strong suppressor cell activity. Antitumor effector mechanisms will be reduced by the presence of suppressor cell activity.

▶ Investigators at UCLA have identified what is apparently a "zoned" immunosuppression associated with the presence of suppressor T cells in the most proximal draining lymph nodes. The balance between killer cell and cytotoxic antibody formation in the immune response to a tumor, and the suppressor activity as manifested by immunoregulatory cells in regional lymph nodes, often seem tipped in favor of regulation rather than enhancement of the immune response. This may prove a fertile area for clinical intervention.—O. Jonasson, M.D.

Immunochemical and Functional Analysis of HLA Class II Antigens Induced by Recombinant Immune Interferon on Normal Epidermal Melanocytes
Masayuki Tsujisaki, Muneo Igarashi, Kohsaku Sakaguchi, Magdalena Eisinger, Meenhard Herlyn, and Soldano Ferrone (New York Med. College, Valhalla; Memorial Sloan Kettering Cancer Ctr., New York; and Wistar Inst. of Biology and Medicine, Philadelphia)
J. Immunol. 138:1310–1316, Feb. 15, 1987   9–12

HLA class II antigens may be acquired by cells undergoing malignant transformation, such as melanoma cells. A study was made of the effects of recombinant interferon (IFN-γ) on the expression and shedding of HLA antigens and of melanoma-associated antigens (MAA) by epidermal melanocytes. IFN-γ enhances the expression or shedding, or both, of HLA I antigens and that of the cytoplasmic MAA defined by monoclonal antibody 465.12S.

Melanocytes incubated with IFN-γ acquired HLA-DR, DQ, and DP antigens. In addition, incubation induced expression of the 96-kDa MAA recognized by MoAb CL203. Recombinant leukocyte interferon did not affect the expression of either type of antigen. Treated melanocytes did not become able to stimulate the proliferation of allogeneic lymphocytes. The HLA-DR antigens were most susceptible to induction by IFN-γ.

It appears that recombinant IFN-γ can induce the expression of HLA-DR antigens by normal melanocytes, but the effect is not specific for these antigens. Differential sensitivity of melanocytes to IFN-γ might explain the defection of HLA II antigens in only some primary lesions. The expression of HLA II antigens cannot induce proliferation of allogeneic T lymphocytes.

▶ Tumors and normal tissues show a heterogeneity of expression of HLA class II antigens and of response to enhancement of antigen production by immune interferon. These studies, conducted in normal cultured melanocytes, seek to identify the cells expressing HLA class II antigens and the mechanisms of bringing out this expression with the use of interferon. As is also true in current work on transplantation immunobiology reviewed in this volume, the antigenicity of the tissue involved and the regulation of antigen expression has become an area of intense interest and investigation. The complex interaction of viral infections, normal host defense mechanisms such as interferon, and antigen expression on either tumor or transplanted tissue seems a particularly productive avenue of research.—O. Jonasson, M.D.

Modulation of Estrogen Receptor by Insulin and Its Biologic Significance
Prabir K. Chaudhuri, Bina Chaudhuri, and Nili Patel (Loyola Univ. of Chicago, Maywood, Ill., and Hinsdale Hosp., Hinsdale, Ill.)
Arch. Surg. 121:1322–1325, November 1986   9–13

Insulin is involved in the maintenance and function of estrogen receptors and may influence the behavior of receptor-containing tissue. To assess the effect of insulin on an estrogen receptor-positive tumor, a hamster endometrial carcinoma cell line, receptor-positive, was studied in vitro and in vivo.

Endometrial carcinoma cells were grown for 72 hours in low- or high-insulin-containing medium. The cells in the high-insulin medium maintained their estrogen receptors, but no estrogen receptors were detectable in the cells that were maintained in the low-insulin medium.

The uptake of radioactive thymidine was much greater in cells which were grown in the low-insulin medium, thus implying an increased growth rate for these cells.

Streptozocin was used to induce diabetes in nine Golden Syrian hamsters, which were then inoculated with tumor cells. Ten normal hamsters were also inoculated. At 42 days the tumors in the diabetic animals were significantly larger than those in normal animals. Tumors from normal animals contained estrogen receptors; tumors from diabetic animals did not.

In vitro and in vivo studies demonstrate that insulin affects the maintenance of the estrogen receptor. Lower levels of insulin, such as those that are seen in diabetes, may lead to loss of the insulin receptor and faster growth of tumors.

▶ The potential effect of peptide hormones on steroid receptors is an interesting area of new investigation. In these experiments, the influence of insulin, a peptide hormone, on the estrogen receptor of a hamster endometrial carcinoma cell line, was examined in vitro and in vivo. Low levels of insulin in the medium or a diabetic insulin deficient host was associated with increased tumor growth, implying that insulin did affect the biologic behavior of this tumor. The control of antigen expression and of tumor cell growth is certainly multifactorial and complex and includes peptide hormones in regulation.—O. Jonasson, M.D.

Immunohistological Analysis of Lymphocyte Subpopulations Infiltrating Breast Carcinomas and Benign Lesions
S. von Kleist, J. Berling, W. Bohle, and C. Witterkind (Univ. of Freiburg and Hanover Med. School, West Germany)
Int. J. Cancer 40:18–23, July 1987   9–14

Inflammation and mononuclear cell infiltration often are taken as indicating host resistance against malignant growth. A series of monoclonal antibodies and serial cryosections of breast tissue from 84 cancer patients were utilized to characterize the infiltrating mononuclear cells. Thirty-two cases of benign breast disease also were studied (Table 1). Immunoperoxidase staining was carried out, and mononuclear infiltrates were quantified planimetrically.

T cell infiltration was classed as moderate in half the benign lesions, and as strong or very strong in 10% of cases. Such infiltrates were considerably more pronounced in malignant tumors (Table 2). T helper/inducer cells predominated in malignant tumors, while in benign samples the T helper/suppressor ratios were well balanced. A few monoclonal antibody Leu-7-reactive natural killer cells were found in stroma of breast tumors, but none were found in benign tissues.

Breast cancers often are infiltrated by T lymphocytes, but such cells are present chiefly in the stroma. Natural killer cells are not an impressive finding. Follow-up of patients with breast cancer will indicate whether it is prognostically useful to characterize subsets of mononuclear cells.

▶ It has long been assumed that the intensity of the lymphocyte response surrounding certain types of breast cancer is associated with outcome, with the implication that the more dense the mononuclear cell infiltrate, the greater the host defense mechanisms and the better the prognosis. This hypothesis has been examined in this paper, and scarce evidence is found to substantiate this old belief. NK cells, the cells presumably involved in tumor cell surveillance, were present in inverse proportion to the level of estrogen receptors, a relationship that could be further examined and, perhaps, exploited.—O. Jonasson, M.D.

TABLE 1.—LYMPHOCYTIC INFILTRATION OF BREAST LESIONS
IN RELATION TO THE HISTOLOGICAL TYPE OF THE TUMOR, AXILLARY
LYMPH-NODE METASTASES, ORGAN METASTASES, CLINICAL STAGE,
RECEPTORS FOR ESTROGENS, AND AGE OF PATIENTS*

	ICDO	Number of cases	O^1 *	$+^2$	$++^3$
Histological type					
Benign tissue		32	12	15	5
Gynecomastia		1	1	0	0
Hyperplasia		4	1	3	0
Mastopathy grade I		14	7	5	2
Mastopathy grade II		8	2	5	1
Fibroadenoma		3	1	2	0
Mastitis		2	0	0	2
Malignant tumors		85	7	34	44
Intraductal carcinoma	8500/2	2	0	0	2
Invasive mucinous carcinoma	8480/3	2	1	1	0
Invasive lobular carcinoma	8520/3	9	1	4	4
Invasive ductal carcinoma	8500/3	72	5	29	38
Axillary lymph-node metastases					
No LN metastases		42	10	15	17
Less than 3 LN metastases		29	2	15	12
3 or more LN metastases		14	0	6	8
Organ metastases					
+		8	0	6	2
Clinical stage					
I		21	2	10	9
II		40	4	11	25
IIIa		13	1	5	7
IIIb		3	0	2	1
IV		8	0	6	2
Receptors for estrogen					
< 10 fmol		21	0	5	16
10–30 fmol		10	0	7	3
> 30 fmol		49	8	20	21
Age in years					
<45		21	3	9	9
>45		96	16	40	40

*O_1, None: $+_2$, slight or moderate; $++_3$, strong or very strong lymphocytic infiltration.
(Courtesy of von Kleist, S., et al.: Int. J. Cancer 40:18–23, July 1987.)

TABLE 2.—INTENSITY OF T-CELL INFILTRATION (LEU-4)
IN BENIGN AND MALIGNANT BREAST LESIONS*

	T-cell infiltration			
	Slight	Moderate	Strong or very strong	Total
Benign lesions†	12	15	3	30
Carcinoma‡	7	34	42	83

*The difference between benign and malignant strong or very strong infiltrations
was statistically significant, e.g. $P < 0.001$.
†Without mastitis; (n=2).
‡Without carcinoma in situ; (n=2).
(Courtesy of von Kliest, S., et al.: Int. J. Cancer 40:18–23, July 1987.)

Alcohol Consumption and Breast Cancer in the Epidemiologic Follow-Up Study of the First National Health and Nutrition Examination Survey

Arthur Schatzkin, D. Yvonne Jones, Robert N. Hoover, Philip R. Taylor, Louise A. Brinton, Regina G. Ziegler, Elizabeth B. Harvey, Christine L. Carter, Lisa M. Licitra, Mary C. Dufour, and David B. Larson (Natl. Insts. of Health, Bethesda, Md.)
N. Engl. J. Med. 316:1169–1173, May 1987 9–15

Several epidemiologic studies have shown a correlation between alcohol consumption and breast cancer. This article presents the results of a cohort study, based on a sample of the U.S. population, that investigated the relation between moderate alcohol consumption and breast cancer incidence.

The study comprised 7,188 women, aged 25 to 74 years (mean age 49 years), who were examined during a 5-year period. Examination included a sociodemographic and medical history, a standardized medical examination, a dietary questionnaire, hematologic and biochemical tests, and anthropometry. The participants were traced and interviewed again about 10 years later. At follow-up, 121 cases of breast cancer that developed after the baseline examination were identified through hospital records or death certificates.

Results show that consumption of any amount of alcohol increased the risk of breast cancer by 50%–100%. There was a 40%–50% increase in risk among women who drank less than 5 gm of alcohol per day, equivalent to about three drinks per week. This finding is in contrast with the findings from two previously published reports that showed no increased risk for breast cancer at this low level of alcohol intake. The greatest risk in this study was noted among women who drank 5 gm of alcohol or more per day.

The authors suggest further epidemiologic studies of alcohol consumption and breast cancer; these should include data on the type of alcohol consumed and the timing of drinking during a woman's life.

▶ In this large study from the National Institutes of Health and a similar companion study from Harvard Medical School and School of Public Health (W. C. Willett, M. J. Stampfer, G. A. Colditz, et al.: *N. Engl. J. Med.,* 1987; 316:1174–1180) powerful statistical evidence is presented implicating alcohol ingestion with the development of breast cancer. How or what the causal relationship is between ingestion of alcohol and development of breast cancer has not been determined, but the association seems real and appropriate data should be sought when obtaining the history from patients with breast cancer.—O. Jonasson, M.D.

Presence of In Vivo-Activated T-Cells Expressing HLA-DR Molecules and IL-2 Receptors in Peripheral Blood of Patients With Nasopharyngeal Carcinoma

M. Lakhdar, R. Ellouz, H. Kammoun, S. Ben H'Tira, N. Khedhiri, R. Kastally, and W.H. Fridman (Lab. d'Immunologie Cellulaire Hôp. Habib Thameur, Tunis, Tunisia, Inst. Salah Azaiez, Tunis; and Inst. Curie, Paris)
Int. J. Cancer 39:663–669, June 1987   9–16

Epstein-Barr virus (EBV) is associated with both African Burkitt's lymphoma and undifferentiated nasopharyngeal carcinoma (NPC). Cell-mediated immunity was examined in patients with undifferentiated and differentiated NPC in North Africa, where the incidence of NPC is high. Thirty-seven newly diagnosed patients participated in the study. Immunofluorescence staining employed OKT3, OKT4, and OKT8 monoclonal antibodies. Lectin-induced lymphocyte proliferation was quantified. Increased proportions of OKT8 cells and large granular lymphocytes were present in patients with NPC, compared with healthy matched subjects. About one third of peripheral blood lymphocytes from patients were HLA-DR-positive and interleukin-2 receptor-positive cells. The cells proliferated normally when exposed to T cell lectins (PHA and concanavalin A); the response to pokeweed mitogen was increased. Natural killer activity against K562 cells was low, and the cells did not lyse HLA-matched EBV-transformed B cells.

Increased circulating T lymphocytes are present in patients with both differentiated and undifferentiated NPC. The activated T cells are not EBV-specific cytotoxic T lymphocytes or natural killer cells. They might be cytotoxic T cells directed against tumor-related antigens expressed on malignant epithelial cells. They might also be EBV-specific T suppressor cells, reported to be contained in the OKT8 subpopulation of T cells.

▶ In these investigations of the peripheral blood lymphocytes of patients with nasopharyngeal carcinoma associated with EBV, activated T cells of the OKT8-positive variety were found. The role of these activated lymphocytes and of antibody to EBV in patients with nasopharyngeal carcinoma is uncertain. Since these cells did not appear to be cytotoxic to EBV-infected cells, one of the possible conclusions is that these cells are EBV-specific suppressor cells. This particular model is interesting because of the spectrum of disease, from infectious mononucleosis through nasopharyngeal carcinoma, that is clearly associated with viral infection.—O. Jonasson, M.D.

Influence of Cellular DNA Content on Survival in Differentiated Thyroid Cancer

Heikki Joensuu, Pekka Klemi, Erkki Eerola, and Juhani Tuominen (Univ. of Turku, Finland)
Cancer 58:2462–2467, Dec. 1, 1986   9–17

Patients with several types of cancer do better with diploid than with aneuploid cancers. The import of cellular DNA content of differentiated thyroid cancer was explored in 125 patients, using a new flow cytometric

ANEUPLOIDY, DNA INDEX, AND CUMULATIVE SURVIVAL
CORRECTED FOR INTERCURRENT DEATHS IN 125 PATIENTS
WITH DIFFERENTIATED THYROID CANCER

Histologic type	Cumulative corrected survival at 5 years	Cumulative corrected survival at 10 years
Papillary (n = 82)		
Diploid n = 62 (75%)	95.7%	95.7%
Aneuploid n = 20 (24%)	90.5%	75.4%
Mean DNA index 1.34		
Follicular (n = 36)		
Diploid n = 16 (44%)	85.1%	85.1%
Aneuploid n = 20 (56%)	60.3%	53.6%
Mean DNA index 1.76		
Medullary (n = 7)		
Diploid n = 3 (43%)	1/1 (100%)	—
Aneuploid n = 20 (24%)	1/4 (25%)	0/3 (0%)
Mean DNA index 2.24		
Papillary, follicular, and medullary combined (n = 125)		
Diploid n = 81 (65%)	93.6%	93.6%
Aneuploid n = 44 (35%)	70.4%	61.1%
Mean DNA index 1.61		

(Courtesy of Joensuu, H., et al.: Cancer 58:2462–2467, Dec. 1, 1986.)

method that can be applied to archival paraffin-embedded material. The mean patient follow-up was 78 months.

One fourth of papillary tumors and more than half of follicular and medullary cancers were aneuploid (table). Aneuploidy was more frequent

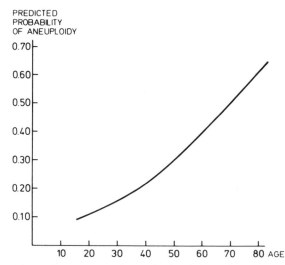

Fig 9–5.—Probability of DNA aneuploidy correlated with age at diagnosis. (Courtesy of Joensuu, H., et al.: Cancer 58:2462–2467, Dec. 1, 1986.)

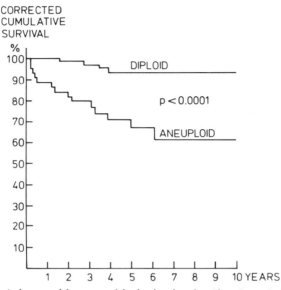

CORRECTED
CUMULATIVE
SURVIVAL

Fig 9–6.—Survival corrected for causes of death other than thyroid carcinoma in 81 diploid and 44 aneuploid differentiated thyroid carcinomas. (Courtesy of Joensuu, H., et al.: Cancer 58:2462–2467, Dec. 1, 1986.)

with advancing age (Fig 9–5) and was more common in moderately and poorly differentiated tumors and in large infiltrating primary tumors. Patients with diploid tumors had much better survival than those with aneuploid cancers. The survival advantage of diploid cancers persisted after correcting for other causes of death (Fig 9–6). Statistical analysis showed that age, follicular histology, and tumor size independently influenced survival. Tumor ploidy and histologic grade were prognostic factors only when analyzed alone.

Patients having aneuploid thyroid tumors have a poorer outlook than those with diploid tumors. The increased likelihood of aneuploidy in older patients helps explain the poor prognosis of such patients.

▶ These studies were very well done. The histologic material was carefully classified, the clinical information was complete, and the multivariant statistical analysis with the use of Cox's proportional hazard model, was thorough and important. The authors clearly demonstrated that aneuploidy and advancing age of the patient are closely linked, especially over the age of 45, and that these factors taken together convey substantial prognostic implications.—O. Jonasson, M.D.

Phenotypic Characterization of Lung Cancers in Fine Needle Aspiration Biopsies Using Monoclonal Antibody B72.3
William W. Johnston, Cheryl A. Szpak, Ann Thor, and Jeffrey Schlom (Duke Univ. and Natl. Cancer Inst., Bethesda, Md.)
Cancer Res. 46:6462–6470, December 1986   9–18

Fine needle aspiration biopsy has significant limitations and pitfalls in spite of its current effectiveness and accuracy. When interpreted in experienced laboratories, its reliability lies somewhat midway between that of tissue section from an open biopsy and that of purely exfoliated cells. A study was undertaken to determine the usefulness of monoclonal antibody B72.3, an IgGI immunoglobulin raised against a membrane-enriched extract of a human metastatic breast carcinoma, which recognizes a high-molecular weight, oncofetal tumor-associated glycoprotein, TAG-72, found in most adenocarcinomas. Of 318 fine needle aspirates from primary lung neoplasms, neoplasms metastatic to the lungs, and neoplasms metastatic from the lungs submitted for diagnostic cytologic interpretation, 127 (40%) contained tumor cells in the cell block. These were examined with monoclonal antibody B72.3. Eighteen randomly selected cases of benign lung lesions with adequate cellular material in the cell block were also evaluated.

In all of 14 acinar adenocarcinomas, all of five bronchioloalveolar carcinomas, and all of eight adenosquamous carcinomas, TAG-72 antigen was expressed. The monoclonal antibody B72.3 failed to stain cell blocks from 21 small cell carcinomas and one carcinoid tumor. There was positive antigen expression in the squamous cell carcinoma group in 4 of 6 well-differentiated lesions, 3 of 3 moderately differentiated lesions, and in 17 of 22 poorly differentiated lesions.

Primary lung tumors appear to fall into three antigenic groups on the basis of TAG-72 expression: (1) adenocarcinoma and adenosquamous carcinoma group, in which TAG-72 could be detected in all 27 tumors and was expressed strongly in 22 of 27 (81%); (2) a small cell tumor group, where no expression of TAG-72 could be detected in any of 22 tumors; and (3) squamous cell carcinomas and large cell carcinomas, in which TAG-72 was present in varying numbers. While it was expressed in 24 of 31 (77%) squamous cell carcinomas, its expression in at least 10% of tumor cells dropped to 11 of 31 cases (35%).

These studies with monoclonal antibody B72.3 have defined a tumor-associated glycoprotein antigen, TAG-72, expressed in certain neoplastic cells but absent or rare in benign lesions and in lung normal cells. In adenocarcinoma and the adenosquamous group of tumors it is most selectively expressed, and it is not expressed at all in small cell carcinoma. Examination of a cellular specimen obtained by fine needle aspiration biopsy of a lung tumor and examined by immunoperoxidase staining with monoclonal antibody B72.3 will accurately predict the phenotypic expression of TAG-72 and is a potentially useful tool in the differential diagnosis of lung neoplasms prior to surgical resection.

▶ The development of a panel of monoclonal antibodies detecting various tumor-associated antigens has permitted considerable application in diagnosis and perhaps in treatment of many malignancies. The monoclonal antibody B72.3, which recognizes an oncofetal tumor associated glycoprotein (TAG-72), has been of particular interest especially to this group at the National Cancer Institute. This antibody seems to quite specifically recognize adenocarcinomas and stains these cells strongly without staining normal mucus-producing or glandular epithelium. In these studies the antibody is used in an immunoperoxidase staining technique for histology and has enabled the histopathologist to clearly differentiate between mesothelial and other cells and carcinoma cells of many types.

This antibody has also been used by other investigators to carry isotopes to tumor site for localization of the tumor and even for delivery of cytotoxic agents. Specificity of the monoclonal antibodies is crucial in determining their usefulness as agents, and in this study the B72.3 antibody appeared to have a high degree of specificity.—O. Jonasson, M.D.

Increased Expression of the Epidermal Growth Factor Receptor on Human Colon Carcinoma Cells
Stephen J. Bradley, Geri Garfinkle, Elizabeth Walker, Ronald Salem, Lan Bo Chen, and Glenn Steele, Jr. (New England Deaconess Hosp. and Dana Farber Cancer Inst., Boston)
Arch. Surg. 121:1242–1247, November 1986   9–19

Epidermal growth factor (EGF) is a small polypeptide hormone that stimulates the growth of several types of cells and elicits the differentiation of some epithelial tissues. Several types of tumor cells express increased amounts of the EGF receptor. A monoclonal antibody to the EGF receptor was used to study its expression and function in human colon carcinoma cell lines and frozen tissue sections.

By indirect immunofluorescence, Western blotting, and I^{125} I-labeled EGF binding assays, all eight of the moderately well differentiated colon carcinoma cell lines showed increased expression of the EGF receptor, whereas five poorly differentiated colon carcinoma cell lines did not. Several frozen sections from moderately well differentiated colon carcinomas demonstrated elevated levels of the EGF receptor. Sections from normal colon tissue did not show elevated expression of the EGF receptor. Live cell immunofluorescent staining of a moderately well differentiated human carcinoma cell line demonstrated internalization of the EGF receptor-antibody complex.

Moderately well differentiated human carcinoma cells express increased amounts of the EGF receptor, as compared to normal colon tissue and poorly differentiated human carcinoma cells. The receptor appears to be intact and grossly functional. Increased expression of the EGF receptor, which bears a 90% sequence homology to the v-erb B oncogene product, may play a role in the generation of a transformed state. Internalization of the monoclonal antibody-receptor complex may present a target for immunotherapy.

▶ In these elegant studies, the investigators have used a monoclonal antibody to the EGF receptor and have demonstrated that increased expression of this receptor is found in well-differentiated human colon cancer cells and that this receptor appears to be functional and is internalized into the cell when the antibody attaches.

The role of increased epidermal growth factor on well-differentiated colon tissues but not on normal colonic epithelium or poorly differentiated cell lines raises questions concerning the possible role of EGF in causing transformation from a hyperplastic to a malignant lesion such as in polyposis or chronic inflammatory bowel disease. The results of further studies of colon tumor oncogenesis and possible relationships to the EGF receptor will be of considerable interest.—O. Jonasson, M.D.

Prevalence of *ras* Gene Mutations in Human Colorectal Cancers
Johannes L. Bos, Eric R. Fearon, Stanley R. Hamilton, Matty Verlaan-de Vries, Jacques H. van Boom, Alex J. van der Eb, and Bert Vogelstein (State Univ. of Leiden, The Netherlands, and Johns Hopkins Univ.)
Nature 327:293–297, May 1987   9–20

Activated *ras* genes in human tumors may go undetected in the NIH 3T3 transfection assay. A study was done using a combination of DNA hybridization methods and tissue sectioning techniques to show that *ras* gene mutations occur in more than one third of human colorectal cancers.

Twenty-seven tumors with large areas of tumor cells and relatively small numbers of nonneoplastic cells were studied. Studies of some tumors suggested that *ras* mutations might arise during the development of carcinoma from a preexisting adenoma. Of six tumors containing *ras* mutations and areas of adenoma and carcinoma, five had the mutation in both the adenoma and carcinoma. Mutations were present in 11 tumors in all; all occurred somatically. Ten were in the c-Ki-*ras* gene; nine, at codon 12 of the gene.

Most *ras* gene mutations in colorectal cancers are at codon 12 of the c-Ki-*ras* gene. The mutations usually precede the development of malignancy. Mutations in *ras* genes may occur frequently in adenomas, with only a small fraction of these progressing to malignancy.

Alternately, *ras* gene mutations may occur infrequently in adenomas, while those with such mutations have a high likelihood of progressing to malignancy. It is possible that the step promoting the adenoma-carcinoma sequence sometimes may be a mutation in the c-Ki-*ras* gene.

Detection of High Incidence of K-*ras* Oncogenes During Human Colon Tumorigenesis
Kathleen Forrester, Concepcion Almoguera, Kyuhyung Han, William E. Grizzle, and Manuel Perucho (State Univ. of New York at Stony Brook and Univ. of Alabama at Birmingham)
Nature 327:298–303, May 1987   9–21

A role for *ras* oncogenes in mammalian tumorigenesis is well documented in various carcinogen-induced animal tumor models. Activation of *ras* oncogenes by somatic mutation appears related to the initiation of carcinogenesis in these models. In addition, activated *ras* oncogenes are found in a significant proportion of human tumors.

The ribonuclease A mismatch cleavage method was used to detect point mutations in the first coding exon of the c-K-*ras* gene in a large panel of primary human colon tumors. Mutant genes were present at codon 12 in about 40% of 66 tumors. Mutations were not detected at other positions of the first coding exon. The presence of mutant oncogenes could not be related to the stage of progression. *Ras* oncogenes were, however, frequent in premalignant villous adenomas and in cancers arising in villous adenomas. Seven of eight colon tumors originating in villous adenomas contained c-K-*ras* genes mutant at the first coding exon, five at the first base of codon 12, and two at the second.

The association of somatic mutations at codon 12 of the c-K-*ras* gene with human colon tumors is more frequent than previously estimated using the NIH 3T3 transfection assay. Activated *ras* oncogenes apparently contribute importantly to tumor progression in this setting. The findings support a frequent association of *ras* mutational activation with the early stages of human tumorigenesis.

▶ These two studies (Abstracts 9–20 and 9–21), appearing simultaneously in *Nature,* describe the preliminary and very interesting observations of the role of certain oncogenes in the genesis of colon cancer in humans. The particular gene group that is studied encodes for proteins in the plasma membrane of cells in the colon and other tissues and is associated with specific point mutations in human tumor cells.

Both of these papers demonstrate the occurrence of *ras* gene mutations in human colorectal cancers, and both also document the presence of these findings in villous adenomas and other nonmalignant adenomas coexisting with the colon cancer. This suggests that the oncogene activation precedes the development of the adenoma and the carcinoma and is responsible for tumor progression.—O. Jonasson, M.D.

Inhibition of Established Rat Fibrosarcoma Growth by the Glucose Antagonist 2-Deoxy-D-Glucose
Kenneth A. Kern and Jeffrey A. Norton (Natl. Cancer Inst., Bethesda, Md.)
Surgery 102:380–385, August 1987   9–22

Sarcomas have high rates of glycolysis, suggesting a dependence on glucose for growth. It is possible that antimetabolites such as 2-deoxy-D-glucose (2-DG) will prevent tumor growth. The efficacy of 2-DG was studied in rats bearing methylcholanthrene-induced (MCA) rat fibrosarcoma. Animals inoculated subcutaneously with varying burdens of tumor cells received 2-DG in doses of 0.75, 1.5, or 1.75 gm/kg or saline, starting 3 days after tumor implantation and continuing for 10 days. Tissue levels of [^{14}C]-2-DG were estimated in tumor, brain, liver, and muscle tissue.

Tumor weights were lowered by 50%–70% in 2-DG-treated rats.

Toxicity was minimal at dose levels lower than 1.75 gm/kg. Tumor tissue had the highest level of radioactive 2-DG at 1 hour. Liver had the highest glucose-5-phosphatase activity, followed in order by brain, tumor, and muscle.

Growth of MCA fibrosarcoma is glucose-dependent, and the glucose antimetabolite 2-DG inhibits its growth. Treatment with 2-DG might prove useful in patients having unresectable, recurrent high-grade sarcomas. Toxicity to glucose-sensitive tissues might be lowered by supplying glycerol as a substrate. Accelerated glycolysis in malignant tissues may be a marker of altered gene expression for enzymes supporting the production of substrates for nucleic acid biosynthesis.

▶ These investigators have taken advantage of a particular biologic phenomenon of high glucose requirements in sarcomatous tumor growth and have demonstrated that deprivation of usable glucose is associated with inhibition of tumor growth in experimental models. These investigations have already been carried forward into clinical trials, and the approach seems quite reasonable if the toxicity of the glucose analogues can be managed satisfactorily.—O. Jonasson, M.D.

10 Skin, Subcutaneous Tissue, and the Hand

Conservative Treatment of Fingertip Injuries
Tune Ipsen, Peter Alex Frandsen, and Troels Barfred (Odense Univ., Denmark)
Injury 18:203–205, May 1987   10–1

Traumatic fingertip amputations are common injuries that frequently lead to long periods of discomfort and convalescence. Many surgical procedures have been described. The authors evaluated conservative treatment in a prospective series of 81 patients with loss of fingertip of at least 1 sq cm or at least 0.5 sq cm in children. Only patients seen within 6 hours of injury were included. Fifty-three patients with 61 injuries were evaluable. Group A patients with no bone exposed were managed by washing with aqueous solution of quaternary ammonium compound and dressing with Vaseline gauze. Group B patients, with bone exposed or covered by less than 2 mm of subcutaneous tissue, had loose bone and nail fragments excised and any protruding bone nibbled down until at least 3 mm of soft tissue covered the bone. These patients received antibiotics for 1 week.

The average healing time was 25 days and was similar for patients in both groups. Sharp injuries and crush injuries healed in similar periods. An average of 22 working days were lost. Cold intolerance was present at 6 months in 36% of fingertips, and tender stumps occurred in 26%. Two-point discrimination was slightly increased in the injured fingers. No patient complained of stiffness. The appearances were considered good in 67% of patients and poor in 5%. No patient underwent secondary surgery. Two patients in each group had superficial infection.

Conservative treatment is recommended as a simple, safe approach to fingertip loss, even if bone is exposed in the wound. The treatment is inexpensive, and special surgical skill is not required. The results are cosmetically acceptable to patients. Surgery is performed if associated hand injury precludes open treatment or if finger length or nail shape is critical.

▶ There is no question that too much surgery is performed for fingertip injuries. Only rarely is a complex flap or even a free graft indicated. Loss of a few millimeters of length is a small price to pay for rapid healing and return to full activity. The old principle, "If it is hard, it is wrong," is generally applicable.—E.E. Peacock, Jr., M.D.

The Venous Skin Graft Method for Repairing Skin Defects of the Fingers

Mitsuo Yoshimura, Takao Shimada, Shinichi Imura, Koji Shimamura, and Shigeki Yamauchi (Fukui Med. School and Kanazawa Univ., Japan)
Plast. Reconstr. Surg. 79:243–248, February 1987   10–2

A new skin graft method has been developed for use where conventional reconstructive methods are difficult to apply, as with multidigital injuries, long and narrow skin defects, or defects on the radial side of the index finger or the ulnar side of the little finger. Skin from the forearm or dorsal aspect of the foot is taken along with the subcutaneous small vein and subcutaneous tissues, and both ends of the vein are joined to the dig-

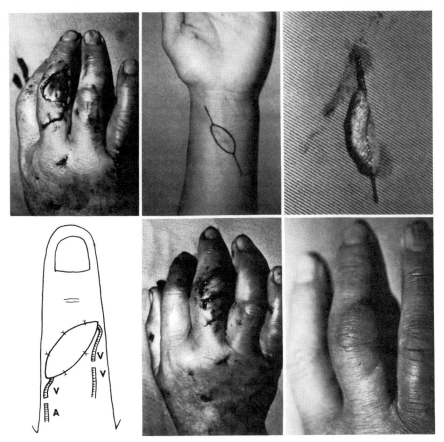

Fig 10–1.—A 45-year-old woman with open dislocation of the proximal interphalangeal joint of the right middle finger. The right index and ring fingers also sustained crushing injury. *Above, left:* the 3- × 1-cm skin defect on dorsal aspect of middle finger proximal interphalangeal joint. *Above, center:* the design of the 3.1- × 1.3-cm flap and 6-cm length vein. *Above, right:* venous skin raised from the forearm, ready for transfer. *Below, left:* the distal end of the vein is anatomosed with a digital artery, and the proximal end of the vein is sutured to the subcutaneous vein of the middle finger. *Below, center:* flap grafted over skin defect immediately after skin graft. *Below, right:* 6 months postoperatively, grafted flap is matched to the skin of the finger. (Courtesy of Yoshimura, M., et al.: Plast. Reconstr. Surg. 79:243–248, February 1987.)

ital vessels. Either both ends of the vein are joined to the digital veins, in a "cutaneous vein graft" procedure, or one end of the vein is anastomosed to a digital artery and the other to the subcutaneous vein in a "venous skin graft" or "venous free flap" procedure (Fig 10–1). Microsurgical technique is used with both methods. Anticoagulants generally are not given systemically after operation.

Venous skin grafts were done on 13 digits of 11 patients, and complete survival was achieved in 12 instances. Partial superficial necrosis developed in one digit. The distal part of the flexor forearm served as the donor site in the successful cases. Ten wounds healed within 3 weeks of operation. The thin subcutaneous fat of the grafted skin takes well to the finger. Any aspect of the finger can be managed in this way. Immobilization is not necessary postoperatively. The wound is completely resurfaced in a single operation. Injured digital arteries may be used, although this is not preferable.

▶ Because cellular organs such as kidney and spleen cannot be perfused in a retrograde manner, it should not be assumed that primarily fibrous structures such as skin have similar circulation. Arteriolized venous perfusion has been shown to be possible by several investigators. This paper reinforces the principle that nonconventional vascular perfusion of a composite graft such as skin can be performed when indicated.—E.E. Peacock, Jr., M.D.

Long-Term Follow-Up on Tendon Transfers to the Extensors of the Wrist and Fingers in Patients With Cerebral Palsy

M. Mark Hoffer, Maxine Lehman, and Margaret Mitani (Univ. of California, Irvine)
J. Hand. Surg. 11A:836–840, November 1986 10–3

Tendon transfers to improve hand function in selected cerebral palsy patients with active finger extension have given good results for many years. The long-term follow-up in a group of cerebral palsy patients who underwent tendon transfers to the extensors of the wrist and fingers is described.

The study comprised 38 patients, including ten who had poor hand placement, sensibility, or motor control and 28 patients who had better preoperative criteria. Each patient was evaluated preoperatively and postoperatively for intelligence, sensibility, hand placement, range of motion, muscle control, and hand function. The patients were divided into three groups. Group A included ten patients who had no functional gain. Group B included 11 patients who had 12 tendon transfers to the extensor carpi radialis brevis muscle, which resulted in functional gains. Group C included 17 patients who had tendon transfers to the extensor digitorum communis muscle, which resulted in functional gains.

The ten patients in Group A who had no functional gains already had poor preoperative criteria. Of the 11 patients in Group B, five patients developed wrist extension postures with difficulty in release that ultimately required division of the transferred tendon in two of these patients. Division decreased extension contracture, but it did not increase the patients' ability to open their hands. All patients in Group C had improved release and improved overall hand function.

It appears that only patients with active finger extension should be selected if good results with transfer operations are to be achieved. Preoperative electromyography should be performed to eliminate the selection of any continuously active or out-of-phase muscle for transfer.

▶ It is probably time to stop talking about the value of reconstructive hand surgery in patients with cerebral palsy. Cerebral palsy is not a clinical diagnosis specific enough to be meaningful in discussing reconstructive hand surgery. The problems are varied and complex. Each patient must be looked at and analyzed as an individual problem. The results of large groups of patients are not meaningful in individual analysis and planning.—E.E. Peacock, Jr., M.D.

The Treatment of Amputation Neuromas in Fingers With a Centrocentral Nerve Union
Moshe Kon and Joannis J.A.M. Bloem (Soroka Univ., Israel; Ben-Gurion Univ. of the Negev, Israel; and Free Univ. Hosp., Amsterdam)
Ann. Plast. Surg. 18:506–510, June 1987   10–4

The treatment of painful neuromas in the hand and fingers remains difficult. The authors have used a method of centrocentral union with an autologous nerve graft to treat digital neuromas. The neuromas are mobilized under tourniquet control, using an operating microscope, and the nerve is transected proximally enough so that no intraneural scar binds the fascicles. An end-to-end repair is then carried out between the two proximal digital nerve stumps, using 10–0 nylon sutures. One of the nerves is severed proximally to provide a 5–10-mm autologous graft. A second tension-free end-to-end repair is then done (Fig 10–2).

Eighteen males with 32 symptomatic neuromas of the fingers and disabling symptoms underwent this operation. Seven patients had been operated on previously. Two patients required revision of a centrocentral union done without nerve grafting because of recurrent neuroma formation. One patient has required reexploration for recurrent neuroma. Decreased sensation was the rule, and some patients had mild sensitivity to percussion at the site of nerve union. Nevertheless, all patients were definitely improved and had relief of disabling pain.

This method of treating symptomatic neuromas in the digits has proved generally successful. Careful approximation of the epineurium is very important. A study of the value of centrocentral union in preventing neuroma formation after finger amputation is in progress.

▶ The reason why a cross nerve neurorrhaphy should reduce neuroma formation is not clear but there is no question about it doing so. A similar effect can be obtained by using a small segment of free nerve graft and reversing the po-

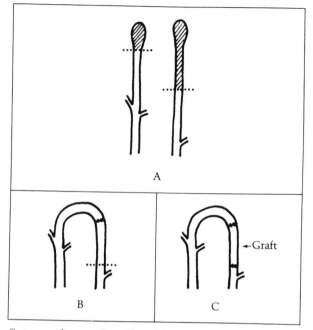

Fig 10–2.—Centrocentral nerve union with graft for bilateral neuromas. **A,** transection of both digital nerves. **B,** end-to-end repair and proximal transection of one nerve. **C,** second end-to-end repair completed. (Courtesy of Kon, M., and Bloem, J.J.A.M.: Ann. Plast. Surg. 18:506–510, June 1987.)

larity. There is probably an important principle of peripheral neurobiology involved; it is yet to be elucidated.—E.E. Peacock, Jr., M.D.

Symptomatic Relief Following Carpal Tunnel Decompression With Normal Electroneuromyographic Studies

Dean S. Louis and Fred M. Hankin (Univ. of Michigan)
Orthopedics 10:434–436, March 1987

10–5

   Normal electrodiagnostic findings sometimes cause surgeons not to operate for carpal tunnel syndrome even if classic symptoms are present. A review of 174 patients with a presumptive diagnosis of carpal tunnel syndrome showed that 88% of patients had electrodiagnostic evidence of median nerve entrapment. Twenty-two patients had normal nerve conduction studies and electromyographic (EMG) findings. Marked symptomatic improvement followed carpal tunnel release, which was done as an outpatient procedure. Epineurotomies and internal neurolyses were not routinely done. Despite the absence of electrodiagnostic abnormality, patients were relieved of pain, numbness, and tingling. The average time to resumption of usual work and vocational activities was about 6 weeks.
   The decision to perform carpal tunnel release should be based on the history, physical findings, radiographic assessment and, at times, the electrodiagnostic findings. The history and examination will suffice for diag-

nosis in 90% of cases. Electrodiagnostic studies should not be relied on in deciding whether to operate. They may, however, be helpful in diagnosing a concomitant peripheral neuropathy or in localizing a more proximal site of compression as in pronator teres syndrome.

▶ Electroneuromyographic studies are of little value except in relieving anxiety in some patients. Experienced hand surgeons know that the results of decompression of the median nerve in the carpal canal do not correlate with either positive or negative electroneuromyographic study. Clinical evidence of compression of the median nerve should be treated regardless of the electroneuromyographic findings and such studies are probably best reserved for patients who require complimentary studies before agreeing to surgery.—E.E. Peacock, Jr., M.D.

A Combined Regimen of Controlled Motion Following Flexor Tendon Repair in "No Man's Land"
Jimmy A. Chow, Linwood J. Thomes, Sam Dovelle, William H. Milnor, Alan E. Seyfer, and Allan C. Smith (Walter Reed Army Med. Ctr.)
Plast. Reconstr. Surg. 79:447–455, March 1987   10–6

Since 1981 the authors have used the "Washington regimen," which incorporates the features of active extension against rubber band passive flexion with those of therapist-assisted passive extension and passive flexion after repair of flexor tendons in the hand.

In this prospective study complete lacerations of the flexor digitorum profundus and flexor digitorum superficialis in zone 2 of 44 digits were treated, 29 with delayed primary repairs and 15 with immediate primary repairs. Repair of both the flexor digitorum profundus and the flexor digitorum superficialis tendons was performed in 25 digits; in 21 digits only the flexor digitorum profundus was repaired.

For the first 4 weeks after flexor tendon repair, the Brooke Army Hospital modification of the rubber band passive flexion splint is used in conjunction with voluntary active extension of the interphalangeal joints. Modification of the rubber band traction system includes a "palmar pulley" that is made with a safety pin, which is placed at the distal palmar crease, and a nylon fishing line that is attached to a fingernail hook, which runs through the eye of the safety pin to a rubber band which is anchored at the proximal forearm (Fig 10–3).

Modifications by the authors have changed the direction of the fingernail traction, thereby increasing passive flexion of the interphalangeal joints by pulling the fingertip to the distal palmar crease of the hand. By increasing joint flexion tendon excursion in the flexor sheath is maximized.

For the first 2 weeks after tenorrhaphy full passive extension and passive flexion exercises of the proximal and distal interphalangeal joints are performed daily to safeguard against contracture at the interphalangeal joints. On the 28th day rubber band traction is discontinued, and for 2

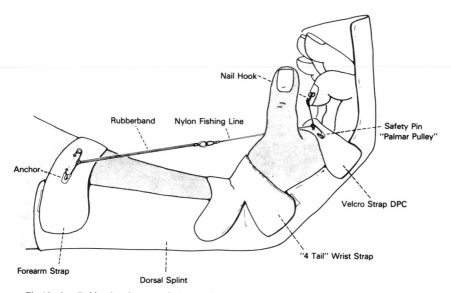

Fig 10–3.—Rubber-band passive flexion orthosis (Brooke Army Hosp. modification) with "palmar pulley" at distal palmar crease and nylon fishing line attached to rubber band. Dorsal splint is fabricated with low-temperature thermoplastic material and extends from upper forearm to tip of fingers. (Courtesy of Chow, J.A., et al.: Plast. Reconstr. Surg. 79:447–455, March 1987.)

weeks the patient performs hourly finger motion exercises of active flexion followed by passive flexion and active extension. Bunnell blocking exercises are instituted to improve the range of active flexion of the fingers 2 months after surgery, if deemed necessary.

By using the Strickland formula of total active motion of the interphalangeal joints, 36 fingers were rated excellent, 7 were rated good, 1 was rated fair, and none was rated poor. With the Louisville system of evaluating pulp-to-palm distance and extension lag, 38 fingers were rated excellent, 5 were rated good, 1 was rated fair, and none was rated poor. There was no statistical difference between results of delayed and immediate primary repair.

The authors believe this study is the first to advocate a combined regimen that uses the technique of rubber band passive flexion with active extension and the technique of controlled passive extension and passive flexion.

The modification of the rubber band traction orthosis provides a greater and more natural range of passive flexion of the fingers with a maximal excursion of the repaired tendons. The authors believe this accounts for the nearly normal range of active flexion in these patients after 6 weeks of rehabilitation. No patient required secondary reconstructive tendon surgery of the tendon.

▶ It is not possible to prevent fibrous adhesions around free flexor tendon grafts or flexor tendon repair by forced motion. It may be possible to influence favorably the length and physical properties of adhesions by controlled motion provided the blood supply is not interrupted. Clinical experience suggests that a rubber band is not needed to exercise good judgement.—E.E. Peacock, Jr., M.D.

Classification of the Main Tenodesis Techniques Used in Hand Surgery
Marc P. Revol and Jean Marie Servant (Hôpital St. Louis, Paris)
Plast. Reconstr. Surg 79:237–242, February 1987   10–7

The authors present a simple classification of the main types of tenodesis, which is based on the theoretical mechanical effects of different techniques. This classification separates simple tenodesis, which overrides only one joint, from dynamic tenodesis, which crosses two or more joints, and also subdivides "direct" and "crossed" dynamic tenodesis.

Simple tenodesis, by overriding only one joint, has a purely passive ligament-like effect. The profundus tenodesis is the simplest example and is sometimes used in chronic zone 1 division with an intact sublimis. "Lasso" tenodesis is another example. It was used by Zancolli to correct clawing of some quadriplegic restored hands.

A dynamic tenodesis, by definition, crosses two or more joints between its origin and insertion, thus having a double effect. One is purely passive, ligament-like, as a simple tenodesis, and the other is "activated" or automatic, being the tenodesis effect and results from active motion in one of the involved joints.

In direct dynamic tenodesis both extremities of the tendon are on the same side, dorsal or volar, of the flexion-extension axes of the involved joints; it is most usually used when the proximal joint still has at least one good motor, flexor or extensor, with the direct tenodesis then replacing the distal joint antagonist motor, extensor or flexor. The flexion of one activates the extension of the other when two adjacent joints are involved.

In crossed dynamic tenodesis the extremities of the tendon are situated on both sides of the flexion-extension axes of the involved joints. This is mostly used when the distal joint still has at least one efficient motor, flexor or extensor, with the crossed dynamic tenodesis then replacing the antagonist motor of the proximal joint. The flexion of one activates the flexion of the other when two adjacent joints are involved.

If the proximal joint retains an active motor opposite the tenodesis fixation also, the reciprocal tenodesis effect tends to replace the distal motor of the joint agonist. One example is provided by the normal lateral retinacular ligaments of the digits, which are called oblique bands by Landsmeer or longitudinal cords by Zancolli. Both have the same physiologic effect as crossed dynamic tenodesis. All other examples are provided by palliative surgical techniques for intrinsic muscle paralysis.

By using a tendinous graft that is sutured proximally on the extensor digitorum communis, the Srinivasan tenodesis uses the crossed dynamic tenodesis effect but is, in fact, a real transfer of the extensor digitorum communis on itself. The authors believe that this technique is more an "autotransfer" than a true tenodesis because its normal extension action on the basis of the proximal phalanx is impeded by the tenodesis, which rather helps with the extension of the distal joints.

▶ The editor is not so concerned about the classification or nomenclature of tenodesis procedures as he is that surgeons be reminded that tenodesis is a superb way to manage a number of tendon and joint afflictions in the upper extremity. Some tenodeses undergo change in length with time but most are stable, extra-articular, permanent solutions to difficult problems. Moreover, they are relatively inexpensive, quick, and dependable. Because many flexor tendon repairs turn out to be a tenodesis in the wrong position, intentional tenodesis in a correct position would not only have been less expensive and quicker than the more complicated reconstructive procedure but would also give a better functional result.—E.E. Peacock, Jr., M.D.

Morbidity in the Forearm Flap Donor Arm
J.G. Boorman, J.A. Brown, and P.J. Sykes (St. Lawrence Hosp., Chepstow, Wales)
Br. J. Plast. Surg. 40:207–212, March 1987   10–8

The authors undertook a retrospective study of morbidity in the donor arm of 27 patients after the use of a radial forearm flap. In a previous study of this procedure disquiet was voiced about the possible deleterious effect on the hand after the radial artery was removed; in another study the cosmetic appearance of the donor site gave concern; and in a third study complications arose in 15 patients after the use of this flap. Twenty-seven of 35 patients who received radial forearm flaps between August 1982 and August 1985 participated in this study. Age ranged from 11 to 80 years (average age, 52 years). Review after surgery ranged from 2 to 36 months, with all but 3 patients being at least 9 months postoperation at time of review.

Bone in the flap was included in 13 patients, and four of the 13 sustained fractures of the radius within 6 weeks of the operation; two were asymptomatic. In 11 of the 13 no difference between the fracture and nonfracture groups was found in either length or cross-sectional area of bone that was removed. There was no loss of range of movement at the elbow in any patient. Except in fracture cases, there was only occasional stiffness of the wrist, and other movements were unaffected.

Patients with fractures fared worst with regard to hand movement; they had an average of 50% weakness of grip and pinch in the operated arm. The patients without bone in the flaps had normal power.

In 12 of 25 free flaps the radial artery was reconstructed, and seven grafts were patent at follow-up. There were no clinical vascular problems in the hand, whether or not there was reconstruction of the artery. No patient admitted any sensory disturbance or intolerance to cold around the donor site. There was no complaint about appearance of the donor arm, but at least one patient had a significant deformity.

The major morbidity was in patients who had sustained a fracture after removal of a segment of radius and had limitation of power and range of movement. It appears that if fractures can be avoided, movement in the donor arm will be little affected. Factors that predispose to fractures may be the amount of bone removed, age, inadequate immobilization, and ischemia. No patient in this study had clinical signs of ischemia, either when the flap was elevated or when the procedure was reviewed. Flaps that contain skin alone produce few complications, but including bone leads to greater defects in contour and risk of fracture.

No benefit to the patient could be found from artery reconstruction, although 60% were patent at follow-up. By placing the skin paddle away from the nerve on the volar aspect, sensory disturbances that are usually related to the radial nerve can be minimized.

▶ Fascination with the fact that a free or pedicle forearm flap can be transplanted to the hand is responsible for a serious drop in standards of what flap coverage of a hand should be. Obsession with the fact that a free transplant can be performed does not make up for the placement of functionally incorrect suture lines, skin of the wrong texture, and hideous donor site deformities in visible sites. In spite of the recent popularity of a free forearm flap to resurface the hand, the editor feels that there are very little, if any, good indications for such a flap and that the procedure is being vastly overused. A split-thickness skin graft covering the donor site on the forearm is an avoidable cosmetic complication.—E.E. Peacock, Jr., M.D.

Malignant Fibrous Histiocytoma Involving a Digit
Fred. M. Hankin, Rebecca C. Hankin, and Dean S. Louis (Univ. of Michigan and William Beaumont Hosp., Royal Oak, Mich.)
J. Hand. Surg. [Am.] 12A:83–86, January 1987   10–9

Malignant fibrous histiocytoma (MFH) involving the upper extremity has been reported, but skeletal involvement of the hand has not. This case report warrants presentation because of the specific location and unusual clinical course of MFH of bone involving the hand.

Man, 42, had caught his right ring finger in a file cabinet drawer. Initial radiographs were read as "consistent with a crushing injury to the distal phalanx." After physical therapy, "pressure point treatments," a program of soaks for a shingles diagnosis, an ointment for a fungal infection diagnosis, and a recommendation of an orally administered antibiotic for treatment of a soft-tissue infection, he was referred to the authors' institution 10 months after the onset of his symptoms. Results of a physical examination showed a markedly enlarged distal phalanx with a 20-degree flexion contracture of the proximal interphalangeal joint. Along the palmar aspect of the fourth web space, there were several small excrescences. Radiographs demonstrated dissolution of the distal phalanx and radial aspect of the middle phalanx. Biopsies of the distal phalanx and proximal satellite lesions were performed, and histopathologic examination showed a spindle cell tumor infiltrating dermis and subcutaneous tissue, which was interpreted as MFH. No evidence of metastatic disease to the lungs was shown on further examination. A fourth ray resection was performed to obtain a wide local excision; the middle phalanx contained the same neoplasm. Ten years later, the patient had no evidence of local recurrence of metastatic disease.

When both soft tissue and bone involvement are present, MFH of soft tissue with secondary extension into osseous structure must be considered. Radiographic changes of the distal phalanx preceded local soft-tissue problems, which indicated bone as the primary tumor site. This case is unusual because of its location, the manner in which the neoplasm was initially managed, and the length of follow-up. Factors in this patient's 10-year survival rate might include the peripheral anatomical location and the histologic characteristics of the specific lesion. Proper and accurate evaluation remains mandatory for all chronic lesions of the hand.

▶ Malignant fibrous histiocytoma seems to turn up once or twice in the experience of every surgeon who takes care of hands. It should be remembered that the histologic evaluation of the degree of malignancy is the most important determination. Generally, it is not necessary to perform procedures that destroy function in patients who have a low grade malignant fibrous histiocytoma. Amputation and radiation are not necessary in low grade malignant tumors.—E.E. Peacock, Jr., M.D.

11 The Breast

Xeromammographic Diagnosis of Carcinoma of the Breast in Office Practice
Linda Warren Burhenne, J. Donald Longley, and H. Joachim Burhenne (Univ. of British Columbia, Vancouver, Canada)
Surg. Gynecol. Obstet. 164:452–456, May 1987   11–1

The authors reviewed data on 12,317 patients referred consecutively for xeromammography to an office consultative practice in 1983–1984. Both craniocaudal and lateral positive-mode xeroroentgenograms were obtained for nearly all patients. Further projections occasionally were obtained. In women aged younger than 30 years, only lateral negative-mode studies were performed, with supplemental frontal views when needed.

A total of 382 histologically proved breast cancers were diagnosed roentgenographically in this population. About 55% of women were symptomatic, while 45% were examined for screening purposes. The detection rate was 33 per 1,000 for all cancers and 7.6 per 1,000 for clinically occult cancers. The yield ratio for biopsy in 93 patients with clinically occult lesions was 36%. The cost for diagnosing one occult breast cancer was $10,657 (Canadian). The cost per cancer diagnosed was about $2,500.

Mammographic screening of women aged older than 40 years can be expected to yield a significant number of occult and potentially curable breast cancers. This can be achieved at a safe radiation dose with a minimum of unnecessary surgical treatment. Mammography was 94% sensitive in the present population. The biopsy yield ratio for mammography was 36%.

▶ The real question is whether xeromammographic diagnosis of carcinoma can reduce the unacceptably high incidence of negative biopsies caused by over-reading classical mammograms. Over 70% negative excisional biopsies is too high in the judgement of the editor.—E.E. Peacock, Jr., M.D.

"For" or "Against" Bone Scintigraphy of Patients With Breast Cancer
Stoyan G. Derimanov (Veliko Turnovo, Bulgaria)
Nucl. Med. Commun. 8:79–86, 1987   11–2

Opinions vary widely regarding the value of bone scintigraphy in evaluating patients with breast cancer. Review was made of the bone scintigraphic findings in 422 patients with breast cancer examined in 1979–1985. The average patient age was 56 years. Scintigraphy was performed using ^{99m}Tc-phosphon and a gamma camera with color display.

Scintigrams were positive in 30.6% of patients with skeletal symptoms and in 6.1% of those without such symptoms. The proportion of positive studies varied from 14% to 42%, depending on the stage of cancer. All patients scanned preoperatively had normal findings. Bone metastases became apparent after periods ranging from 21 to 51 months. Metastases were most prevalent in the spinal column alone, and in both the spine and pelvis.

Bone scintigraphy is appropriate before or after operation in patients with breast cancer if there is clinical or laboratory evidence suggesting skeletal abnormality. Bone scintigraphy is part of the evaluation of patients with stage II or more advanced disease.

▶ Unless the patient is in a drug study that requires baseline data, the case for performing bone scintigraphy in asymptomatic patients does not seem sound to the editor. Since there is no cure for breast cancer which has metastasized to bone, there seems little point in demonstrating questionable lesions that are not causing symptoms, particularly in elderly patients. Where patients are being studied to evaluate experimental treatment, however, bone scintigraphy can produce valuable data and should be performed for that purpose.—E.E. Peacock, Jr., M.D.

Lumpectomy vs Mastectomy: The Costs of Breast Preservation for Cancer
Eric Muñoz, Felix Shamash, Murry Friedman, Ira Teicher, and Leslie Wise (Long Island Jewish Med. Ctr., New Hyde Park, N.Y., and State University of New York at Stony Brook)
Arch. Surg. 121:1297–1301, November 1986   11–3

Conservative treatment of potentially curable breast cancer is rapidly gaining acceptance in this country, and the authors have evaluated the costs which are related to this shift from extensive to minimal surgery plus irradiation. Financial records were obtained on 79 patients who were treated for either stage I or stage II breast carcinoma in 1983 and 1984.

For lumpectomy patients total mean charges for hospital and surgeon were computed and included those for lumpectomy, axillary dissection, and postoperative 6-week radiation therapy, as well as hospital outpatient charges and fees of the radiation therapist. Financial charges to the mastectomy patient included hospital inpatient charges and fees of the surgeon. No fees of other physicians were included in either group.

Of the 79 patients 49 had lumpectomy and 30 had mastectomy; none had complications or required another operation. Mean length of stay for lumpectomy patients was 7.9 days; for mastectomy patients mean stay was 9.9 days.

Mean total physician charges per patient were 49.3% greater for lumpectomy than for mastectomy (Fig 11–1), but mean hospital inpatient charges were 27.6% higher for mastectomy than for lumpectomy patients. Mean total hospital and physician charges were 37% greater for lumpectomy than for mastectomy patients, a significantly higher rate.

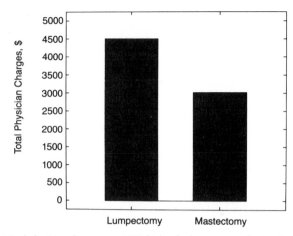

Fig 11–1.—Total physician charges were 50% higher for lumpectomy plus irradiation than for mastectomy. (Courtesy of Muñoz, E., et al.: Arch. Surg. 121:1297–1301, November 1986.)

Although hospital inpatient and surgeons' fees were significantly lower for lumpectomy, postoperative radiation therapy costs made it markedly more expensive than mastectomy. The data suggest the importance of complementing local excision with postoperative irradiation, but it is possible there may be subsets of lumpectomy patients who can be identified that do not benefit from radiation therapy.

Financial incentives which stem from the diagnosis related groups in-hospital payment system may encourage hospital administrators to support lumpectomy over mastectomy. Hospital care for lumpectomy plus axillary dissection may make this procedure more expensive than simple lumpectomy, and hospitals may be entitled to extra reimbursement.

Proposed changes in physician payment, including a system whereby reimbursement would be divided by all practitioners that are involved in the patient care, could also have a marked effect on which therapy is to be used. To be equitable, because there are higher physician costs involved in lumpectomy than in mastectomy patients, the system would have to provide for these costs. This study made it clear that the surgical health payment systems for physicians could provide financial incentives to encourage the use of one or the other of these two breast cancer therapies.

If a subset of lumpectomy patients who need local excision only can be identified, the relatively large expense that is related to radiation therapy can be obviated in certain cases. Hospital inpatient costs may be reducible for both operations by reducing lengths of stay and use of ancillary services. Extended care facilities may be able to provide adequate postoperative management during the latter part of a routine recovery for either procedure, thus improving efficiency.

▶ Charges included in this study did not take into consideration subsequent plastic surgery often needed to make a postlumpectomy acceptable cosmetically. Lumpectomy is a popular slogan now. It seems likely to this editor that it is a fad that will fade when more data are available.—E.E. Peacock, Jr., M.D.

Is It Necessary to Irradiate the Breast After Conservative Surgery for Localized Cancer?

Nemetallah A. Ghossein, Jacques Vilcoq, Patricia Stacey, and Bernard Asselain (Albert Einstein College of Medicine, New York, and Inst. Curie, Paris)
Arch. Surg. 122:913–917, August 1987   11−4

Trends toward less radical surgery for breast cancer make the issue of how much radiotherapy to administer most important. Postoperative radiotherapy was given to 201 patients with breast cancer following limited surgery, and the patients were followed for 5 years. A large majority of patients (187) had T2 lesions and underwent either biopsy excision or segmental resection. The breast and homolateral lymph drainage areas were treated with megavoltage therapy. Another 324 patients with tumors 3 cm or less in size and N0 stage were studied for distant dissemination in relation to local control.

The rate of recurrence at 5 years was 14%, less than half the reported rate for patients having limited surgery but no radiotherapy. Patients with positive margins who were irradiated had a recurrence rate of 13%. In the larger group, patients free of local disease or those who had recurrences more than 5 years after treatment had better survival than those who failed locally within 5 years (Fig 11−2).

It appears that breast irradiation following conservative surgery for breast cancer lowers the rate of local recurrence and reduces the need for

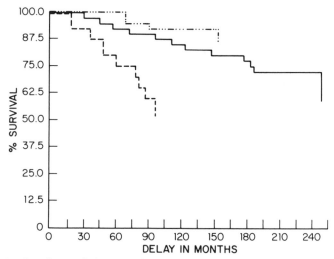

Fig 11−2.—Overall survival of patients who remained free of local disease *(solid line)* and of patients who had local recurrence within 5 years *(dashed line)* and after 5 years *(dashed and dotted line)*. (Courtesy of Ghossein, N.A., et al.: Arch. Surg. 122:913−917, August 1987.)

salvage mastectomy. Some patients may do well after wide local excision alone, but at present it is unwise to take this approach if the goal of conservative treatment is breast preservation.

Extent of Axillary Dissection Preceding Irradiation for Carcinoma of the Breast
Gordon F. Schwartz, Domenico M. D'Ugo, and Anne L. Rosenberg (Jefferson Med. Coll., Philadelphia, and Univ. Cattolica del Sacro Cuore, Rome)
Arch. Surg. 121:1395–1398, December 1986   11–5

The single most important criterion presaging the outcome of a patient with breast cancer is generally accepted to be the status of the axillary lymph nodes. To determine the likelihood of missing "skip metastases," defined as metastases demonstrated in at least one node at level II or III, or in the interpectoral fascia, without concomitant node metastases to even a single node at level I, the records of 127 patients from a single surgical practice who had at least one axillary or interpectoral node demonstrating metastatic disease were studied. Sixty-one patients (mean age, 51 years) had undergone radical mastectomy, and 66 had undergone modified radical mastectomy.

The number of nodes retrieved from the specimens ranged from 12 to 75 (mean, 39), with 34 for radical and 43 for modified radical mastectomies. There were 17 women with skip metastases, representing 13.4% of the women with positive nodes; within this group 15 patients had skip metastases to axillary nodes; two had involvement of interpectoral nodes only. Two patients had metastases to level III only and neither one had involved interpectoral nodes. Only multicentricity incidence and history of contralateral breast cancer suggests the possible chance of encountering skip metastases of all the other criteria analyzed; specifically, patient age, receptor status, number of nodes retrieved, or histologic features of the tumor. Ten of the 17 women with skip metastases had a single node involved at level II or III, including both of the women with skip metastases to level III only.

Because of the 13.4% of women with positive nodes who had metastases beyond level I, the authors currently advocate dissection of both levels I and II. Anything less than meticulous axillary dissection, defined by precise anatomical landmarks, even for patients with small tumors, is interdicted, since the data indicated that the disease in 26% of these women with positive nodes had been considered to be at clinical stage I at the time of diagnosis, and disease in 41% of patients with skip metastases was also at stage I.

Based on information retrieved from the present study, and because incidence of complications related to axillary dissection preceding irradiation is not insignificant, it was purposely chosen not to dissect the complete axilla. The likelihood of missing skip metastases in the usual patient with invasive carcinoma is far outweighed by the occurrence of annoying, although not life-threatening, complications. It would also be misleading to extrapolate and suggest that similar axillary dissection is indicated for women with noninvasive ductal carcinoma, because this study considered women with invasive carcinomas.

▶ It should not be forgotten that cells need oxygen to be most effectively hurt by radiation. Anything that is done to curtail blood supply and reduce oxygen delivery make subsequent radiation less effective. This factor should not be overlooked in the argument about what level of lymph nodes need to be taken when a limited excision of breast tissue has been performed.—E.E. Peacock, Jr., M.D.

Psychological Response to Mastectomy: A Prospective Comparison Study
Joan R. Bloom, Mary Cook, Sophia Fotopoulis, Daphne Flamer, Christopher Gates, Jimmie C. Holland, Larry R. Muenz, Benjamin Murawski, Doris Penman, and Robert D. Ross (Breast Cancer Study Group)
Cancer 59:189–196, Jan. 1, 1987   11–6

The authors report data on 412 women who were studied prospectively at five medical centers over a 1-year period. The study was supported by the National Cancer Institute and was undertaken to obtain systematic data that would compare the emotional effects of breast cancer and its treatment with those of major surgery on another organ or in another life-threatening disease. Assessment was done at four 3-month intervals after initial treatment for stage I or II mastectomy (145 women), for biopsy of benign breast disease (87), for cholecystectomy (90), or no surgical treatment (90); 88% of women were tested at all four time blocks.

Women who had had stage I or II mastectomy experienced greater psychological distress than those in the other three groups. Anxiety, hostility, and concern about the body were found to be consistently greater in these women than among the other groups when any of the three assessment techniques across assessment methods was used. Other constructs that differentiated these women reflected aspects of impaired everyday functioning, leisure time activity, and daily household activities. The findings showed that breast cancer interferes with both intrapersonal and interpersonal functioning, thus confirming other reports.

Women with stage II cancer had more distress initially than those with stage I disease as measured for the somatic distress factor and for the irritability and physical complaint factor at final assessment. These findings were most prominent for somatic complaints and physical limitations.

The women with mastectomy continued to have greater distress during the 1-year follow-up, which is consistent with English studies, but the authors cannot infer whether or not the distress may eventually return to that of a healthy population or whether additional intervention may be appropriate at times more distant from surgery when formal intervention programs and other support are less likely to be offered.

An increased frequency of women with breast cancer who have moderate, albeit transitory, psychopathologic symptoms was found. Although these women are at greater risk of postsurgical psychosocial difficulties, it was clear that diagnosis and treatment for breast cancer is not an etiologic factor in the development of severe and lasting psychopathology.

This study eliminated most problems which have plagued previous research on psychosocial aspects of cancer by using standardized measures with available estimates of reliability and internal validity. Contrary to other reports of dramatic reactive anxiety or depressive disorders after mastectomy, such results were notably absent in this group, which may be due to this sample in which women had less extensive surgery. These data suggest that for women without prior psychiatric disturbance, the risk of developing severe reactive anxiety or depression after mastectomy is low.

▶ The editor is impressed that mastectomy is not nearly so psychologically disturbing to women now as the possibility of having to undergo other types of therapy. Modern surgery, including lumpectomy, immediate or delayed reconstruction, and advanced use of radiation have all reduced the psychological trauma of mastectomy.—E.E. Peacock, Jr., M.D.

Psychological Impact of Adjuvant Chemotherapy in the First Two Years After Mastectomy

A.V.M. Hughson, A.F. Cooper, C.S. McArdle, and D.C. Smith (Univ. of Glasgow, Victoria Infirmary, and Royal Infirmary, Glasgow, Scotland)
Br. Med. J. 293:1268–1271, Nov. 15, 1986   11–7

On the basis of a recent analysis of 10,000 patients which showed that adjuvant chemotherapy reduced the number of early deaths in postmenopausal women by about one sixth and in premenopausal women by about one third, adjuvant chemotherapy is likely to be more widely used. The physical toxicity associated with its use is well documented, but less attention has been paid to the incidence of psychological morbidity.

Psychological symptoms were assessed for 2 years in 74 patients with a mean age of 52.4 years who had had mastectomy for stage II breast cancer; 24 received radiation therapy, 27 had chemotherapy, and 23 had combined treatment. The groups were similar in age, social class, marital status, and previous psychiatric history.

As measured by Maguire's observer scales, at 1 month after mastectomy the group that received only radiation therapy had a prevalence of anxiety and depression of 33% and 38%, respectively, with both falling to 14% at 1 year. In the two groups that were treated with chemotherapy the results were similar at 1, 3, and 6 months, but at 13 months, anxiety and depression were significantly greater in these two groups. At 1 month psychological morbidity was slightly more evident on all self-rating scales in patients with combined treatment. At 13 months both groups who received chemotherapy showed greater psychological morbidity, compared to the control group on radiation therapy alone, with the excess being significant on the Leeds depression and severe depression scales.

The prevalence of psychological morbidity decreased in both groups that were treated with chemotherapy during the second year; at 18 months, in contrast, it apparently increased in the group that was treated with radiation therapy alone, but virtually all the psychological morbidity occurred in patients who had systemic relapse.

After 6 months on chemotherapy, 33% of patients in both groups had conditioned reflex nausea and 13% had conditioned reflex vomiting. At 13 months the prevalence had increased considerably, to 59% and 35%, respectively, and the symptoms persisted after treatment was stopped. All but 2 of 23 patients on combination treatment considered the adverse effects of chemotherapy worse than those of radiation therapy.

This study failed to show appreciable differences in anxiety or depression up to 6 months after mastectomy, but by 13 months nearly all patients on radiation therapy alone seemed to have recovered emotionally whereas depression, anxiety, and conditioned reflex symptoms had risen to a peak in both groups that were treated with chemotherapy, thus indicating that adjuvant chemotherapy has its main psychological impact during the second 6 months of intended treatment. The results of this study suggest that on psychological grounds adjuvant chemotherapy should be restricted to 6 months in the absence of a clear advantage for more prolonged treatment.

▶ There is no question in the editor's judgement that the psychological trauma of having to take chemotherapy is a major factor in reluctance of women to accept modern diagnostic and therapeutic management of breast neoplasms. In the minds of many patients, chemotherapy looms as a greater or at least as great a bête noir as radical mastectomy. It is also likely that chemotherapy is not always beneficial enough to warrant the psychological trauma it causes. Many patients ask the editor if they will have to take chemotherapy before they ask how much breast will have to be removed.—E.E. Peacock, Jr., M.D.

Autogenous Tissue Reconstruction in the Mastectomy Patient: A Critical Review of 300 Patients
Carl R. Hartrampf, Jr., and G. Kristine Bennett (St. Joseph's Hosp. and Emory Univ., Atlanta)
Ann. Surg. 205:508–519, May 1987   11–8

The efficacy, practicality, and safety of the transverse abdominal island flap (TAIF) operation for breast reconstruction after mastectomy were evaluated in 300 consecutive patients. Basically, the procedure involved raising a large transverse ellipse of abdominal skin and subcutaneous fat on one or two rectus muscle pedicles with the superior gastric vessels. The flap was then delivered through a subcutaneous tunnel into the re-created mastectomy defect where it was shaped into the form of a breast. The TAIF method was used to reconstruct a modified radical defect in 207 patients and to salvage a failed previous reconstruction in 54. Follow-up period ranged from 1 to 6 years.

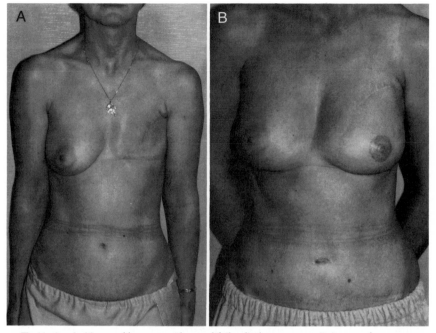

Fig 11–3.—A, 38-year old woman with a modified radical mastectomy. **B,** 2 years after reconstruction. The breast mound was formed in a single operation. No alloplastic material was used in either breast. (Courtesy of Hartrampf, C.R., Jr., and Bennett, G.K.: Ann. Surg. 205:508–519, May 1987.)

The breast mound was formed in a single operation in 221 of 338 breast reconstructions (58%) and these breasts required no further revision. A comparison before and after reconstruction is illustrated in Figure 11–3. Only 18 patients required a revision after 1 year. Of the 217 unilateral reconstructions, symmetry was achieved in 113 (52%) without altering the opposite breast. Breast reduction (30%) was most frequently performed to establish symmetry when a change in the contralateral breast was necessary. Total flap loss occurred in one (0.3%) patient and partial flap loss in 18 (6%). All but three eventually achieved satisfactory results. In retrospect, a preventable cause of flap loss was found in these patients, such as injudicious patient selection, use of flap beyond reasonable limits, and technical errors. Overall abdominal complication rate was 1.6% and included abdominal hernia in one (0.3%) patient; abdominal laxity in two (0.6%), including that one required repair; and small defects in the anterior rectus sheath in two (0.6%). As expected, there was some loss of abdominal wall strength after reconstruction, but this did not affect sports or work performance in more than 90% of patients. The operation was judged worth their time and effort by 266 of 272 (98%) respondents.

The TAIF operation for breast reconstruction is a complex and demanding major operation, and the margin for error is small. This procedure is therefore indicated only in healthy individuals and is contraindicated in the obese patient, the chronic heavy smoker, and in those with major health problems.

▶ This paper presents the supreme standard for reconstruction of the breast in patients with the most difficult problems such as skin loss, radiation dermatitis, and classical radical mastectomy. The procedure is a demanding one and cannot be learned by reading a paper. Fortunately, it is not indicated for most patients who are being treated by modern surgical techniques. When it is indicated it should be performed only by those who have mastered the procedure under the tutelage of others, and the more experience the better.—E.E. Peacock, Jr., M.D.

Surgical Technique and Pitfalls of Breast Reconstruction Immediately After Mastectomy for Carcinoma: Initial Experience
Jon A. van Heerden, Ian T. Jackson, J. Kirk Martin, Jr., and Jack Fisher (Mayo Clinic, Rochester, Minn.)
Mayo Clin. Proc. 62:185–191, March 1987   11–9

The surgical option of immediate breast reconstruction at the time of modified radical mastectomy is being given with increasing frequency in the United States. Of the first 100 consecutive patients who had this procedure, 79 had initial permanent subpectoral implantation of a Silastic prosthesis and 21 had tissue expansion before permanent implantation. All patients were offered immediate breast reconstruction; thus primarily the request of the patient was the indication for the procedure. Patients ranged in age from 29 to 79 years (mean age, 50.5 years).

Necessary changes in the modified radical mastectomy are the use of a transverse or oblique skin incision (a lateral approach is not preferred because it creates a point of weakness through which herniation may occur); development of more extensive skin flaps, inferiorly in particular; and careful protection of the pectoralis major muscle and preservation of the rectus sheath. If a patient wishes subsequent nipple reconstruction, the procedure is usually done 2 to 3 months after the initial reconstruction, or if she is on chemotherapy or radiation therapy, it is delayed until the therapy has been completed. Most patients decided against nipple reconstruction because they were satisfied with the breast mound that had been created.

Only 15% of the patients would not recommend immediate reconstruction, but 85% would. Reasons for dissatisfaction were mainly pain and asymmetry. Of the 21 patients who had nipple reconstruction 11 rated their results as 10 (perfect), seven rated the result as greater than 6, and three rated the result as less than 5. Mean hospital stay for the entire group was 7.8 days, compared with 7.5 days for patients who did not undergo reconstruction.

There was no death in the immediate postoperative period, but there was a major complication in 13 patients, wound infection in 5, partial exposure of the prosthesis in 3, partial flap necrosis in 3, and hematoma in 2. There was no postoperative complication in patients who initially had insertion of a tissue expander. Of the 23 patients who required postoperative adjuvant therapy, no complication ensued because of the presence of the prosthesis, and there was no instance of chemotherapy being delayed because of it.

Although immediate breast reconstruction was offered to all patients, the authors now appreciate that a good result is not obtained in obese patients with large breasts. They now believe that the ideal candidate is a woman with small breasts who desires to undergo the reconstruction and is younger than age 55 years, however, none of these indications is absolute.

The initial experiences with breast reconstruction immediately after mastectomy are encouraging. The authors believe it should be used by every surgical team that deals with breast carcinoma and that the stage of the disease is not a contraindication to immediate reconstruction.

▶ Most bad results from early attempts at immediate breast reconstruction were due and are still due to placing the implant in a subcutaneous position and trying to use too large an implant. By utilizing a carefully prepared submuscular pocket and limiting the size of the implant to 300 or 350 cc, as good a result can be obtained in most patients as can be obtained at a later stage. The overall effect of immediate reconstruction is good, and the procedure should be offered patients with more enthusiasm than was justified following early experience.—E.E. Peacock, Jr., M.D.

Immediate Breast Reconstruction With Tissue Expansion
J. Ward, I.K. Cohen, George A. Knaysi, and Peter W. Brown (Virginia Commonwealth Univ., Richmond)
Plast. Reconstr. Surg. 80:559–566, October 1987   11–10

Thirty-one patients underwent primary breast reconstruction with tissue expansion in 1983–1985, following mastectomy. This approach was used where remaining muscle and skin were inadequate to accommodate a prosthesis matching the opposite breast. The expanders were placed beneath an investing muscle pocket made by elevating the pectoralis major and serratus anterior muscles (Fig 11–4). Expansion began within 1 week of operation, expanding the breast to double the volume of the opposite one. About 3 months are needed for the breast mound to soften. Ptosis is best created by placing the expander below the inframammary fold beneath the rectus fascia. An incision in the area of the new inframammary fold allows direct suturing and fold creation.

Twenty-two patients were followed for a mean of 7 months after the completion of reconstruction. Expansion required a mean of 65 days, and a breast prosthesis was placed an average of nearly 6 months after initial mastectomy and placement of the expander. The total volume of expansion averaged 816 cc. Complications included five deflations and four postoperative infections. Creation of a degree of ptosis was necessary in two thirds of cases.

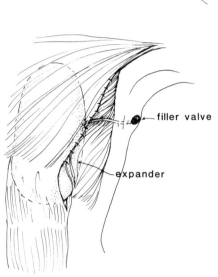

filler valve

expander

Fig 11–4.—Expander covered by muscular pocket: lower border of expander can be placed under rectus fascia or at inframammary fold. Filler valve in subcutaneous tissue, easily palpable, placed laterally or over inferior rib cage. (Courtesy of Ward, J., et al.: Plast. Reconstr. Surg. 80:559–565, October 1987.)

It appears that immediate breast reconstruction with tissue expansion has many advantages. Secondary surgery to place a prosthesis is an outpatient procedure. A very favorable psychological response is encountered. The new permanent Becker prosthesis has been used in recent cases where ptosis is absent or will be corrected on the opposite side. Touch-up procedures may be done at the time of nipple-areola reconstruction.

▶ The only thing wrong with this recommendation is that, in the experience of the editor, it is not necessary. The editor puts in a 300-cc implant at the time modified radical mastectomy is performed. Most patients obtain the contour and even the cleavage they need with a 300-cc implant. For those who do not, replacement 6 weeks later with a 400- or 500-cc implant can be carried out with no difficulty. The primary implant serves as an adequate expander. Thus, one operation suffices for most patients, and no more than two operations are needed even if an expander, which requires two operations, is utilized.—E.E. Peacock, Jr., M.D.

12 The Head and the Neck

The Management of a Neck Mass: Presenting Feature of an Asymptomatic Head and Neck Primary Malignancy?
M. Barakat, L.M. Flood, V.H. Oswal, and R.W. Ruckley (North Riding Infirmary, Middlesbrough, England)
Ann. R. Coll. Surg. Engl. 69:181–184, July 1987   12–1

Adults with a neck mass often present to a general surgeon instead of an otolaryngologist. Unfortunately, inappropriate neck exploration adversely alters the prognosis, if carcinoma is present. The value of otolaryngologic evaluation was studied in a series of 112 patients who presented over a 10-year period with a painless, enlarging neck mass. Only 14 patients had undergone neck exploration and had a diagnosis of metastatic squamous-cell carcinoma.

Initial ear, nose, and throat (ENT) consultation revealed a primary tumor in 72 patients. Eleven of these patients had prior neck surgery. Radiologic screening detected three bronchial cancers and one esophageal malignancy. Panendoscopy revealed three more bronchial cancers and one postcricoid carcinoma. Only 29 previously unoperated patients required neck exploration for diagnosis. Twelve of these 29 patients had a benign lesion. Of all 24 patients ultimately found to have epithelial malignancy, half had never had a primary lesion evident in the head-neck region.

Thorough ENT evaluation frequently is rewarding in adults who present with an enlarging neck mass. Examination under anesthesia should include excision and serial sectioning of the tonsils. Incisional biopsy should be avoided to reduce the risk of sepsis, fungation of tumor, wound necrosis, local recurrence, and distant metastases.

▶ There is no question that specialists are needed to perform examinations of the head and neck when metastatic cancer in the neck is found. The major question, however, is what can be done when the specialist, using all of his specialized techniques, cannot find a primary tumor. The editor has always thought that cancer should be treated where it is found; failure to locate a primary lesion is not an exception. Continued search, including multiple biopsies of areas where microscopic primary lesions are known to occur, usually identifies the primary lesion. Metastases should not be allowed to become untreatable when search for a primary lesion is prolonged.—E.E. Peacock, Jr., M.D.

Is the Treatment for Thyroglossal Duct Cysts Too Extensive?
Keith G. Bennett, Claude H. Organ, Jr., and G. Rainey Williams (Univ. of Oklahoma)
Am. J. Surg. 152:602–605, December 1986   12–2

The thyroglossal duct cyst is a rare cause of benign midline neck mass. It is seen most often in pediatric patients, and it generally is managed by the Sistrunk procedure, which involves removal of the cyst with the infrahyoid tract, body of the hyoid bone, and a tissue core. Some think that excision of the cyst alone is adequate.

Sixty-four patients had treatment of thyroglossal duct cysts in 1970–1985. The mean age was 12 years, and the mean duration of symptoms before operation was 10 months. The mean postoperative follow-up was 5 years. Thirty-seven patients had the classic Sistrunk procedure, 20 had a modified Sistrunk operation with resection of the infrahyoid tract, and seven patients underwent removal of the cyst only.

One fifth of patients had postoperative complications, which were most frequent in patients younger than 10 years of age and those older than age 60. Three of 58 patients followed up had recurrences. One third of patients having removal of the cyst only had recurrences, compared with 3% of patients having the classic operation. Rupture of the cyst at operation was associated with an increased recurrence rate, as was infection or a draining sinus tract.

These findings support Sustrunk's contention that cure of a thyroglossal cyst requires complete removal of the epithelium-lined tract from the cyst to the foramen cecum, including the hyoid bone.

▶ Sistrunk's work has held up through the years. About every decade, however, an inquiring surgeon asks the question, "Why perform such an extensive excision for a cyst? It would not be a cyst if it was not contained within the visible outline of the cyst wall." The answer is still, "Thyroglossal duct cyst is a developmental anomaly of an area; it is not an isolated lesion. Microscopic rests may be present in the entire extent of pouch descent."—E.E. Peacock, Jr., M.D.

The Significance of Incomplete Excision in Patients With Basal Cell Carcinoma
J.D. Richmond and R.M. Davie (Bangour Gen. Hosp., West Lothian, England)
Br. J. Plast. Surg. 40:63–67, January 1987   12–3

The surgeon has a dilemma as to whether to perform immediate wider excision or to reserve further treatment until there is clinical evidence of recurrence when surgically treated basal cell carcinomas are reported as having been incompletely excised. Both philosophies have been followed at the Bangour General Hospital. Data were reviewed on 67 patients who were reported as having tumor cells at the margins of excision in 1970 to

1979. Twenty-eight had not been previously treated; of the 39 who had been treated 20 had had radiation therapy, 12 had surgery and radiation therapy, and 7 had surgery alone.

Seven of the 67 had immediate further treatment, but it is difficult to determine on what grounds they were selected. The defect had been closed directly in 4 cases, 1 had a full-thickness skin graft, and 2 had been covered with local flaps. No patient developed recurrent disease in a minimum follow-up period of 3 years (average follow-up 5 years).

Of the 60 who were not offered immediate further treatment, 23 had not been previously treated, and 23 subsequently developed clinical evidence of recurrent disease. Overall recurrence rate was 38%, representing a 30% recurrence rate for those with new tumors and 43% for those who had been previously treated.

Patients who had both surgery and radiation therapy were at particularly high risk of further recurrence, ten patients out of 11; five were still not cured by another operation. All four who were shown to have incomplete excision at both the lateral and deep margins developed recurrent disease.

Six of ten patients with morpheic tumors developed recurrence. In patients who had grafts, the time from the attempt at curative surgery until recurrence was shorter than the time for those who had had direct closure or had resurfacing with flaps. Once recurrence was detected all 23 patients had supplementary treatment; 21 had a surgical procedure, and ten of the 21 needed more than one further operation; two were considered unsuitable for further surgery.

If problems that are met in controlling recurrent disease beneath flaps were due solely to delay in diagnosis, then similar problems should have also been seen when wounds were directly closed. They were not, which suggests that the opening of tissue planes that were associated with the fashioning of local flaps was more important for those patients in whom recurrent disease proved difficult to control than was a delay in diagnosis.

There would appear to be unacceptable risks in denying immediate further treatment to patients who are already being treated for recurrent disease or in cases in which the excision was incomplete at the deep margin, where flaps had been used to close the defect, or when careful prolonged follow-up poses a problem.

▶ So many technical mistakes during fixation, as well as misinterpretation of the specimen borders, account for basal cell carcinoma appearing to be on the cut section of a surgical specimen that most experienced surgeons do not perform re-excision if gross margins appear safe. It is probably better to wait for a recurrence if the patient can be watched closely and reexcise only the recurrence rather than a large area every time a microscopic section shows tumor at the margin. This, of course, is the antithesis of popular dermatologic excision and reexcision according to frozen section appearance.—E.E. Peacock, Jr., M.D.

Electrocoagulation for Intraoral Cancer

Charles S. Whelan, David E. Marcello, Jr., W. Bradford Patterson, and Peter J. Deckers (Univ. of Massachusetts; Boston Univ.; Brockton (Mass.) Hosp.; Harvard Med. School; Univ. of Connecticut; Hartford (Conn.) Hosp.; and Dana-Farber Cancer Inst., Boston)
Arch. Surg. 122:484–487, April 1987   12–4

Electrocoagulation as an alternative to surgery and irradiation, or a combination of the two, for treating intraoral cancer is a poorly understood technique. Data were reviewed on 58 patients who were treated by electrocoagulation for squamous cell carcinomas of the oral cavity. Twenty-two of the 32 men and 26 women were older than age 70 years. The greatest diameter of the lesions varied from 1 to 6.5 cm. All but one of the operations was done under general anesthesia and with the technique of Franseen.

The 3-year absolute survival was 59%; at 5 years the rate was 52%. All but 3 patients were followed up for at least 2 years. Twenty of 23 patients with T1 lesions (0 to 2 cm), 19 of 29 with T2 lesions (2.2 to 4 cm), and 4 of 6 with T3 lesions (more than 4 cm) had no evidence of recurrent disease or had died of other causes. Electrocoagulation was, therefore, curative in 43 of 58 patients (74%) who were treated.

The overall local failure rate of 19% (11 of 58) was clearly dependent on tumor size, as expected. In five patients with local failure, repeated electrocoagulation provided a cure.

Electrocoagulation has a number of advantages over surgery for appropriate intraoral cancers. Blood loss is less and there is little sacrifice of normal tissue so better postoperative function and cosmesis result. In contrast to the wide, but sometimes uncertain, margins of more aggressive surgery the tumor is destroyed "where it lies." There is minimal disfigurement of the intraoral structures, which allows the surgeon to detect any new lesion earlier. There are fewer associated operative risks because it is an operation of lesser magnitude, which makes it ideal for the elderly or infirm, or both, who make up a large percentage of the patients with intraoral cancer. Contrary to expectations there is little postoperative pain, probably because of the thermal destruction of fine sensory nerve fibers.

There is a real place for radiation therapy in treating large, aggressive lesions and those on the posterior tongue. Electrosurgical removal (debulking) of large intraoral cancers before planned irradiation reduces the anoxic tumor mass in a relatively bloodless procedure. Further trials of this combined treatment when dealing with bulky intraoral cancers are suggested.

It should not be considered a drawback that tumor margins are not monitored because they can be checked histologically in any area if desired. Of prime importance is that electrocoagulation has the advantages of decreased morbidity and conservation of normal, undamaged tissues in other parts of the oral cavity. The authors consider it to be the preferred method of treating many intraoral cancers and to be ideally suited to those patients whose lesions are small, easily seen, mobile, and well differentiated.

▶ General Johnson, founder and president of the Johnson and Johnson Company, had a sign behind his desk which read, "If it is hard, it is wrong." Electrocoagulation does have distinct advantages over other forms of surgery and over irradiation. One is simplicity. Before too much money is spent on lasers and other, more complicated technical devices, it should be remembered that electrocoagulation is a natural refinement of the old soldering iron technique that was successful in obliterating cancer.—E.E. Peacock, Jr., M.D.

Therapeutic Concepts of Brachytherapy/Megavoltage in Sequence for Pharyngeal Wall Cancers: Results of Integrated Dose Therapy
Yung H. Son and Barry M. Kacinski (Yale Univ.)
Cancer 59:1268–1273, April 1, 1987   12–5

The nature of the host site makes pharyngeal wall cancers difficult to control. Most of the authors' cases have been stage II and III lesions. Most lateral, posterior oropharyngeal wall lesions above the epiglottic level were implanted transorally. A megavoltage dose of 5,200 rads and an iridium 192 interstitial dose of 3,000–3,500 rads are recommended. Since 1978, iodine 125 has been used in a dose of 12,000–15,000 rads. Megavoltage therapy is given to lateral opposed neck fields extending from the cranial base to the lowermost echelon of neck nodes. Persistent neck disease may necessitate supplementary electron beam doses.

Twelve of 14 patients having both brachytherapy and craniocervical megavoltage irradiation had locoregional control. All nine patients treated with ^{125}I to the primary site have remained controlled locally, although one had distant failure. Three patients had reversible soft tissue and mucosal injury. There was one patient each with impaired swallowing due to hypoglossal nerve injury and brachial plexopathy. No soft tissue or mucosal necrosis was observed.

Sequential ^{125}I brachytherapy and megavoltage irradiation can be locally curative in cases of pharyngeal wall cancer. This approach has the advantage of organ preservation. Integrated doses of irradiation apparently confer site-specific benefit for oropharyngeal, hypopharyngeal wall tumors.

▶ Megavoltage radiation and ^{192}Ir or ^{125}I brachytherapy are superior to radical surgery, at least as a first attempt to cure. It should be remembered, however, that the posterior and lateral oropharyngeal and hypopharyngeal walls can be excised and reconstructed with free jejunal flaps, even if radiation fails.—E.E. Peacock, Jr., M.D.

Reirradiation of Recurrent Head and Neck Cancers

B. Emami, M. Bignardi, G.J. Spector, V.R. Devineni, and M.A. Hederman (Mallinckrodt Inst. of Radiology, St. Louis; Ospedale Regionale, Varese, Italy; and Washington Univ.)
Laryngoscope 97:85–88, January 1987   12–6

In many cases reirradiation is deemed the only therapeutic possibility for recurrent cancer of the head and neck, which is usually a locoregional recurrence. Of 73 men and 26 women aged 23 to 83 years (mean age, 59 years) who had had head and neck cancer and were treated with surgery, radiation therapy, or a combination of the two, approximately two-thirds had recurrences within 1 year, but some patients developed recurrence 3 years after initial treatment. Follow-up ranged from 18 months to 18 years. Treatment regimens were not homogeneous. Eleven of the recurrent tumors were treated with surgery alone; 52 patients received less than 5,000 rad and 36 received more than 5,000 rad.

There were 67 complete responses (CR), 7 partial responses (PR), and 27 no responses or tumor progressions, but eventually most of the 67 with CR had recurrence at the site of treatment, with only 15 of the 67 complete responders having final tumor control, a finding in sharp contrast with results that were observed with similar lesions that were treated with combination hyperthermia and radiation therapy in which 80% of patients with CR sustained their response or tumor control (50%).

All 11 patients who were treated by surgery alone at the first recurrence had CRs, but eventually all patients in this group died of their recurrence. Thirty-nine of 48 patients who were treated by combination therapy had CRs and 2 had PRs, and eventual tumor control was achieved in 10 of the 48. Eighteen of 40 patients who were treated with radiation alone had CRs and 5 had PRs, with 5 maintaining their CRs. Forty-four of 62 patients with recurrence at the primary site achieved CRs, and 2 achieved PRs.

Among the 52 patients who were treated with radiation therapy in doses of less than 5,000 rads, there were 23 with CRs and 4 with PRs, eventually 6 patients achieved tumor control. In 36 patients who were treated with doses greater than 5,000 rads, 29 achieved CR and 2 achieved PR, with 9 eventually achieving tumor control (statistically significant results). Of the 67 patients who had CRs 11 are alive without evidence of tumor, 2 are alive with persistent tumor, and 5 have died without evidence of disease. Most of those who died had persistent tumors in locoregional sites (74 of 99).

Managing recurrent head and neck carcinoma remains a difficult challenge. In the judgment of the authors the potential higher complication rate is not an adequate reason for treatment. These data indicate that long-term disease-free survival can only arise among that group of patients who had an initial CR, and that perhaps newer modalities, such as hyperthermia in combination with radiation therapy and surgery, appear to be leading in the right direction.

► This report must reflect progress in the type of equipment and the use of such equipment that was not possible two decades ago. Traditionally, a patient who has recurrence after a full therapeutic dose of radiation is in the same situation as a boxer who has swung his best punch and his opponent just laughs at him. Reirradiation has been of very limited usefulness in the past.—E.E. Peacock, Jr., M.D.

Multidrug Chemotherapy Using Bleomycin, Methotrexate, and Cisplatin Combined With Radical Radiotherapy in Advanced Head and Neck Cancer
J. Zidan, A. Kuten, Y. Cohen, and E. Robinson (Technion-Israel Inst. of Technology, Haifa)
Cancer 59:24–26, Jan. 1, 1987   12–7

The authors had suggested in a previous article that by using the bleomycin, methotrexate, and cisplatin (BMP) regimen followed by radical radiation in advanced, previously untreated head and neck cancer, cure rates could be improved over surgery and radiotherapy used as a single treatment modality or in combination. Thirty-one patients with stages III–IV previously untreated head and neck cancer were treated with BMP between May 1980 and May 1984. Twenty-nine patients with a mean age of 53 years were available for follow-up. Half of the patients had nasopharyngeal carcinoma, and the others had carcinoma of oropharynx, larynx, and oral cavity.

After three courses of BMP, 4 patients had complete response (CR), 13 had partial remission (PR), and there was no change in 12. Of the 13 patients who had PR with chemotherapy, 11 achieved complete local control after radiotherapy. Four of the patients who had no change after chemotherapy achieved CR with radiotherapy, and four achieved PR. Two patients with PR after completion of chemotherapy and radiotherapy achieved CR by local excision of residual disease, increasing the overall CR rate to 72%. Calculated from the day chemotherapy was initiated, the actuarial survival of all patients at 30 months was 61%. The patients with CR had a survival rate of 76%, whereas those with residual disease had a survival rate of only 25%. The survival rate of patients with nasopharyngeal cancer was 80%, compared with 37% for patients with squamous malignancies occurring in other sites of the head and neck region. Fourteen of 19 patients were alive and free of disease, 1 was alive with disease, 2 died of intercurrent disease, and 12 died of cancer.

Toxic effects of the chemotherapy were acceptable, with no fatalities. The combination therapy did not increase significantly the amount and severity of radiation side effects. Although no survival advantage could be shown for patients who had PR, those achieving CR with the combined modality therapy had a significant survival benefit at 30 months. This advantage was more obvious in nasopharyngeal carcinoma, most probably because most of those patients had anaplastic carcinoma or lymphoepithelioma. The authors agree in part only, therefore, with Vogl's observation that there will be improved initial control rates using

BMP and radiotherapy, but that there will be no long-term survival benefit.

▶ The effectiveness of radiotherapy combined with even one agent such as cisplatin is obscure enough now so that more reports of multidrug chemotherapy only serve to complicate evaluation of treatment of advanced head and neck cancer. It appears that the combination of cisplatin and radiotherapy is effective and safe in treating patients with advanced head and neck cancer, but no one has performed studies sufficient to ascertain whether cisplatin administered with radiotherapy is significantly better than radiotherapy alone. Adding a number of other agents does not help us make a better determination of where we stand now in nonsurgical treatment of advanced head and neck cancer.—E.E. Peacock, Jr., M.D.

Reconstruction of the Middle Third of Mandible
J.D. Frame, N. Bradley, D.R. James, M.P. Stearns, and M.D. Brough (Univ. College Hosp., London)
Br. J. Plast. Surg. 40:274–277, May 1987   12–8

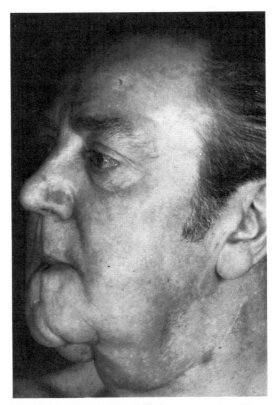

Fig 12–1.—Semi-lateral view after anterior mandibular reconstruction. (Courtesy of Frame, J.D., et al.: Br. J. Plast. Surg. 40:274–277, May 1987.)

The free radial forearm flap, or "Chinese flap," makes it possible to harvest about 14 cm of radius for use in reconstructing the mandible. The authors have used a simple method or riberration of the hemiradius within the free flap, combined with Champy plate fixation, to satisfactorily reconstruct the anterior mandible in two patients.

Man, 61, presented with a floor-of-mouth ulcer and a history of both smoking and alcohol abuse. He was discovered to have a necrotic, fungating carcinoma beneath the tongue base, involving most of the floor of the mouth. Right neck block dissection and en bloc excision of tumor with a segment of mandible were carried out.

A vascularized left radial forearm flap containing 14 cm of radius was raised, and the bone was riberrated vertically on the proposed buccal surface while still in situ. The radial segment with attached soft tissue was molded and held in position using a long Champy plate screwed to the buccal aspect of the hemiradius segment. The contoured hemiradius was then attached to the remaining mandibular segments using two miniature plates, and the flap was revascularized. The skin paddle provided lining to the floor of the mouth; it also acted as a flap monitor. A good chin contour was achieved (Fig 12–1).

The radial forearm flap with hemiradius provides good-quality skin and a thin layer of subcutaneous fat. Revascularization is possible well away from the site of previous surgery or irradiation. A skin-grafted forearm donor site is the chief disadvantage. In addition, complications may result from the use of miniplates. The present patients have had a good outcome on follow-up for 28 and 22 months, respectively.

▶ There is no question that a free bone, muscle, and skin flap is the best technique available for restoring the anterior arch of the mandible. An osteomyocutaneous flap using the trapezius and part of the spine of the scapula is one of several other procedures that are generally more acceptable from a donor site standpoint than the skin flap and radius described in this paper.—E.E. Peacock, Jr., M.D.

Some Ancillary Procedures for Correction of Depressed Adherent Tracheostomy Scars and Associated Tracheocutaneous Fistulae
Victor L. Lewis, Jr., Paul N. Manson, and Michael C. Stalnecker (Northwestern Univ. and Johns Hopkins Univ.)
J. Trauma 27:651–655, June 1987   12–9

Most posttracheostomy patients can gain an improved appearance from fistula closure and scar revision. Such measures as removal of atrophic skin, reapproximation of the strap muscles, and release of contractures will prove helpful. Selective use of a Z-plasty involving the subcutaneous tissue and platysma will improve the contour in patients having atrophic subcutaneous tissues.

After the fistula or adherent atrophic skin is circumscribed and the surrounding scar is de-epithelialized, pretracheal fascia and the skin are turned over as marginally based flaps to close a fistulous opening or, if there is no fistula, to provide bulk. The strap muscles are then sutured together over the de-epithelialized scar. The subcutaneous tissue and skin are widely mobilized to release contractures. If necessary, a Z-plasty is performed with interposed flaps of platysma or subcutaneous tissue, or both. Multiple Z-plasties in the skin are rarely used.

Thirty-three patients had subcutaneous Z-plasty procedures within a 3-year period. Uniform healing occurred in all cases. One air leak into the neck sealed without reoperation or intubation. The appearances improved in all patients. Three tracheocutaneous fistulas were closed at the time of scar release and revision. This approach may be used to repair defects up to 5 cm in width. Significant sacrifice of local muscle function is not necessary.

▶ Ugly tracheostomy scars that move with the trachea are caused by failure of repair of subcutaneous tissue, including platysma, and allowing skin to heal to the trachea. It is not a difficult procedure to fill up the suprasternal notch with local fat and interpose muscle between the trachea and the skin to prevent or correct an ugly scar that moves when the patient swallows.—E.E. Peacock, Jr., M.D.

MR Imaging of the Intraparotid Facial Nerve: Normal Anatomy and Pathology

Louis M. Teresi, Elliot Kolin, Robert B. Lufkin, and William N. Hanafee (Univ. of California, Los Angeles, and Mt. Sinai School of Medicine, New York)
AJR 148:995–1000, May 1987   12–10

The value of computed tomography (CT) in studying the facial nerve is limited by the variability of landmarks and the difficulty of visualizing them at different levels. Magnetic resonance (MR) imaging therefore was used to directly image the intraparotid facial nerve. Such imaging with surface receiver coils produces better contrast resolution than CT, with comparable spatial resolution. A multislice rapid spin-echo technique was utilized. Control images were recorded in 58 subjects in the sagittal, axial, and coronal planes.

On T1-weighted images the facial nerve appeared as a curvilinear structure of relatively low signal intensity within the high-signal parotid parenchyma. Specially angled axial scans demonstrated the major divisions and branches of the nerve. Several variations in the normal appearance and course of the nerve were observed. Three patients with parotid tumors were studied. The MR imaging technique demonstrated the relation of the nerve and its branches to the tumor in these cases and helped in planning surgery.

Magnetic resonance imaging can directly display the facial nerve within the parotid gland and can show the relation of the nerve to parotid tumor. The MR imaging technique may be of significant help in planning the surgical management of parotid tumors.

▶ MR imaging will be overused in the head and neck area (as elsewhere); the recommendations in this report may make the increased cost of such presurgical work-up seem justified. A parotid tumor deep to the facial nerve, unrecognized before surgery, can be disastrous for an inexperienced surgeon. Localization of such a tumor preoperatively can help prevent damage to the facial nerve and seeding of the tumor, particularly for those who are unaccustomed to performing simultaneous nerve tumor dissection of a deep lobe tumor.—E.E. Peacock, Jr., M.D.

13 The Thorax

Incisional Herniae Following Median Sternotomy Incisions: Their Incidence and Etiology
B.R. Davidson and J.S. Bailey (Groby Road Hosp., Leicester, U.K.)
Br. J. Surg. 73:995–996, December 1986   13–1

Hernias occurring in association with median sternotomy for cardiac surgery were studied in a series of 582 operations in an 8-year period. Incisional epigastric hernia complicated the procedure in 20 patients (4.2%). Only patients older than age 16 years were included in the study. Follow-up information was available in 82% of cases.

Seven of the 20 patients with incisional hernia were symptomatic and underwent repair. No single factor was associated with hernia formation. Two thirds of hernias were apparent within 3 months of operation. No patient with a hernia had repair with polypropylene sutures. A disproportionate number of hernias followed sternotomy for aortic valve replacement. Fifteen patients had major postoperative complications. Five required further surgery through the median sternotomy incision. Wound infection occurred in one fourth of cases. As a group, the patients were significantly overweight.

Incisional epigastric hernia follows median sternotomy for cardiac surgery in a significant number of patients. Obese patients, those having aortic valve replacement, and those requiring reoperation through the sternotomy incision are particularly at risk. Nonabsorbable sutures may be best for closing the sternal wound.

▶ This retrospective study of 582 patients undergoing median sternotomy over a period of 8 years found a 4% frequency of incisional hernia. Although the series was not randomized, it seemed most significant that Dexon sutures were used in all of the patients who subsequently developed a hernia, while Prolene sutures were used in those who did not. Other complicating factors, of uncertain statistical significance, included obesity and postoperative complications of wound infection or left ventricular failure.—F.C. Spencer, M.D.

Management of Airway Trauma II: Combined Injuries of the Trachea and Esophagus
James P. Kelly, Watts R. Webb, Peter V. Moulder, Nicholas M. Moustouakas, and Mitchell Lirtzman (Tulane Univ., New Orleans)
Ann. Thorac. Surg. 43:160–163, February 1987   13–2

Twenty-four patients were treated for combined tracheal and esophageal injuries in 1967–1983. Their mean age was 32 years. Twenty-one

213

penetrating wounds, most due to gunshot injuries, and three blunt wounds were treated. The cervical esophagus was involved in 20 cases and the thoracic esophagus, in four. The presenting findings were quite variable. Subcutaneous emphysema and hemoptysis were relatively frequent. Twenty patients had respiratory difficulty at presentation; five required immediate tracheostomy. Two of 16 patients had false-negative esophagographic findings.

Eleven of the tracheal injuries were "through-and-through" injuries. Primary tracheal repair was undertaken in 23 patients. Suture lines were reinforced with strap muscle or sternocleidomastoid muscle flaps in the cervical region, and with pericardium or pleura in the thorax. Esophageal injuries were repaired in standard manner using two layers of nonresorbable sutures. Two patients had surgery for late tracheoesophageal fistulas. The operative mortality was 21%. Four of the 20 patients with combined cervical injuries died postoperatively. Two patients with missed cervical esophageal injuries due to inaccurate esophagography died. Two other deaths were in patients with extensive combined wounds and a vascular component.

Patients with severe associated injuries may require emergency intervention before tracheal/esophageal evaluation is possible. Tracheal wounds are aggressively explored. Endoscopic evaluation in place of esophagography would have lowered mortality in the present series.

▶ This report describes experiences with 24 patients treated at the Charity Hospital in New Orleans over a period of 16 years who had the unusual combination of injuries to both the trachea and esophagus. Twenty-one of the 24 injuries resulted from penetrating trauma.

Appropriate diagnostic measures to identify all sites of injury seemed to be the key message from the data. Esophagoscopy has been adopted as a routine procedure because of the significant false-negative rate with esophagograms. Three of the five deaths that occurred resulted from missed injuries to the esophagus or trachea.—F.C. Spencer, M.D.

Laryngotracheal Trauma
Douglas J. Mathisen and Hermes Grillo (Harvard Univ.)
Ann. Thorac. Surg. 43:254–262, March 1987   13–3

Failure to diagnose laryngotracheal injury may lead to cicatrization and later airway obstruction. Data on ten cases of acute laryngotracheal trauma and 17 patients presenting for late management were reviewed.

In acute cases, subcutaneous emphysema was the most frequent finding. Most of these injuries involved the laryngotracheal junction. Eight patients had repair through a collar incision. Two patients with tears in the distal membranous trachea were explored transthoracically. Two patients required laryngeal stenting and tracheostomy. The sternohyoid muscle may be used to prevent fistula formation (Fig 13–1). Primary repair was successful in all cases. No patient yet has developed tracheal

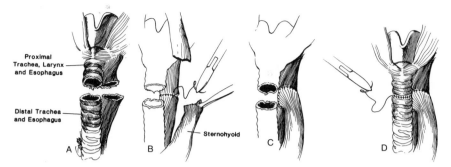

Fig 13–1.—A, view of transected trachea and esophagus. **B,** esophagus closed in two layers. **C,** strap muscle interposed between the esophageal and tracheal suture line. **D,** completed repair. (Courtesy of Mathisen, D.J., and Grillo, H.: Ann. Thorac. Surg. 43:254–262, March 1987.)

stenosis. The two patients with recurrent nerve injuries have very good voices.

Patients seen for delayed treatment usually had injuries at the laryngotracheal junction or upper trachea, but there were three middle tra-

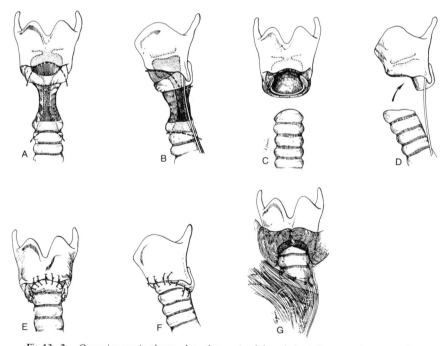

Fig 13–2.—Operative repair of anterolateral stenosis of the subglottic larynx and upper trachea. **A,** anteroposterior view. **B,** lateral view showing the extent of disease involvement and the ultimate lines of transection. **C** and **D,** larynx and trachea after removal of the specimen. Recurrent nerves have been left intact. Mucous membrane of larynx has been transected sharply at same level of division as cartilage. **E,** anteroposterior and (**F**) lateral views of reconstruction. **G,** thyroid isthmus has been approximated to cover the anastomosis. Strap muscle, and occasionally thymus, is brought over to shield innominate artery from open area of anterior tracheal wall. Area is walled off for possible placement of tracheostomy tube. (Courtesy of Mathisen, D.J., and Grillo, H.: Ann. Thorac. Surg. 43:254–262, March 1987.)

cheal and three lower tracheal injuries. Seven patients required procedures to achieve an adequate laryngeal airway before definitive repair of stenosis. The stenotic segment was removed, and primary repair was carried out in all cases (Fig 13–2). All patients but one were successfully decannulated. Ten patients had good voices, and six had husky but very functional voices. There was only one vocal failure.

Conservation of viable trachea and avoidance of tracheostomy are important in the management of acute laryngotracheal trauma. Delayed treatment involves initial repair of the larynx, the resolution of inflammation and scarring, and separation of the tracheal and esophageal suture lines in the definitive repair.

▶ This report describes experiences with 27 patients with serious trauma to the larynx and trachea. Grillo, of course, is surely the most experienced person in the world with the repair of these complex problems. Hence, the paper is a valuable source of information for the surgical treatment of both acute and chronic problems from this devastating injury.—F.C. Spencer, M.D.

Surgery for Total Congenital Tracheal Stenosis
David N. Campbell and John R. Lilly (Univ. of Colorado)
J. Pediatr. Surg. 21:934–935, November 1986   13–4

Complete congenital tracheal stenosis is a rare and lethal anomaly. The authors inserted a cartilaginous strut through the entire length of the trachea and had a successful result.

Male, 4½ months, with agenesis of the right lung, presented with advancing respiratory distress. A 3.5-mm tube could not be advanced beyond the subglottic region, but a 2.5-mm tube was placed. Bronchoscopy showed stenosis extending from the first tracheal ring to the left mainstem bronchus. The right bronchus was represented by a tiny diverticulum. The trachea was split anteriorly in a stepwise manner to the midportion of the left main stem bronchus, and a cartilaginous rib graft with perichondrium intact on one side was wedged into the trachea and bronchus with the perichondrium facing the lumen. An endotracheal tube was left for 3 weeks when a widely patent and stable tracheoplasty was present. At 5 months, only minimal narrowing was noted; the mucosal lining was normal. The patient was asymptomatic and growing well 9 months postoperatively.

More severe lesions of congenital tracheal stenosis present at younger ages. Conservative management does not reliably prevent death in respiratory insufficiency when tracheal stenosis is complete. More aggressive treatment may, however, succeed, and this lesion should no longer be viewed as uncorrectable and uniformly fatal. Gradual incision of the trachea with advancement of an endotracheal tube into the distal segment provides maximal airway control and placement of a tracheal strut.

▶ This remarkable report describes the successful treatment of a 4½ month-old boy with complete tracheal rings throughout the trachea, a condition that is almost always uniformly fatal. At the time of the report, 9 months following operation, the child was doing well. Hopefully, this favorable experience can be duplicated by others. The basic operative technique was to incise the entire trachea and widen it with a cartilaginous rib graft, leaving pericardium on the surface of the graft that became intraluminal. Hopefully, others can duplicate this remarkable experience with this uncommon but highly lethal condition.—F.C. Spencer, M.D.

A Modified Pectoralis Muscle Flap for Closure of Postpneumonectomy Esophagopleural Fistula: Technique and Results
H.J. Mud, H. van Houten, R. Slingerland, P. Sonneveld, and S. Kho (Univ. of Rotterdam, the Netherlands)
Ann. Thorac. Surg. 43:359–362, April 1987

13–5

Esophagopleural fistula should be suspected in patients with recurrent empyema after pneumonectomy when bronchopleural fistula is excluded. If thoracentesis with antibiotic instillation and nasogastric feeding fail to control the fistula, surgery is indicated.

The goal of operation is to obliterate the postpneumonectomy space. A pectoralis major muscle flap can be used to obliterate the entire empyema cavity if a wide thoracoplasty is performed, and ample decapitation of the empyema cavity is carried out. An adequate medial attachment must be left in order not to damage the large perforating internal mammary artery branches that vascularize the muscle. If necessary, the pectoralis minor may be detected from the coracoid process and inserted simultaneously in the empyema cavity. The empyema cavity and subcutaneous space are drained at the end of the operation.

Two cases of esophagopleural fistula, 3 and 16 years with pneumonectomy, were successfully managed with this operation. Endoscopic cannulation of the fistula, if possible, facilitates its identification at operation. Direct closure of the fistula is probably not very important as long as the empyema space is closed.

▶ This short report describes the successful treatment of two patients with one of the most dread complications in thoracic surgery: development of an esophagopleural fistula after a pneumonectomy. Both were successfully treated with a combination of the pectoralis muscle flap with a thoracoplasty. With present supportive techniques, the proper combination of a thoracoplasty with a muscle flap procedure should make it feasible to successfully treat many patients who develop this rare but highly lethal complication.—F.C. Spencer, M.D.

Legionnaires' Disease: An Emerging Surgical Problem
Joyce A. Korvick and Victor L. Yu (Univ. of Pittsburgh)
Ann. Thorac. Surg. 43:341–347, March 1987

13–6

Legionnaires' disease is an important complication in surgical patients but frequently is overlooked. More than fifty outbreaks of nosocomial legionellosis have been reported since 1980. The most obvious risk factors are advancing age, smoking, and chronic lung disease. Up to 40% of patients have been immunosuppressed. Water distribution systems are the primary source of most, if not all, occurrences of nosocomial Legionnaires' disease. The mode of transmission is uncertain, but aerosolization is the most widely accepted hypothesis. Legionnaires' disease most often presents as pneumonia, but wound infection, perirectal abscess, pericarditis, and endocarditis have been described. Failure to respond to β-lactam and aminoglycoside antimicrobials may suggest the diagnosis. Culture, direct-fluorescent antibody staining, and serology together comprise the most sensitive diagnostic approach.

Legionnaires' disease is treated with erythromycin, preferably by the intravenous route. Treatment generally lasts 10 to 14 days. Surgical patients represent one fourth to half of all hospital patients with *Legionella* pneumonia. Transplant recipients may be most frequently affected. Attack rates as high as 55% have been reported in renal transplant recipients. Surgeons may have to persuade personnel at microbiology laboratories to make available specialized testing for *Legionella* for working up patients with postoperative pneumonia. Specialized laboratory testing must be available if environmental surveillance shows that *Legionella* is present in the hospital water supply. Preventive measures are available.

▶ The clinical and diagnostic characteristics of legionnaires' disease are summarized in this review article. As the disease is uncommon, often occurring as epidemics in hospitals with a contaminated water supply, the diagnosis may not initially be considered. To compound the problem further, many hospitals may not have the complex facilities required to establish the diagnosis, including fluorescent antibody staining and serology. Hence, the progressive pneumonia could easily become fatal without ever establishing a precise diagnosis. As intravenous erythromycin is a specific treatment, the importance of considering the diagnosis in puzzling refractory pneumonias is particularly important.—F.C. Spencer, M.D.

Surgical Intervention in Histoplasmosis
H. Edward Garrett, Jr., and Charles L. Roper (Washington Univ., St. Louis)
Ann. Thorac. Surg. 42:711–722, December 1986   13–7

Histoplasmosis is frequent in endemic regions. It generally follows a subclinical course, but excessive inflammation may lead some patients to present to the thoracic surgeon to rule out malignancy or to relieve compression of specific structures. Mediastinal granulomatosis or fibrosing mediastinitis can involve the superior vena cava, pulmonary vessels, pericardium and heart, tracheobronchial tree, or esophagus.

Data on 94 patients seen in 1975–1984 with diagnoses of histoplasmosis, excluding ocular cases, were reviewed. Seventy-five of these patients had surgery or endoscopy to establish the diagnosis or to relieve obstructive symptoms. Fifteen patients had an asymptomatic noncalcified pulmonary mass; most underwent wedge resection for diagnosis. Nineteen patients had an asymptomatic noncalcified mediastinal mass, and 16 of them underwent biopsy, most often by mediastinoscopy. Six dyspneic patients had pulmonary artery obstruction secondary to histoplasmosis. Seven patients had superior vena caval syndrome, and one presented with constrictive pericarditis. Thirteen patients had narrowing of bronchi by compression. Eleven others had hemoptysis or recurrent pneumonia due to bronchial erosion by calcified hilar nodes. Pneumonia was diagnosed in six patients. Nine patients had dysphagia, odynophagia, or chest pain due to esophageal histoplasmosis. Four patients had systemic disease.

Thoracic histoplasmosis has a wide clinical spectrum. Asymptomatic patients with mediastinal granuloma may be observed, but antifungal agents, such as ketoconazole, are used in cases of chronic cavitary pulmonary histoplasmosis or active systemic disease. Fibrosing mediastinitis and broncholithiasis generally do not respond to antifungal therapy or steroids.

► This review article summarizes experiences with 94 patients treated for different complications of histoplasmosis, a disease concentrated around the Ohio and Mississippi river valleys in the central eastern United States.—F.C. Spencer, M.D.

Pulmonary Aspergilloma: Results of Surgical Treatment

Richard C. Daly, Peter C. Pairolero, Jeffrey M. Piehler, Victor F. Trastek, W. Spencer Payne, and Philip E. Bernatz (Mayo Clinic and Found., Rochester, Minn.)

J. Thorac. Cardiovasc. Surg. 92:981–988, December 1986   13–8

There is much controversy over whether and when to operate on patients who have been diagnosed with pulmonary aspergillosis. While some authors believe that surgical excision of pulmonary aspergillomas should be avoided entirely because of the reported high incidence of postoperative complications, others hold the opinion that all such tumors should be excised because of potential hemoptysis. Still others believe that excision should be done only if hemoptysis occurs. In light of this controversy, the authors reviewed their experience with the surgical management of pulmonary aspergilloma.

The study population included 40 men and 13 women, aged 4 to 86 years (median, 58 years), who underwent thoracotomy for treatment of pulmonary aspergilloma. Of 53 patients, 49 (92%) had underlying lung disease or immunologic risk factors. Twenty-one patients (31%) had simple aspergilloma (SA) (Fig 13–3), while 32 (47%) had complex aspergilloma (CA). Symptoms included cough, hemoptysis, fever, weight loss, dyspnea, and chest pain. The most common indications for operation included the presence of an indeterminate mass, hemoptysis, or chronic severe cough. The most frequently performed operations were lobectomy, edge excision, and pneumonectomy. Early postoperative com-

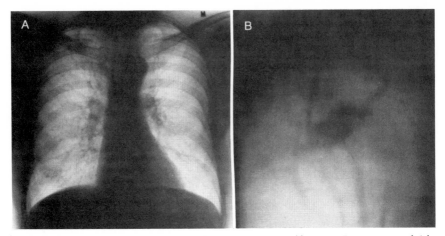

Fig 13–3.—**A,** complex aspergilloma in right apex in a 66-year-old woman. **B,** tomograms of right apex. Note extensive pulmonary infiltrate and thick-walled cyst. (Courtesy of Daly, R.C., et al.: J. Thorac. Cardiovasc. Surg. 92:981–988, December 1986.)

plications occurred in 7 patients (33%) with SA and in 25 patients (78%) with CA. One (5%) of 21 SA patients and 11 (34%) of 32 CA patients died of postoperative complications. Twenty-five of the 41 surviving patients required subsequent procedures. At follow-up, 16 of 20 surviving SA patients and 9 of 21 surviving CA patients were still alive and were asymptomatic. Two surviving CA patients were symptomatic at follow-up. The observed 5-year survival rate for SA patients was 83%, compared with 44% for patients with CA.

It is concluded that patients with SA can safely undergo elective pulmonary resection: their chances for a long-term cure are excellent.

▶ Fifty-three patients underwent thoracotomy for aspergilloma at the Mayo Clinic over a period of 31 years. Operative mortality was 5% in simple cases, 34% in complex cases. The paper is a good reference source for treating patients with this unusual complication of chronic cavitary pulmonary disease.—F.C. Spencer, M.D.

Tube Drainage of Lung Abscesses
T.W. Rice, Robert J. Ginsberg, and Thomas R.J. Todd (Cleveland Clinic Found. and Univ. of Toronto)
Ann. Thorac. Surg. 44:356–359, October 1987   13–9

The treatment of lung abscesses has changed considerably in the past 40 years. Because of improved respiratory management in intensive care units and the emergence of necrotizing anaerobic and gram-negative bacteria, patients with large lung abscesses who are not candidates for extensive pulmonary resections must now be managed. In the past, drainage of such abscesses was considered too hazardous.

The authors describe experience with 14 patients with complicated lung abscesses that were more than 4 cm in diameter or were associated with respiratory failure and required mechanical ventilation. The nine men and five women had a mean age of 57.6 years. A percutaneous tube was inserted in 11 patients, three of whom subsequently underwent rib resection, and three patients underwent rib resection with operative insertion of the tube. The resultant bronchopleural fistulas did not interfere with respiratory management, despite the use of mechanical ventilation. Only two patients needed subsequent surgical closure. Eleven patients could be discharged from the hospital.

Complications were minimal and included two episodes of hemorrhage, one during surgical débridement of the abscess and one delayed. Both episodes were successfully treated. Of the three patients who died in the hospital, only one died from complications of the lung abscess.

This experience shows that tube drainage of complicated abscesses can be safe, simple, and effective. The authors recommend it for treating complicated lung abscesses, even when they are associated with respiratory failure and mechanical ventilatory support.

▶ This report reminds one that tube drainage of lung abscesses is an acceptable compromise form of therapy when more definitive therapy is not possible. Experiences with 14 patients are described, 11 of whom were subsequently discharged from the hospital. Two of this group required further surgical operation for treatment. Drainage of a lung abscess was the basic form of therapy for years, virtually abandoned after the superiority of pulmonary resection was demonstrated. However, with complicated problems, it remains a valuable reasonable alternative.—F.C. Spencer, M.D.

The Thoracic Surgical Spectrum of Acquired Immune Deficiency Syndrome

Joseph I. Miller (Emory Univ., Atlanta)
J. Thorac. Cardiovasc. Surg. 92:977–980, December 1986   13–10

Thirty-eight patients with acquired immunodeficiency syndrome (AIDS) underwent 49 operations in 1983–1986. Their mean age was 32 years. Eleven patients had open lung biopsy, and 14 had closed chest tube thoracostomy. Six patients underwent fiberoptic bronchoscopy with transbronchial lung biopsy and bronchoalveolar lavage. An air leak was closed surgically in five patients. Seven patients underwent tracheostomy, and three had mediastinoscopy. Thirty patients had confirmed pulmonary infection. Two others had Kaposi's sarcoma.

Only four patients had surgical complications, usually persistent air leakage. Operative mortality, however, was 26%. All seven patients requiring tracheostomy died; four of them also had closed chest tube placement. Two thirds of all patients were dead 1 year after surgery.

Open lung biopsy is considered for AIDS patients who have an infectious course, but not definitive diagnosis by fiberoptic bronchoscopy. The AIDS patient should not be placed on mechanical ventilation. Tracheostomy should be avoided. If an air leak persists for longer than a week and it is thought that the patient can be discharged from the hospital, surgical closure with pleurodesis may be safely performed.

► This short report summarizes experiences with thoracic procedures upon 38 patients with the acquired immune deficiency syndrome. Most procedures were lung biopsies, closure of air leaks, or open lung biopsies. *Pneumocystis carinii* was the most common cause of a pulmonary infection, fatal in 30%, with a mortality of 30%. Tracheostomy and ventilatory support was rarely performed after 1985, as all seven patients previously treated with this approach died. The report is a useful summary of evolving experiences with this grim disease on a thoracic surgical service. With improvement in diagnostic techniques, fortunately, thoracic operations are seldom required.—F.C. Spencer, M.D.

Non-Small Cell Lung Cancer
Charles M. Haskell and E. Carmack Holmes (Univ. of California, Los Angeles)
Curr. Probl. Cancer 11:1–53, January–February 1987   13–11

Lung cancer is the most important malignancy in the United States, partly because of the great potential for prevention that exists through controlling cigarette smoking. Early diagnosis by screening of high-risk persons is the key to effective treatment. Surgery has a pivotal role in the management of local nonsmall cell lung carcinoma (NSCLC). Patients should be treated in the setting of clinical trials of new modalities whenever possible.

A wide range of operations has been used to treat NSCLC. Lobectomy is the most frequent procedure, but pneumonectomy is required in a varying proportion of cases. The trend today is toward the minimal operation that encompasses all known areas of disease. Lung spirometry and arterial blood gas estimates are used to determine physiologic operability. The use of radiotherapy remains controversial, but preoperative treatment is not indicated in patients having operable lung cancer. Postoperative adjuvant radiotherapy is used only in patients with node involvement; it is avoided where potentially curative resection has been done. The role of chemotherapy in the treatment of NSCLC is controversial, but some reviews have been cautiously optimistic.

Stage I NSCLC is managed by resection of the primary tumor and careful intraoperative node staging; more than two thirds of patients are cured. Experimental postoperative measures may be tried in properly informed patients with positive intrapulmonary or hilar nodes. Stage IIIa disease is resected if possible, and chemotherapy is used postoperatively. Patients with stage IIIb disease generally receive radiotherapy. Stage IV cases are managed palliatively.

► This important monograph summarizes current concepts concerning non-small cell carcinomas, including squamous cell, adenocarcinoma, and large cell carcinoma. The importance of the problem is well summarized in the Introduction, stating that lung cancer is the most common lethal neoplasm in the United States, accounting for 28% of all cancer deaths. Regarding etiology, the interesting statement is made that the difference in frequency over the world is primarily related to the use of tobacco, which is now thought to have a significant influence on etiology in over 90% of all lung cancers. Another significant statement is that it has been estimated that 90% of American smokers would like to quit but only 10–30% succeed, well delineating the major goal with preventive methods.—F.C. Spencer, M.D.

Bronchoplastic and Angioplastic Operation in Bronchial Carcinoma: Long-Term Results of a Retrospective Analysis From 1973 to 1983
I. Vogt-Moykopf, T. Fritz, G. Meyer, H. Bülzerbruck, and G. Daskos (Heidelberg, West Germany)
Int. Surg. 71:211–220, 1986   13–12

Both bronchial sleeve resection and angioplastic procedures are used to avoid pneumonectomy in patients with bronchial carcinoma. A total of 248 such operations was done in 1973–1983. Bronchoplastic operations ranged from removal of part of a bronchus alone to sleeve segmental resection and sleeve lobectomy. Tumors of the bronchus often infiltrate adjacent parts of the pulmonary artery. Areas of lung parenchyma may be preserved by circumscribed resection of the part of the artery involved. Combined sleeve resection of the bronchus and pulmonary artery (Fig 13–4) usually is done in conjunction with upper lobectomy.

Bronchial sleeve resection was the most frequent procedure. Nearly as many patients had small bronchoplastic procedures, and 17% of patients had small angioplastic procedures. Pulmonary arterial sleeve resection was done, alone or with bronchial resection, in 15% of cases (Fig 13–5). Twelve percent of patients received radiotherapy, and 10% had chemotherapy. The 3-year survival for bronchial sleeve cases of stage I and II disease was 46%. The 5-year survival for all stages I and II patients having bronchoplastic operations was 42%. Seven patients died of acute pul-

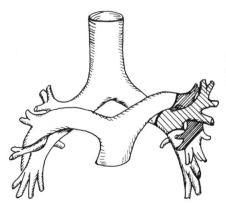

Fig 13–4.—Principle of the combined bronchial and arterial sleeve resection, e.g., left upper lobe. (Courtesy of Vogt-Moykopf, I., et al.: Int. Surg. 71:211–220, 1986.)

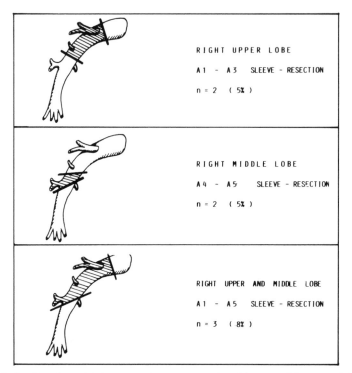

Fig 13–5.—List of arterial sleeve resections accompanying right upper lobectomy, right middle lobectomies, and right upper bilobectomies. (Courtesy of Vogt-Moykopf, I., et al.: Int. Surg. 71:211–220, 1986.)

monary bleeding, and four of anastomotic insufficiency in the postoperative period.

Partial sleeve resection no longer is done, but sleeve lobectomy has a definite role in the surgical treatment of bronchial carcinoma. It is especially useful where pulmonary reserve is restricted.

▶ This important article summarizes experiences with 248 bronchoplastic and angioplastic procedures performed over a period of 10 years. Five-year survival was 35%. A particularly significant aspect of the report is that some type of pulmonary arterial sleeve resection was performed in about 37 of the 248 patients, often in conjunction with a bronchial sleeve resection. The authors well emphasize that indications should be strict; otherwise the local recurrence rate is prohibitive. However, with appropriate indications, the technique is a valuable one, intermediate between lobectomy and pneumonectomy.—F.C. Spencer, M.D.

Small Cell Carcinoma of the Lung: A Progress Report of 15 Years' Experience

Noah C. Choi, Robert W. Carey, S. Donald Kaufman, Hermes C. Grillo, Jerry

Younger, and Earle W. Wilkins, Jr. (Harvard Univ. and Massachusetts Gen. Hosp., Boston)
Cancer 59:6–14, Jan. 1, 1987   13–13

Treatment of small-cell carcinoma of the lung (SCCL) remains difficult. The value of therapeutic advances was assessed in a series of 508 patients treated at a single institution from 1968 to 1982. Sixty-six earlier patients with limited-stage disease and 91 with extensive disease received low-dose small-volume irradiation and either cyclophosphamide alone or cyclophosphamide, vincristine, procarbazine, and prednisone chemotherapy. The later patients, 180 with limited and 171 with extensive disease, received multidrug chemotherapy and high-dose large-volume radiotherapy. Radiotherapy in the former cases was limited to 3,000–4,000 cGy, whereas later patients received up to 5,400 cGy. Elective cranial irradiation was used in one third of the later patients with limited-stage disease.

The earlier and later groups with limited disease had respective 5-year actuarial survival rates of 3% and 7%. Patients with extensive disease had actuarial 2-year survival rates of 2% and 4%, respectively, and median survival times of 5 and 7 months. Early thoracic irradiation appeared to lower the rate of local relapse and improve survival, compared with chemotherapy alone in patients with limited-stage disease.

At present, patients with SCCL are best managed by the judicious use of chemotherapy and radiotherapy. Early thoracic irradiation will improve long-term survival in patients presenting with limited-stage disease. Elective cranial irradiation is an important aspect of the treatment of limited-stage SCCL.

▶ This significant report evaluated results with 508 patients treated over a period of 15 years at the Massachusetts General Hospital. Despite encouraging short-term results with the combination of multiple chemotherapy and radiotherapy, long-term survival remained disappointing, about 8% with a localized small cell neoplasm and only a very rare 5-year survival with an extensive small cell neoplasm.—F.C. Spencer, M.D.

Superior Sulcus Lung Tumors: Results of Combined Treatment (Irradiation and Radical Resection)
Cameron D. Wright, Ashby C. Moncure, Jo-Anne O. Shepard, Earle W. Wilkins, Jr., Douglas J. Mathisen, and Hermes C. Grillo (Massachusetts Gen. Hosp. and Harvard Univ., Boston)
J. Thorac. Cardiovasc. Surg. 94:69–74, July 1987   13–14

Twenty-one patients had surgery for Pancoast tumor of the superior sulcus in 1976–1985. These patients had a small apical lung mass involving the apex of the chest, usually causing pain in the shoulder, arm, or both. All patients but one received radiotherapy before en bloc removal of the apical chest wall with underlying lung tissue. Eighteen lobectomies and four segmentectomies or wedge excisions were done.

Removal of the lower brachial plexus was necessary in 13 cases, and removal of the subclavian artery, in four cases. Three patients died postoperatively, one of empyema and bronchopleural fistula that probably was preventable. The median survival was 24 months. Actuarial survival was 63% at 1 year and 27% at 5 years. Pain was relieved in more than two thirds of patients for as long as they lived. Four of five patients with radionecrosis of the tumor lived longer than 2 years after operation.

Pancoast tumor is best managed by a combined surgical and radiotherapeutic approach. Even tumors involving the vertebral column or subclavian artery can be effectively treated. Irradiation alone is less effective than combined treatment. Needle biopsy is a helpful adjunct, but computed tomography may not definitively demonstrate or exclude invasion of chest wall structures.

▶ This report describes a more radical resection for the Pancoast tumor than is usually reported. Among 21 patients treated, the subclavian artery was resected in four, and a portion of the vertebral body, in five. The actuarial survival rates of 55% at 3 years and 27% at 5 years are clearly better than those usually achieved with radiation for these advanced lesions.—F.C. Spencer, M.D.

Pancoast Tumors: Improved Survival With Preoperative and Postoperative Radiotherapy
David M. Shahian, Wilford B. Neptune, and F. Henry Ellis, Jr. (Lahey Clinic, Burlington, Mass.; New England Deaconess Hosp., Boston; Overholt Thoracic Clinic, Boston; and Harvard Univ.)
Ann. Thorac. Surg. 43:32–38, January 1987   13–15

Pancoast tumors of the lung often are curable because local invasion produces symptoms before metastasis takes place. Preoperative irradiation, radical resection, and aggressive postoperative radiotherapy were used to treat patients seen with Pancoast tumor in 1972–1985. The average duration of symptoms preoperatively in 18 cases was 5 months. All patients but one presented with severe shoulder or scapular pain. Seventeen patients received 3,000–4,000 rads of treatment preoperatively; one had previously been treated. Half the patients had wedge or segmental resection. One pneumonectomy was performed.

There were no hospital deaths. Fourteen patients were given postoperative radiotherapy because of positive nodes or margins. External beam irradiation was used most often. The overall 5-year survival was 56%. Only two deaths resulted from local recurrence in the chest. Nine patients are alive without disease 6 months or longer after resection. Nine of ten long-term survivors had good or excellent pain relief. Eight patients had adequate shoulder mobility.

Postoperative radiotherapy is indicated for patients with Pancoast tumors who have unfavorable operative findings. These tumors may be resected even if positive lymph nodes are present. Deaths usually result from distant disease that is present but undetected at the time of operation. Better detection of occult metastasis and adjunctive chemotherapy may improve the survival of patients with pancoast tumors.

▶ This report summarizes experiences with 18 patients treated with preoperative radiation, resection, and postoperative radiotherapy in 14. There were no hospital deaths.

It is remarkable that there were only two late deaths from local recurrence. Ten of the 18 patients are alive 6 months to 13 years following operation, nine of whom have no evidence of recurrence. Hence, this paper fully supports the radical approach to a Pancoast tumor as originally proposed by Paulsen and Shaw in 1961. This contribution is best recognized by the fact that prior to 1961, 5-year survivors following any types of treatment were virtually unknown.—F.C. Spencer, M.D.

Chylothorax: A Review of 18 Cases

A.J. Fairfax, W.R. McNabb, and S.G. Spiro (Brompton Hosp., London)
Thorax 41:880–885, November 1986   13–16

Chylothorax is characterized by the accumulation of thoracic duct lymph in the pleural space. Chylothorax may occur following trauma to the thoracic duct; or it may occur as a postoperative complication of cardiothoracic surgery, as a complication of malignant disease of the thoracic lymphatic system, or spontaneously. The case histories of all patients treated for chylothorax at this institution during a 25-year period were reviewed.

The study comprised 18 patients, including 11 who developed a chylothorax following operation and seven who spontaneously developed a chylothorax. Of 11 patients with postoperative chylothorax, eight were children younger than 10 years. Five children developed chylothorax following resection of a coarctation of the aorta, and two children developed effusions after repair for Fallot's tetralogy. Nine patients showed evidence of chylothorax within 48 hours of operation, while the other two patients developed chylothorax 7 and 10 days, respectively, after operation. The duration of continuing cycle accumulation in the pleural space ranged from 2–56 days.

All 7 patients with spontaneous chylothorax were adults, ranging in age from 34 to 78 years, and all had a poor prognosis. Five patients had bilateral spontaneous chylothorax. Three developed chylothorax as a feature of malignant lymphoma; two developed chylothorax as a secondary complication of pulmonary lymphangioleiomyomatosis, while the cause could not be detected in the remaining two patients. Five patients died within 2 years of the occurrence of chylothorax of the underlying disease.

It is concluded that chylothorax is a rare condition that frequently goes undetected, especially in patients with idiopathic chylothorax.

▶ This significant report summarizes experiences with 18 patients who developed chylothorax over a period of 25 years at the Bromptom Hospital in London. The chylothorax followed a thoracic operation in 11 patients and developed from other causes in seven. Seven of the surgical cases were subsequently operated upon. All eventually recovered. A particularly important point in the data is that the frequency of chylothorax following operations for coarctation was about 1%, almost certainly due to inadvertent division of a large thoracic lymphatic during dissection.

The data show that operation, when performed, was uniformly successful. In the editor's experience, if spontaneous closure does not occur within a few days, the patient should be promptly operated upon. With modern techniques the lacerated lymphatic in almost all cases can be easily identified and ligated.—F.C. Spencer, M.D.

Pleural Mesothelioma
Nael Martini, Patricia M. McCormack, Manjit S. Bains, Larry R. Kaiser, Michael E. Burt, and Basil S. Hilaris (Memorial Sloan-Kettering Cancer Ctr., New York)
Ann. Thorac. Surg. 43:113–120, January 1987   13–17

Benign pleural mesotheliomas may be cured surgically, but malignant tumors are locally aggressive and very difficult to treat. Benign lesions are important chiefly because they are difficult to differentiate from malignant mesothelioma before operation. Malignant mesotheliomas may present as localized tumors or as diffuse pleural disease with effusion and encasement of the lung. In the latter cases, the pleural space may be obliterated. Both local and diffuse tumors frequently cause chest pain and dyspnea. Localized malignant mesothelioma usually is fibrosarcomatous. Asbestos exposure correlates with diffuse epithelial mesothelioma. Most patients with the latter form of tumor die within a year of diagnosis; long-term survivals are rare.

Radiotherapy alone will not eliminate diffuse mesothelioma. Patients who receive operations seem to live longer than those managed less aggressively. The value of chemotherapy remains uncertain. Diffuse mesothelioma has been treated by both radical extrapleural pneumonectomy and pleurectomy. Subtotal parietal pleurectomy preserves functioning lung tissue, removes the bulk of disease, and controls effusion. Residual disease may be treated with both external radiotherapy or implantation of radioactive material. Most patients also receive chemotherapy, but systemic agents are best reserved for patients having recurrent disease.

▶ This article reviews current data with this rare highly lethal neoplasm. The extensive experience at Memorial Hospital over the previous 35 years is described, during which time a total of 226 patients were seen.—F.C. Spencer, M.D.

Technique of Successful Lung Transplantation in Humans
Joel D. Cooper, F.G. Pearson, G.A. Patterson, T.R.J. Todd, R.J. Ginsberg, M. Goldberg, and W.A.P. DeMajo (Univ. of Toronto)
J. Thorac. Cardiovasc. Surg. 93:173–181, February 1987   13–18

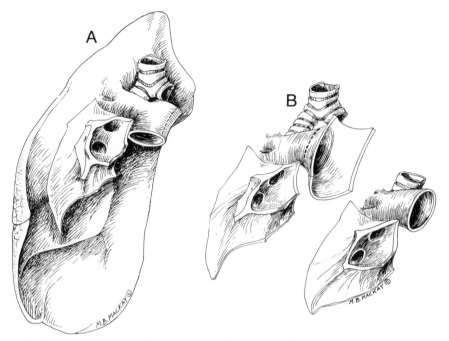

Fig 13–6.—A, preparation of right donor lung. The heart-lung block is removed intact, after which the right lung is dissected free. The airway is initially divided at the distal trachea and the left main bronchus. The main pulmonary artery and the left pulmonary artery are divided, with a cuff of the main artery left attached to the right pulmonary artery. A large flap of pericardium is left attached to the hilum of the lung. **B,** the donor bronchus is transected two rings above the right upper lobe bronchus. A large cuff of main pulmonary artery is left attached to the right pulmonary artery, if necessary. Otherwise, the right pulmonary artery is transected just at its origin. (Courtesy of Cooper, J.D., et al.: J. Thorac. Cardiovasc. Surg. 93:173–181, February 1987.)

The authors have performed five single-lung transplantations for end-stage pulmonary fibrosis with four long-term survivors. Two patients had right and two had left lung transplantation. The operation is limited to cases of end-stage fibrotic disease, in which both ventilation and perfusion are preferentially diverted to the transplanted lung.

The operation is done using one-lung anesthesia, but cardiopulmonary bypass is available on standby. The donor and recipient operations are done in adjoining rooms. A lack of suitable donors is the chief obstacle to more widespread lung transplantation. Preparation of the donor lung is illustrated in Figure 13–6, and its implantation is shown in Figure 13–7. A pedicle of omentum is wrapped about the bronchial anastomosis in order to restore bronchial artery circulation and protect the anastomosis.

Four of the five operated patients were discharged well 4–6 weeks after surgery. Ventilatory assistance was necessary for up to 6 days after transplantation. Three of the four long-term survivors required reintubation for ventilatory assistance, usually in association with rejection. The one failure occurred when an unsuitable donor lung was used in a desperate attempt to save a patient's life. Both cyclosporine and azathioprine were used for immunosuppression.

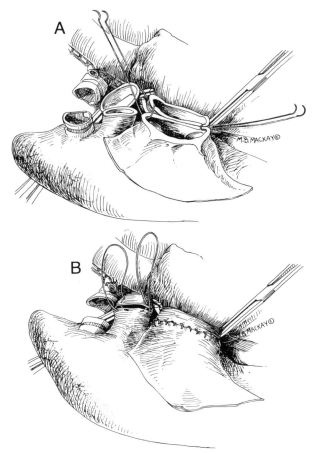

Fig 13–7.—A, the donor lung has been positioned in the recipient's chest and the back wall of the atrial anastomosis is performed with running monofilament suture material. **B,** after completion of the venous anastomosis, the pulmonary artery is anastomosed without the need to reposition in the lung. Before completion of the pulmonary anastomosis, the venous clamp is temporarily removed to provide back bleeding out the pulmonary artery, after which the anastomosis is completed and the vascular clamps are removed. (Courtesy of Cooper, J.D., et al.: J. Thorac. Cardiovasc. Surg. 93:173–181, February 1987.)

Careful patient selection and the use of cyclosporine will enhance the success of single lung transplantation. Avoidance of daily steroid therapy in the early postoperative period also is helpful.

▶ This impressive report describes five lung transplantations with four long-term survivors. Key technical features include the use of omentum around the bronchial anastomosis and immunosuppression with cyclosporine. This impressive achievement is well illustrated by the fact that previously only one patient in the previous 20 years was discharged from the hospital following lung transplantation. This patient, operated upon by Denom in Europe in 1968, lived for 10 months.—F.C. Spencer, M.D.

14 Congenital Heart Disease

Myocardial Protection in the Neonatal Heart: A Comparison of Topical Hypothermia and Crystalloid and Blood Cardioplegic Solutions
Antonio F. Corno, Daniel M. Bethencourt, Hillel Laks, Gary S. Haas, Sunita Bhuta, Hakob G. Davtyan, William M. Flynn, Davis C. Drinkwater, Craig Laidig, and Paul Chang (Univ. of California, Los Angeles)
J. Thorac. Cardiovasc. Surg. 93:163–172, February 1987   14–1

Congenital heart defects are increasingly being repaired in early infancy. The protection afforded by topical hypothermia was compared with that afforded by crystalloid and blood cardioplegia during 2 hours of ischemic arrest in 45 isolated, blood-perfused, neonatal piglet hearts. Topical cooling was compared with the use of hyperosmolar low-calcium crystalloid cardioplegic solution; St. Thomas' Hospital solution; cold blood cardioplegia with potassium, citrate-phosphate-dextrose, and tromethamine; and cold blood cardioplegia with potassium alone.

Hemodynamic recovery, as assessed from the percent of preischemic stroke work, was highest and essentially normal when cold blood cardioplegia with potassium alone was used. Recovery was lowest when the hyperosmolar low-calcium crystalloid solution was used. More than 85% recovery occurred at 1 hour with topical cooling.

Topical cooling is an effective means of myocardial protection in the neonatal pig. Optimal functional recovery is obtained by using cold blood cardioplegia with potassium added. The neonatal heart may be relatively sensitive to calcium in cardioplegic solution. Hyperosmolar low-calcium crystalloid cardioplegia provided poor functional protection in the present study.

▶ The findings in this important report are impressive and significant. The experimental model included two hours of ischemic arrest in 45 neonatal piglet hearts. Topical hypothermia alone gave much better results than crystalloid cardioplegia. In addition, blood cardioplegia with potassium was far superior to blood cardioplegia with a lowered calcium, suggesting a sensitivity of the neonatal myocardium to a low calcium concentration.

The original concept for lowering calcium concentration in cardioplegia solutions was to minimize intracellular migration of calcium when the cellular membrane was injured from anoxia. Unless the calcium concentration was reduced to a very low level, simply lowering calcium concentration did not result in membrane injury. This report suggests that these observations are not valid in neonatal hearts, a most important finding.—F.C. Spencer, M.D.

231

Extracorporeal Membrane Oxygenation for Postoperative Cardiac Support in Children

Kirk R. Kenter, D. Glenn Pennington, Thomas R. Weber, Miriam A. Zambie, Paul Braun, and Victor Martychenko (St. Louis Univ.)

J. Thorac. Cardiovasc. Surg. 93:27–35, January 1987   14–2

Because of technical considerations and size limitations, the application of various methods and devices for prolonged circulatory support for cardiac failure has very limited use in children. During a 3-year period, 13 children were treated with extracorporeal membrane oxygenation (ECMO) for severe postoperative cardiopulmonary failure refractory to conventional therapy. Their ages ranged from 9 days to 17.6 years (mean, 3.8 years) and weights ranged from 2.8 kg to 50 kg (mean, 13.8). Seven patients had obstructive lesions of the right ventricle, such as pulmonary stenosis and tetralogy; the other patients had tricuspid atresia, truncus arteriosus, complete transposition, total anomalous pulmonary venous connection, pericardial tamponade, and a drug reaction after heart transplantation. Groin cannulation using the femoral or iliac vessels was used early in the study; chest cannulation with venous return from a single right atrial cannula and arterial inflow through an ascending aortic cannula were performed in the latter patients. The interval between operation and institution of ECMO ranged from 9 hours to 50 hours (mean, 22.2), while one patient, who could not be weaned from cardiopulmonary bypass, required ECMO in the operating room.

Peak flows ranged from 1.05 L/min/sq m to 2.74 L/min/sq m (mean, 1.92), and duration on ECMO ranged from 12 hours to 9 days (mean, 3.4 days). In five children (38%) severe renal insufficiency developed, and in three, irreversible brain damage: both complications resulted from prolonged periods of hypotension and inadequate cardiac support prior to ECMO. Thrombosis during the oxygenator circuit occurred in two patients, and seven patients required reexploration for bleeding. Seven patients (54%) were successfully weaned from ECMO, and mediastinitis developed in three of these patients. Causes of death in patients not weaned from ECMO was related to neurologic sequelae of prolonged hypotension in three, irreversible cardiac failure in two, and sepsis and bleeding in one. One hospital death occurred 74 days after the patient was weaned from ECMO. Of the six hospital survivors (46%), one died 6 months after ECMO was withdrawn, and the remaining were well with normal cardiac function 7 months to 4.3 years postoperatively (mean, 32 months).

Despite the high incidence of complications, severe cardiac insufficiency after cardiac surgery in children can be managed successfully with ECMO, with an excellent chance for functional recovery.

▶ Thirteen children with postoperative refractory cardiac failure were treated with extracorporeal membrane oxygenation for 12 hours to 9 days (average, 3½ days). There were five long-term survivors with normal cardiac function.

Activated clotting times were maintained between 175 and 200 seconds. Nonetheless, severe bleeding problems occurred in over one half the patients; thrombi developed in the oxygenator circuit in at least two patients. Other complications were common. This report well illustrates both the potential of salvage with this extreme form of circulatory support as well as the serious complications associated with continued heparinization.—F.C. Spencer, M.D.

Phrenic Nerve Paralysis After Pediatric Cardiac Surgery: Retrospective Study of 125 Cases
Takashi Watanabe, George A. Trusler, William G. Williams, John F. Edmonds, John G. Coles, and Yuhei Hosokawa (Hosp. for Sick Children and Univ. of Toronto)
J. Thorac. Cardiovasc. Surg. 94:383–388, September 1987   14–3

Phrenic nerve paralysis developing after cardiac surgery can cause severe respiratory distress to infants and children. Paralysis was diagnosed in 1.6% of 7,670 cardiac operations performed in pediatric patients between 1974 and 1985. The incidence was 1.9% after open heart surgery and 1.3% after closed heart operations. The most frequent open-heart procedures associated with phrenic paralysis were the Mustard procedure and right ventricular outflow tract reconstruction. Among closed heart operations the Glenn anastomosis and Blalock-Hanlon atrial septectomy were most often implicated. Phrenic nerve paralysis was nearly twice as frequent after repeat surgery.

Seven patients with phrenic paralysis, 5.6% of the total, died. Twelve patients underwent diaphragmatic plication, with no deaths, and were extubated an average of 2.3 days after plication. Patients not operated on who were younger than 2 years were intubated for 16 days on average, while older patients were intubated for an average of 7 days.

Phrenic nerve paralysis occurs most often after dissection near the nerve, or after secondary surgery where the phrenic nerve anatomy is obscured by adhesions. Initial treatment is ventilatory assistance, with continuous positive airway pressure to normalize lung volumes and stabilize the rib cage. If ventilatory assistance remains necessary after 2 weeks, diaphragmatic plication is considered, especially in children younger than 2 years.

▶ This important report from one of the large children's hospitals in the world describes experiences with phrenic nerve paralysis in 125 children, resulting from a series of over 7,600 cardiac operations over a period of 12 years. Morbidity with phrenic paralysis can be especially severe with small children. Caution is particularly indicated with reoperations, probably because mediastinal scarring makes the phrenic nerve more vulnerable to injury by traction. Traction is probably the most common cause of injury because eventual recovery of phrenic nerve function occurred in 84% of the group.—F.C. Spencer, M.D.

Surgical Intervention in Neonates With Critical Pulmonary Stenosis
Walter H. Merrill, Todd A. Shuman, Thomas P. Graham, Jr., John W. Hammon, Jr., and Harvey W. Bender, Jr. (Vanderbilt Univ., Nashville, Tenn.)
Ann. Surg. 205:712–717, June 1987   14–4

Neonates with critical pulmonary stenosis and an intact ventricular septum have marked right ventricular hypertension and a right-to-left shunt. Severe systemic arterial desaturation results. The mortality is high. Eighteen consecutive infants with critical stenosis, all aged 2 weeks or younger, were studied in 1972–1986. Eight infants had a right ventricular end-diastolic volume (RVEDV) less than 72% of predicted, whereas ten others had a normal or increased volume.

All the infants underwent closed pulmonary valvotomy. Five of the eight with a low RVEDV required a systemic-pulmonary shunt or postoperative prostaglandin₁ treatment. One patient died. Nine of the ten patients with a normal or high RVEDV did well after valvotomy, and one, who was moribund, died after valvotomy and shunting. Six patients required reoperation; four underwent valvectomy, and two had takedown of a shunt. Four reoperated patients also had a transanular patch placed. All the long-term survivors are free of symptoms. Recatheterization of four patients who initially had a small right ventricle showed significant ventricular growth. Most patients had mild pulmonary insufficiency at follow-up.

Most young infants with critical pulmonary stenosis and intact ventricular septum can be managed by closed transventricular valvotomy. If there is a diminutive right ventricle, prostaglandin should be infused. Shunt surgery is reserved for patients who have hypoxemia and inadequate pulmonary blood flow despite prostaglandin infusion.

▶ Experiences with 18 neonates surgically treated for critical pulmonic stenosis at Vanderbilt University over a period of 14 years are summarized in this report. A cogent argument is presented for simply doing a closed pulmonic valvulotomy rather than an open approach with temporary circulatory arrest. Sixteen of the 18 patients survived but six required reoperation, including valvectomy in four. Four of the six patients reoperated upon also had a transannular patch. These data indicate the severity of the pathology, which required valvectomy in some patients, patch outflow reconstruction in others. Hence, it seems evident that the objective with the semiemergency operation in the neonate should be to preserve life, recognizing that a significant percentage will require reoperation because of the extensive pathology.—F.C. Spencer, M.D.

Surgical Repair of Acquired Ventricular Septal Defect: Determinants of Early and Late Outcome
M.T. Jones, P.M. Schofield, J.F. Dark, H. Moussali, A.K. Deiraniya, R.A.M. Lawson, C. Ward, and C.L. Bray (Wythenshawe Hosp., Manchester, England)
J. Thorac. Cardiovasc. Surg. 93:680–686, May 1987   14–5

Because of the high incidence of preoperative death when repair of ventricular septal defect (VSD) is delayed, this procedure is generally considered a surgical emergency. The early and long-term results of surgical repair of postinfarction VSD was investigated and outcome related to preoperative right and left ventricular function in a group of patients operated on between 1970 and 1985.

A group of 60 patients who underwent surgery for repair of postinfarction VSD were reviewed. Preoperative cineangiograms were studied to measure left ventricular ejection fraction and to assess right ventricular function by determining the percentage reduction in right ventricular midcavity diameter.

There were 23 early deaths; in 7, death was caused by failure to wean from cardiopulmonary bypass; in 4, death resulted from failed VSD procedure; 8 patients died from myocardial failure; and the others died of renal failure, reinfarction, or cerebrovascular accident. There were also 14 late deaths. Early mortality was more than twice as high for inferior infarction than for anterior infarction. The time interval between infarction and operation also influenced survival. Early survival was improved by good preoperative right ventricular function but was unaffected by left ventricular function before operation. Nevertheless, long-term survival was enhanced by preserved preoperative left ventricular function and unaffected by preoperative right ventricular function. Of the 23 long-term survivors, 87% are in the New York Heart Association class I or II.

To date, this is the largest study of surgical repair of postinfarction VSD. Results have improved between two successive time frames in this series.

▶ This series of 60 patients undergoing surgical repair of postinfarction ventricular septal defects must be one of the largest in the world. The surgical mortality remains high, although it improved with experience over this period of 15 years.

Patients requiring operation within less than 1 week had a mortality of 22%, with the rate gradually decreasing for those able to survive a longer period before operation. The inferior infarcts continue to account for the highest mortality: 86% in the early part of the series, but still 57% among 17 patients operated upon in the previous five years.—F.C. Spencer, M.D.

Ventricular Septal Defect Associated With Aortic Regurgitation
Kouichi Hisatomi, Kenichi Kosuga, Tadashi Isomura, Haruo Akagawa, Kiroku Ohishi, and Michihiro Koga (Kurume Univ., Japan)
Ann. Thorac. Surg. 43:363–367, April 1987   14–6

The best surgical approach to ventricular septal defect (VSD) associated with aortic regurgitation remains uncertain. Data on 76 patients having 1+ or greater regurgitation were reviewed. The mean age was 15 years. Most VSDs were just beneath the pulmonary valve. Seventeen patients had closure of the VSD alone, and 49 had aortic valve repair. Forty operations involved plication or appositioning. Aortoplasty was done as an additional procedure in nine patients. Ten patients required a prosthetic valve.

Pulsed Doppler studies indicated postoperative improvement in more than 70% of patients having valvuloplasty and aortoplasty. The overall rate of improvement after valvuloplasty alone was 65%; all patients having combined valvuloplasty and aortoplasty improved. Four patients were reoperated on because of worsening aortic regurgitation. Two failed to improve, and one died of perforation of the free edge of a bicuspid valve.

Combined aortic valvuloplasty and aortoplasty appears to be the best approach to VSD associated with aortic regurgitation, especially in patients younger than age 15 years. Early closure of the VSD alone may be indicated in younger patients with mild aortic regurgitation. If further surgery proves necessary, the defect may be closed by aortic valvuloplasty or prosthetic replacement carried out. Valvuloplasty is necessary in a patient younger than age 10 years with more than mild aortic regurgitation.

▶ This unusually large series of patients (76) reflects the increased frequency of this problem in congenital heart disease in Japan. Aortic valve repairs were performed in 40 patients; in nine others an aortoplasty was done as well. A new method of aortoplasty is described, used for severe cases when valvuloplasty itself was inadequate. Good results were obtained in 70%–80% of patients.—F.C. Spencer, M.D.

Results With the Mustard Operation in Simple Transposition of the Great Arteries: 1963–1985
George A. Trusler, William G. Williams, Kim F. Duncan, Peter S. Hesslein, Lee N. Benson, Robert M. Freedom, Teruo Izukawa, and Peter M. Olley (Hosp. for Sick Children and Univ. of Toronto)
Ann. Surg. 206:251–260, September 1987   14–7

The results of repair of simple transposition by the Mustard technique were compared in 106 patients undergoing surgery between 1963 and 1973 (group I) and 223 operated on between 1974 and 1985 (group II). Operative mortality was 10% in group I, but only 0.9% in group II. The 10-year actuarial survival rates were 73% and 94%, respectively. Baffle complications were similar in the two groups. The latest ECG showed that fewer than half of group I patients but more than two thirds of group II patients were in normal sinus rhythm. Most patients, however, had sinus node dysfunction or other dysrhythmias on ambulatory ECG study. Right ventricular contractility was definitely reduced in 11% of the children studied. About 75% of the children were in New York Heart Association functional class I at late follow-up, and the rest were in class II. About 20% were taking medication, chiefly for dysrhythmia.

Mortality associated with the Mustard operation has declined significantly. Serious baffle-related complications are infrequent, but dysrhythmia remains a major problem. Such complications are expected to occur less frequently with arterial repair, but it remains to be learned whether the good early results obtained by a few surgeons can be reproduced without excessive risk.

▶ This classic report describes operative experiences over a period of 22 years with 329 patients in whom the Mustard technique was employed. This is particularly significant as the report is from the institution in which Mustard performed his first operation in May 1963. In the last 10 years of the study, the results are most impressive. Operative mortality was 1% with a 10-year actuarial survival of 94%. Significant baffle complications continued to occur throughout the study. Quite important is the fact that with observations now covering two decades, significant right ventricular dysfunction remains uncommon.—F.C. Spencer, M.D.

The Fontan Operation: Ventricular Hypertrophy, Age, and Date of Operation as Risk Factors
James K. Kirklin, Eugene H. Blackstone, John W. Kirklin, Albert D. Pacifico, and Lionel M. Bargeron, Jr. (Univ. of Alabama at Birmingham)
J. Thorac. Cardiovasc. Surg. 92:1049–1064, December 1986   14–8

Results of the Fontan procedure have been puzzling in some instances. For no apparent reason, the outcome appears to be better in patients with tricuspid atresia than in patients with other cardiac defects. Younger patients seem to have increased risk of mortality, yet infants have successfully recovered from the operation. Overall outlook seems to be improving, but some survivors still die a few months postoperatively. The results of several variations of the Fontan operation performed on patients with a variety of cardiac defects were reviewed to identify factors that predispose toward success.

Records of 102 patients who had undergone the Fontan operation were studied. Patient ages ranged from 0.7 to 38 years. Several modifications of the procedure were involved, and most patients had had at least one palliative operation.

Overall survival rate was 63% at 6 years; but in patients with tricuspid atresia, survival was 81% at 9 years. These patients also had lower hospital and late death rates. Risk of mortality was greatest immediately postoperatively. Most patients died of acute or subacute cardiac failure. Younger age was a risk factor for death in the early years of experience, while older age was not. Nevertheless, when other factors were considered, a decreased rate of death was apparent in the current era, especially in younger patients.

It appears that the Fontàn operation should be performed as early in life as prudent to avoid increased ventricular hypertrophy, but older age alone does not contraindicate the procedure.

▶ Experiences with 102 patients operated upon at the University of Alabama over a period of 10 years are summarized. Survival rate at 6 years following operation was 63%, including operative mortality; it was 81% for operations for tricuspid atresia. The data indicated a much higher mortality with significant elevation of right atrial pressure following operation, especially above 14 mm Hg. With current techniques, young age is no longer associated with an increased risk of operation. Hence, the report is a valuable summary of current techniques and results with this important congenital cardiac operation.—F.C. Spencer, M.D.

Apicoaortic Conduits for Complex Left Ventricular Outflow Obstruction: 10-Year Experience
Michael S. Sweeney, William E. Walker, Denton A. Cooley, and George J. Reul (Texas Heart Institute and Univ. of Texas, Houston)
Ann. Thorac. Surg. 42:609–611, December 1986   14–9

Some patients with left ventricular (LV) outflow obstruction may be candidates for creation of a new outflow tract from the LV apex to the aorta at the diaphragmatic level. Indications include fibrous tunnel obstruction of the LV outflow tract; severe hypoplasia of the aortic anulus; and tubular hypoplasia of the ascending aorta. Valved conduits were placed in 38 such patients in a 10-year period. Severe classification of the ascending aorta was another indication. A porcine-valved Dacron conduit was used in each case. All operations but two were done under total cardiopulmonary bypass with cold cardioplegia.

Four hospital deaths occurred. Four of eight late deaths were shunt-related, three resulting from disruption of the conduit from its LV attachment. Three children have required replacement of the porcine valve 3 to 8 years after initial surgery. Two fatal infections occurred. All 26 long-term survivors were asymptomatic without cardiac medications. No thromboembolism has occurred, despite the omission of anticoagulation. None of the surviving patients is restricted physically.

The apicoaortic conduit operation is a useful approach to some patients having complex LV outflow tract obstruction. The operation seems most suited to patients having multiple attempts to open the aortic root, those with a failed Konno or Rastan procedure, and those with some major complication of a previous aortic root operation.

▶ Experiences with valve conduits interposed between the left ventricular apex and aorta in 38 patients over a period of 10 years are described. Seventy-eight percent of the survivors were alive at 5 years, about two thirds of whom had had no major complications. Hence, the technique remains a useful one if alternative methods of treatment are unsuccessful. Significant complications in approximately 25% of patients, however, must be anticipated within the first 5 years after operation.—F.C. Spencer, M.D.

Current Risks and Protocols for Operations for Double-Outlet Right Ventricle: Derivation From an 18 Year Experience

John W. Kirklin, Albert D. Pacifico, Eugene H. Blackstone, James K. Kirklin, and L.M. Bargeron, Jr. (Univ. of Alabama at Birmingham)
J. Thorac. Cardiovasc. Surg. 92:913–930, November 1986   14–10

The cases of 127 patients undergoing initial intracardiac repair of double-outlet right ventricle (DORV) were reviewed. The DORV was defined as a ventriculoarterial connection where the aorta and pulmonary artery both arose more than 50% from the right ventricle. The median follow-up was 51 months.

Fifty-eight patients failed to survive the early and late postoperative periods. The actuarial survival at 12 years was 38%. Six deaths followed reoperation. Acute heart failure was responsible for nearly half the remaining deaths. Eight patients had complete heart block after repair. Most surviving patients were fully active and asymptomatic at follow-up. Reoperation was carried out in 17 patients. Operative mortality after reoperation (at the authors' center) was 31%.

The DORV should be repaired at age 6–12 months—sooner, if necessary. Preliminary pulmonary artery banding is not indicated. The DORV with subpulmonary ventricular septal defect is managed by closure of the septal defect and an arterial switch operation. Shunting may be indicated, if pulmonary stenosis is present. The Fontan operation is technically feasible in DORV with noncommitted ventricular septal defect associated with pulmonary stenosis. The septal defect should be enlarged, if restrictive, and the tricuspid valve closed.

▶ This report describes experiences with 127 patients with a double-outlet right ventricle operated upon over a period of 18 years. The influence of type of double-outlet right ventricle on operative results is impressive. Those with a subaortic ventricular septal defect treated with an intraventricular tunnel had a survival near 98%, whereas those with a noncommitted ventricular septal defect had only a 22% overall 10-year survival.—F.C. Spencer, M.D.

Identification of Risk Factors for Spinal Cord Ischemia by the Use of Monitoring of Somatosensory Evoked Potentials During Coarctation Repair
Himansu K. Dasmahapatra, John G. Coles, Margot J. Taylor, Daniel Cass, Greg Couper, Sharon Adler, Fredrick Burrows, Henriette Sherret, George A. Trusler, and William G. Williams (Hosp. for Sick Children, Toronto)
Circulation 76 (Suppl. III):III-14–III-18, September 1987   14–11

Spinal cord infarction and paraplegia after occlusion of the descending thoracic aorta are infrequent; thus, statistical identification of risk factors is difficult. Reversible spinal cord ischemia (SCI), however, is more common and is detectable by intraoperative neurophysiologic monitoring. It can also lead to irreversible damage to the spinal cord.

The authors examined the potential influence of selected perioperative variables on the development of spinal cord ischemia during coarctation repair. Spinal somatosensory evoked potentials (SEPs) were monitored during operation in 38 patients aged 18 days to 18 years in 1982 to 1986.

No patient sustained perioperative neurologic dysfunction, but ten (26%) developed reversible SCI, which was reflected in a greater than 75% loss of SEP N_1-P_1 interpeak amplitude during aortic occlusion. During occlusion seven patients (18%) sustained complete loss of the SEP. Uniform and prompt recovery of the signal occurred with reperfusion after completion of the repair in six patients and temporary institution of partial occlusion in one patient.

Multiple regression analysis showed that the degree of SCI was negatively related to the distal aortic pressure and the occlusion PCO_2 but was positively related to the change in proximal systolic pressure with aortic occlusion. It was concluded that distal hypotension and SCI commonly occur during aortic occlusion for coarctation repair and that intraoperative interventions that may influence distal aortic perfusion or PCO_2, or both, should be used judiciously.

▶ This report describes experiences with monitoring of somatosensory evoked potentials in 38 patients operated upon for coarctation of the aorta. The mean distal aortic pressure was 30 mm; average cross-clamp time was 29 minutes. Fortunately, no neurologic problems occurred, but 25% of the patients developed reversible spinal cord ischemia, seven of whom lost all sensory potentials.

At the editor's institution, this subject had been studied in some detail since 1982. The safe upper time limit for spinal cord ischemia with loss of sensory potentials is unknown. In a publication from the editor's institution (Krieger, K. H., Spencer, F. C.: Surgery 97:2, 1985) five of six patients in whom potentials remained absent for longer then 30 minutes (patients operated upon for aortic aneurysms) developed paraplegia.

In this report the authors refer to experimental studies demonstrating that ischemic loss of sensory potentials for more than 15 minutes resulted in spinal cord injury. In this series, the duration of complete loss ranged from 1 to 14 minutes. Undoubtedly, this type of monitoring led to effective modification of the operative technique when necessary, avoiding any neurologic injury whatever. More widespread use of this type of monitoring during operation for coarctation of the aorta is clearly indicated.—F.C. Spencer, M.D.

Spinal Cord Damage and Operations for Coarctation of the Aorta: Aetiology, Practice, and Prospects
G. Keen (Bristol Royal Infirmary, Bristol, England)
Thorax 42:11–18, 1987   14–12

The variable and uncertain blood supply to the spinal cord creates a risk of damage at surgery for coarctation of the aorta. A survey of surgeons in the United Kingdom and Ireland revealed paraplegia in 0.3% of operations, or once in 343 operations. Two of 16 cases followed repeat operations for coarctation. Three further patients had temporary postoperative paraplegia. An unknown number of patients may have had less obvious or transient lesions of the spinal cord or cauda equina.

Monitoring of cord function by somatosensory evoked potential recording is an effective means of assessing cord function during surgery. If distal aortic perfusion is inadequate, distal bypass is necessary. Left atriofemoral bypass, a heparin-bonded shunt, and femoral vein to femoral artery bypass all have been used. Special attention is needed for patients in whom there is appreciable blood flow through the coarctation, which will be lost to the lower aorta during cross-clamping.

Somatosensory potential monitoring will be routinely practiced if its reliability is established. Thoracic surgeons, orthopedic surgeons, and neurophysiologists should collaborate in developing evoked potential monitoring systems.

▶ A wide survey of operations for coarctation found paraplegia developing in 16 patients following nearly 5,500 operations, an incidence near 0.3%. This is slightly less than the frequency of 0.5% found in an extensive review by Lyman Brewer over a decade ago.

The author quotes the work by Laschinger and Cunningham in our institution. Routine monitoring of somatosensory potentials should be encouraged with these operations because to date no neurologic problems have occurred in patients in whom the somatosensory potentials remained intact while the aorta was occluded. This has been uniformly associated with a distal aortic pressure above 60 mm. If somatosensory potential monitoring is not available, simple use of an intravascular catheter in the distal aorta to display distal aortic pressure while the aorta is occluded, similar to monitoring of electrocardiogram, provides a valuable guide to adequacy of collateral circulation. Neurologic problems almost never occur unless the distal aortic segment is hypotensive for more than 30 minutes.—F.C. Spencer, M.D.

A New Technique for Repair of Aortic Coarctation: Subclavian Flap Aortoplasty With Preservation of Arterial Blood Flow to the Left Arm
Milton A. Meier, Fernando A. Lucchese, Waldir Jazbik, Ivo A. Nesralla, and José Teles Mendonça (State Univ. of Rio de Janeiro and other Brazilian med. insts.)
J. Thorac. Cardiovasc. Surg. 92:1005–1012, December 1986   14–13

There is controversy as to the appropriate surgical technique for repair of coarctation of the aorta. A procedure is described that uses the subclavian artery as a flap, preserving arterial blood flow to the left arm.

The technique completely mobilizes the left subclavian artery (LSCA) to the origin of its first branches. At this point, before any incision is made, the distance from the origin of the LSCA to the coarctation site should be determined to assess the feasibility of the operation. If the decision is made to proceed, it is not necessary to mobilize the aorta extensively; intercostal arteries are individually controlled with snares. The LSCA is detached from the aorta at its source and incised longitudinally

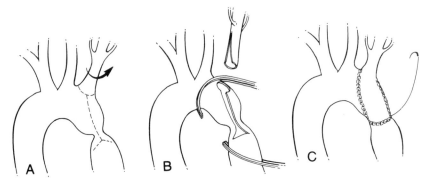

Fig 14–1.—A, the incisions to detach the LSCA and open the descending aorta are made according to the *interrupted lines*. **B,** the LSCA is opened in its posterior wall. The incision in the aorta goes 12 to 15 mm below the site of coarctation and is extended 3 to 4 mm laterally. **C,** the LSCA is sutured over the coarctation site, widening the obstruction and preserving the blood flow to the arm. (Courtesy of Meier, M.A., et al.: J. Thorac. Cardiovasc. Surg. 92:1005–1012, December 1986.)

on the posterior aspect. Beginning with the opening at the origin of the LSCA, the anterior wall of the aorta is incised distally to the descending aorta past the coarctation, the coarctation membrane is excised, and the ductus is ligated and divided. The flap formed by the opened LSCA is sutured to the edges of the aorta, thus widening the coarctation site and preserving blood flow to the left arm (Fig 14–1). When there is a long narrowing of the isthmus, the LSCA is detached together with a portion of the anterior wall of the aorta to form a longer, wider flap.

In 28 patients (from 2 months to 25 years old) who were treated with this technique, there were no hospital deaths. At postoperative follow-up, patients showed satisfactory correction, normal blood flow through the LSCA, and no gradients through the isthmus area. Normal growth of the aorta at the coarctation site was strongly suggested. Findings indicate that the procedure is feasible and preferable to other techniques in most cases of discrete isthmic coarctation—and in some cases of long narrowing of the isthmus—in patients ranging widely in age and weight.

▶ A technical variation of use of the subclavian artery for repair of coarctation is described that preserves blood flow to the left arm. Rather than the reverse subclavian flap, as described by Waldhausen, the aortic origin of the subclavian artery is detached with an oval opening and the intact subclavian artery brought downward and used to patch the site of correction of coarctation. Initial short-term results were uniformly good. Most discussants of the paper expressed satisfaction with the standard Waldhausen subclavian flap procedure. Cooley, by contrast, stated that he preferred the standard synthetic patch repair and had not recognized a single instance of false aneurysm.—F.C. Spencer, M.D.

Anomalous Origin of Left Coronary Artery From Pulmonary Artery: Ligation Versus Establishment of a Two Coronary Artery System

Richard Bunton, Richard A. Jonas, Peter Lang, Azaria J.J.T. Rein, and Aldo R. Castaneda (Children's Hosp. and Harvard Univ., Boston)
J. Thorac. Cardiovasc. Surg. 93:103–108, January 1987   14–14

The preferred management of anomalous left coronary artery arising from the pulmonary artery (ALCAPA) is establishment of a two-coronary artery system. Twenty-four patients seen in 1959–1985 with ALCAPA as an isolated lesion were operated on. Their mean age was 38 months. All patients but one had impaired left ventricular contraction. Eleven earlier patients had ligation or osteal closure of the anomalous left coronary artery. Eleven seen later underwent the Takeuchi procedure: creation of an aorticopulmonary window with an intrapulmonary baffle. These groups were similar, except that the Takeuchi patients tended to be younger when seen for treatment.

Coronary ligation or osteal closure carried an early mortality of 27% and a late mortality of 25% during a mean follow-up of 10½ years. Two patients required surgery for a residual shunt. One patient each had severe mitral regurgitation and recurrent angina. There were no deaths in the Takeuchi group during a mean follow-up of 18 months. One patient was reoperated on for supravalvular pulmonary stenosis. One patient with an obstructed baffle was asymptomatic.

The Takeuchi procedure is the best operation for patients with ALCAPA, particularly young infants in whom other forms of myocardial revascularization are unsuitable. The Takeuchi operation is especially recommended over coronary ligation for patients with congestive heart failure.

▶ This important report describes experiences at the Boston Children's Hospital with 24 patients with anomalous origin of the left coronary artery from the pulmonary artery who were treated over a period of 26 years. In 11 cases, a left coronary–aortic tunnel was created using the Takeuchi procedure with no early or late mortality. In 11 other cases coronary ligation or osteal closure was used with a 27% early mortality. These data dramatically indicate the value and effectiveness of the Takeuchi procedure.—F.C. Spencer, M.D.

15 Valvular Heart Disease

Mechanical Failure of the Björk-Shiley Valve: Incidence, Clinical Presentation, and Management
Dan Lindblom, Viking O. Björk, Bjarne K.H. Semb (Karolinska Hosp., Stockholm)
J. Thorac. Cardiovasc. Surg. 92:894–907, November 1986   15–1

Mechanical disruption has been described in many mechanical heart valves. Even biologic valves may require emergency treatment. Recently, there has been an interest in the increased incidence of strut fractures among convexo-concave Björk-Shiley valves. The manufacturer has recalled these valves several times. The experience after implantation of 3,334 Björk-Shiley valves in a 15-year period is described.

The follow-up rate was 99.2%, covering 17,511 patient-years. The mean follow-up time was 6.3 years. The autopsy rate was 75% among all fatalities. A total of 19 cases of mechanical failure was documented. There were no mechanical failures among the 271 patients with standard Delrin Björk-Shiley valves, the 739 patients with the aortic standard Pyrolyte Björk-Shiley valves, or the 377 patients with the Monostrut Björk-Shiley valves. One of the 430 mitral standard Pyrolyte valves fractured. Eighteen of the 1,461 convexo-concave valves fractured, 6 of the 884 with an opening angle of 60 degrees, and 12 of 577 with an opening angle of 70 degrees. The actuarial incidence of mechanical failure at 5 years for the 60-degree convexo-concave valve was 0.6%; for the 70-degree convexo-concave valve, it was 2.8%. Two groups of valves were found to be especially affected by this complication: the 23-mm aortic 60-degree convexo-concave valve, with a 5-year actuarial incidence of 2.2%, and the 29- to 31-mm mitral 70-degree convexo-concave valve, with a 5-year actuarial incidence of 8.3%. The hazard function indicates a constant or decreasing tendency for mechanical failure in the 60-degree convexo-concave valve and the 70-degree convexo-concave valve, respectively. The time interval between the first symptom of mechanical failure and circulatory collapse was noted to be significantly shorter after aortic failure than after mitral failure. No patient with a fractured aortic prosthesis survived long enough to undergo reoperation. The incidence of mechanical failure among patients dying suddenly who underwent autopsy was 9.6%. Most cases of sudden death were unrelated to the prosthesis.

These results confirm that the incidence of mechanical failure increased with the introduction of the convexo-concave valves. This increase was especially marked among the 70-degree valves, which are not used in the United States. Mechanical failure was found to be responsible for death in a minor fraction of patients dying suddenly after valve replacement. Aortic mechanical failure was associated with almost instantaneous death; mitral mechanical failure allowed patients to live long enough for repair. The diagnosis of patients with suspected mechanical failure must be based on plain chest x-ray films; invasive investigations should not be done. Prophylactic re-replacement was not recommended at this time.

▶ This important paper describes experiences with implantation of 3,334 Björk-Shiley valves over a period of 15 years. Nineteen cases of mechanical failure occurred. No failures occurred among 739 aortic standard Pyrolyte prostheses. Among 1,461 convexo-concave valves, 15 fractured, a higher frequency occurring in those with an opening angle of 70 degrees rather than 60 degrees. Hence, this important paper clearly localizes the hazard of mechanical fracture to the convexo-concave prostheses. Although the frequency of mechanical failure is small, the editor seriously doubts that the minor advantages of the convexo-concave prostheses justify this increased risk. At New York University the standard Pyrolyte valve has been used for many years with excellent results.—F.C. Spencer, M.D.

Reparative Operations for Mitral Valve Incompetence: An Emerging Treatment of Choice
Tali T. Bashour, George E. Andreae, Elias S. Hanna, and Dean T. Mason (St. Mary's Hosp. and Med. Ctr., and Univ. of California, San Francisco)
Am. Heart J. 113:1199–1206, May 1987   15–2

Synthetic heart valves still carry risks of thromboembolism and anticoagulant-related bleeding. Available bioprostheses still degenerate relatively rapidly, prompting current interest in valve repair. It is now possible to design the repair technique to the particular anatomical abnormalities encountered in a given case. A wide range of anatomical lesions can cause mitral regurgitation, necessitating a versatile approach to repair.

Review of reparative operations indicates a favorable trend in mortality, morbidity, long-term survival, and the need for reoperation. Reconstructive operations have consistently proved superior to valve replacement using either synthetic or tissue valves. Fewer thromboembolic complications are expected with valve repair, especially when contrasted with the use of synthetic prosthetic valves. Valve-related complications have been less frequent with repair than with replacement by either bioprostheses or mechanical valves. Actuarial survival rates often have exceeded 90% at 4 to 10 years.

Mitral valve repair now is the treatment of choice for most cases of pure mitral incompetence. Eventually surgery may be recommended at an earlier stage of mitral regurgitation before marked chamber dilatation develops. Surgery probably should be done at centers where experienced surgeons are available.

▶ This review article summarizes concisely the current trend toward increased repair of mitral insufficiency rather than prosthetic replacement. Available data are nicely summarized. The author emphasizes clearly that repair has been used much more widely in Europe in the past decade than in the United States. The editor fully agrees. The data from our institution indicate that probably well over 90% of patients with nonrheumatic mitral insufficiency in the United States can be treated by reconstruction.—F.C. Spencer, M.D.

Posterior Wall Disruption of the Left Ventricle After Mitral Valve Replacement: Management of Bleeding and Cardiac Enlargement
Walter V.A. Vincente, Samuel V. Lichtenstein, Haysam El-Dalati, James Mahoney, and Tomas A. Salerno (St. Michael's Hosp. and Univ. of Toronto)
Can. J. Surg. 30:249–251, July 1987   15–3

Ventricular disruption is a serious complication of mitral valve replacement, and it is associated with a high death rate mostly because of bleeding and heart failure. Two cases are described in which successful surgical repair was achieved without removing the mitral prosthesis.

The patients were a thin woman aged 75 years who had a mitral valve replacement with a 27-mm Ionescu-Shiley prosthesis for calcific mitral stenosis and insufficiency and an obese woman aged 65 years who had replacement of a 29-mm Omniscience mitral valve prosthesis that had been implanted 8 months earlier for mitral stenosis and insufficiency. Both women sustained posterior left ventricular disruption after operation.

Management involved repair from outside the heart without removing the mitral prosthesis. This was done with a running Prolene suture in the atrioventricular junction in one patient and with pledgeted sutures in the other, who had transverse midventricular disruption. Biologic glue was crucial in controlling residual hemorrhage. Bilateral placement of the pectoralis muscle flaps to close the sternal wound was necessary in the patient who had suffered transverse midventricular disruption because of swelling and dilation of the heart.

When posterior left ventricular disruption occurs after mitral valve replacement, the surgeon should consider repair without removing the prosthesis and the use of biologic glue to achieve hemostasis. Mobilization of a muscle flap to accommodate an edematous, dilated heart should also be considered if sternal closure is not possible.

▶ This report describes successful surgical repair of two patients with the highly lethal complication of posterior left ventricular disruption. It is significant that in both patients a successful surgical repair was achieved by suture placed from outside the heart, a method the editor would have considered unlikely to succeed.

This serious complication has been studied in some detail at the editor's institution (NYU) (Spencer, F.C., et al.: *Ann Surg* 202:673–680, 1985). As emphasized in the report by J.M. Craver et al. from Emory University (Ann. Thorac.

Surg. 40:163–171, 1985), routine preservation of some chordae to the annulus of the mural leaflet has been associated with virtual disappearance of this complication in the past 5 years.—F.C. Spencer, M.D.

Traumatic Tricuspid Insufficiency: An Underdiagnosed Disease
Christian Gayet, Bernard Pierre, Jean-Pierre Delahaye, Gerard Champsaur, Xavier Andre-Fouet, and Patrice Rueff (Hôpital de la Croix-Rousse and Hôpital Cardiovasculaire et Pneumologique Louis Pradel, Lyon, France)
Chest 92:429–432, September 1987   15–4

Traumatic tricuspid insufficiency (TI) is considered rare. However, the frequency of this condition may have been underestimated. Twelve cases were recently found in a medium-sized city. These cases are described, and the available diagnostic approaches and treatments are discussed.

The ten men and two women were aged 22 to 64 years at diagnosis, between 1972 and 1984. All but one had sustained multiple lesions in a motor vehicle accident. Ten had rib fractures and nine had cranial trauma with loss of consciousness. Abdominal trauma and fractures of extremities occurred less frequently. In four cases TI was diagnosed within 5 days of trauma because of right heart failure, which led promptly to operation, or development of an obvious tricuspid regurgitant murmur. In three other patients TI was recognized in 15 to 40 days after trauma, also because a regurgitant murmur became evident. In the remaining five cases the diagnosis was delayed 6 months to 19 years after the trauma. In these patients TI was finally recognized because of the development of symptoms, usually dyspnea, or other cardiac abnormalities such as cardiomegaly or right bundle-branch block.

A murmur of tricuspid regurgitation was present in all patients, but it was heard only during deep inspiration in two. The most frequently observed other physical signs were hepatomegaly, occasionally with systolic pulsations; jugular venous distention; and marked venous V waves. The heart was enlarged in nine of 12 chest radiographs. All patients showed sinus rhythm on ECGs. Right bundle-branch block was noted in eight cases and was complete in six. Four patients underwent tricuspid valve replacement, and traumatic TI was confirmed.

This experience suggests that the frequency of traumatic TI is much higher than originally thought. Systematic research of the signs and symptoms of TI and the availability of noninvasive tools, particularly echocardiography and Doppler ultrasound, should lead to more frequent recognition of this condition.

▶ This significant paper from Lyon, France, quite properly emphasizes that traumatic tricuspid insufficiency is not an extremely rare condition. The authors were able to collect 12 cases from their own city.

With modern techniques, diagnosis can be made easily by echocardiography. At the editor's institution, experiences gained from use of the Carpentier techniques of mitral valve reconstruction were successfully applied to a recent patient with traumatic tricuspid insufficiency in whom an automobile accident a few months earlier had ruptured the anterior papillary muscle. Almost surely, similar experiences can be readily duplicated by others, but there is a paucity of published information at this time.—F.C. Spencer, M.D.

Long-Term Follow-up of Patients With the Antibiotic-Sterilized Aortic Homograft Valve Inserted Freehand in the Aortic Position

Brian G. Barratt-Boyes, A.H.G. Roche, R. Subramanyan, J.R. Pemberton, and R.M.L. Whitlock (Green Lane Hosp. and Univ. of Auckland, New Zealand)
Circulation 75:768–777, April 1987   15–5

The antibiotic sterilized aortic homograft valve (ASAHV) has provided better short-term and midterm results than chemical sterilization. The authors describe the long-term follow-up results of the ASAHV and analyze the incidence and causes of homograft failure.

In 248 patients, a series of 252 aortic homograft valves were followed up for a mean period of 10.8 years. All valves were nonvital and were sterilized in antibiotic solution and maintained in a nutrient medium at 4 C.

There were 15 hospital deaths; of these, most were class V patients. In patients undergoing elective first operation, the death rate was 2.7%. The reoperation death rate was 13%, and for class V patients overall, the death rate was 50%. Most patients died of myocardial failure and cerebral damage. Survival rate was 57% at 10 years and 38% at 14 years, with the valve in situ. Homograph valve failure was responsible for 8.4% of late deaths. Valve failure was caused solely by incompetence, either from valve wear or endocarditis. Valves were 95% significantly free from incompetence at 5 years, 78% at 10 years, and 42% at 14 years. The incidence of significant incompetence was significantly lower than for chemically treated valves. Increasing donor valve age, recipient age younger than 14 years, and aortic root diameter greater than 30 mm increased the risk of significant incompetence.

The ASAHV was demonstrated to be a satisfactory device for aortic valve replacement and is recommended over other valves for almost all patients. The results may be less satisfactory in children, but the ASAHV is still preferred in this age group.

▶ This significant report from New Zealand describes results with 248 patients followed from 9 to 16 years following operation. Ninety-five percent were free from valvular incompetence at five years; 78% at 10 years; and 42% at 14 years. From their review of published reports, the authors concluded that the frequency of complications with the aortic homograft valve were far smaller than with porcine prostheses. Recent changes in technique of preservation are described.—F.C. Spencer, M.D.

Aspirin Anticoagulation in Children With Mechanical Aortic Valves

Edward D. Verrier, Robert F. Tranbaugh, Scott J. Soifer, Edward S. Yee, Kevin Turley, and Paul A. Ebert (Univ of California, San Francisco, and State Univ. of New York, Brooklyn)
J. Thorac. Cardiovasc. Surg. 92:1013–1020, December 1986   15–6

The best means of anticoagulation for children with mechanical heart valves remains uncertain. Aspirin, alone or combined with dipyridamole, was given to 51 such children (mean age, 13 years) who were followed up for a mean of 36.5 months after heart valve insertion. Forty-five patients received aspirin alone in doses of 6 mg/kg daily up to 600 mg daily. Six patients received dipyridamole as well, in doses of 25 or 50 mg daily. Fifty Björk-Shiley tilting spherical disc valves and a St. Jude bileaflet valve were placed.

There were few early complications, and the late mortality was 8%. No late deaths were related to thrombosis or embolism. There were no postoperative thromboembolic events. Eleven asymptomatic patients who had brain computed tomography (CT) or magnetic resonance (MR) imaging had no evidence of silent cerebral thromboembolism. Minor hemorrhagic complications occurred in 6% of patients. Treatment for five patients was changed to warfarin. No mechanical valve failures occurred. All patients have remained in normal sinus or paced rhythm.

Children with mechanical valve prostheses in normal sinus rhythm can safely be given aspirin, alone or with dipyridamole. Hemorrhagic complications of aspirin are not serious and are easily managed. Antiplatelet drugs are relatively inexpensive, are easily administered, and do not require laboratory monitoring.

▶ Aspirin was used as the method for anticoagulation in 51 children with mechanical heart valves at the University of California over a period of 6 years. It is most impressive that no major thromboembolic episodes occurred. One perioperative neurologic event occurred and resolved spontaneously. The hazards of anticoagulation in a child constitute the major problem with mechanical heart valves. Hopefully, others can duplicate these favorable results.—F.C. Spencer, M.D.

Aortic Valve Replacement With Concomitant Aortoventriculoplasty in Children and Young Adults: Long-Term Follow-up

William H. Fleming and Lynne B. Sarafian (Univ. of Nebraska, Omaha)
Ann. Thorac. Surg. 43:575–578, June 1987   15–7

Aortic valve replacement (AVR) in young patients with a small aortic root or a disproportionate hypoplastic aortic root can be technically difficult. Numerous reports have described various methods of enlarging the aortic anulus.

To accommodate an adequate-sized prosthetic valve, AVR and aortoventriculoplasty were done in seven female and nine male patients aged 2 to 23 years with aortic stenosis or insufficiency, or both. All procedures were performed between August 1976 and May 1986.

Two patients had rheumatic heart disease, and 14 had congenital heart disease. Twelve had undergone 19 cardiovascular operative procedures before having AVR with a Konno aortoventriculoplasty. The size of the aortic anulus ranged from 10 to less than 21 mm. The valves that were inserted ranged from 21 to 29 mm; 81% were 25 mm or larger.

One patient died during surgery shortly after he was weaned from cardiopulmonary bypass. No operative deaths have occurred since 1977. Another patient died from unknown causes 51 months after surgery. Fourteen patients were followed up from 9 to 120 months.

Twelve of the 16 patients had previous cardiovascular procedures. Degenerated tissue valves in two patients were replaced with mechanical valves at 33 and 110 months. Currently, all patients are classified in New York Heart Association Functional Class I.

These findings show that AVR with a concomitant Konno aortoventriculoplasty can be safely performed in children and young adults. Results were satisfactory during a follow-up of up to 10 years.

▶ This report describes experiences with the Konno aortoventriculoplasty in 16 patients at the University of Nebraska. The only death occurred early in the series. The report was selected because there is a paucity of significant data regarding both the safety and effectiveness of the Konno procedure. These results are excellent.—F.C. Spencer, M.D.

16 Coronary Heart Disease

Long-Term Follow-Up After Percutaneous Transluminal Coronary Angioplasty: The Early Zurich Experience
Andreas R. Gruentzig, Spencer B. King III, Maria Schlumpf, and Walter Siegenthaler (Emory Univ. and Univ. of Zurich, Switzerland)
N. Engl. J. Med. 316:1127–1132, April 30, 1987   16–1

Long-term follow-up has been completed on the first 169 patients having percutaneous transluminal coronary angioplasty. Gruentzig performed these operations in 1977–1980, and the patients have been followed for 5 to 8 years. Patients with multivessel coronary disease were included in the series. Nineteen patients had previously had bypass surgery. All patients were symptomatic, and all but 3% had positive exercise stress tests.

Angioplasty was technically successful in 79% of cases. The actuarial cardiac survival was 96% at 6 years. Two thirds of patients with technically successful results were without symptoms at last follow-up. Only 10% of this group had positive exercise stress tests at follow-up. Stenosis recurred within 6 months of angioplasty in 30% of patients, and subsequently in six more patients. Twenty-seven patients had a second angioplasty, and 19 required bypass surgery. The actuarial survival without infarction or bypass surgery was 79% at 6 years. Patients with multivessel disease had higher cardiac mortality and a lower long-term success rate than those with single-vessel disease.

Patients with single-vessel coronary disease have the best long-term outcome after transluminal angioplasty. Randomized trials are under way to determine the value of angioplasty in patients with multivessel disease.

▶ This significant report describes long-term results in the first 133 patients successfully undergoing angioplasty by Gruentzig in Zurich, beginning in 1977. Actuarial cardiac survival was 96% at 6 years. Stenosis recurred in 30% of patients in the first 6 months after angioplasty; only six more recurrences were detected later among 41 patients who had follow-up angiograms. A second angioplasty was required in 27 patients; coronary bypass surgery, in 19. These data indicate that most recurrences following angioplasty are seen within 6 months. These data are probably some of the most favorable that can be obtained because the early patients were carefully selected and had predominantly single vessel disease.—F.C. Spencer, M.D.

Long-Term Outcome of Revascularization of the Anterior Coronary Arteries With Crossed Double Internal Mammary Versus Saphenous Vein Grafts

Alexander S. Geha, Graeme L. Hammond, Rabie N. Stephan, Robert K. Kleiger, and Ronald J. Krone (Case Western Reserve Univ., Yale Univ., Michigan State Univ., and Washington Univ.)

Surgery 102:667–673, October 1987   16–2

In simultaneous revascularization of the left anterior descending (LAD) artery and the proximal segments of the diagonal LAD and marginal coronary arteries the direction and location of the vessels allow excellent alignment of the left internal mammary artery (IMA) with the LAD and the right IMA with the diagonal LAD or marginal arteries. This approach was originally described in 1976. The authors analyzed and compared the long-term outcome of this approach with the saphenous vein bypass graft (SVG) approach for anterior coronary artery revascularization.

Data were reviewed on 43 patients with crossed double IMAs and 53 patients with SVGs to the same obstructed anterior coronary arteries who were treated from 1973 to 1978. Thirty-two patients in the first group and 43 in the second also had SVGs to other diseased vessels. Demographic and epidemiologic characteristics were comparable between the two groups.

In the group with crossed double IMAs the linearized incidences of late cardiac death, reoperation, recurrent angina, and infarction were 0.2%, 0.7%, 1.4%, and 0% per patient-year, respectively. In the SVG group the incidences were 1.6%, 2.4%, 7.8%, and 1.8%, respectively.

At 5 years the actuarial percentage of patients with crossed double IMAs who were free of late cardiac death was 100%. Ninety-eight percent of such patients were free of reoperation, 98% were free of recurrent angina, and 100% were free of infarction. These values in the SVG group were 94%, 98%, 84%, and 94%, respectively. At 10 years the actuarial incidence of all events was significantly lower in patients with crossed double IMAs than in those with SVGs.

These findings demonstrate that crossed double IMAs have significantly better prognostic effects than SVGs when revascularization of the anterior coronary arteries is necessary. Thus, the former approach is strongly recommended in suitable circumstances.

▶ This short report describes 10-year results in a retrospective comparison of 43 patients who had double mammary grafts and 53 patients who had saphenous vein grafts. Significantly better results were apparent within 5 years after operation and became quite striking at 10 years. Among several factors compared, the most striking was the freedom from late cardiac death. One hundred percent of patients survived 5 years, and 98% 10 years. These data are similar to reports from other institutions and reaffirm the excellent 10-year prognosis in patients with double mammary grafts.—F.C. Spencer, M.D.

Early and Late Results Following Emergency Isolated Myocardial Revascularization During Hypothermic Fibrillatory Arrest
Cary W. Akins (Massachusetts Gen. Hosp., Boston)
Ann. Thorac. Surg. 43:131–137, February 1987   16–3

Although the results have improved, the need to revascularize the myocardium on an emergency basis remains an important incremental operative risk factor. The authors reviewed data on 127 consecutive patients having emergency isolated myocardial revascularization during hypothermic fibrillatory arrest in 1982–1985. The mean age was 62 years, and 27 patients were older than age 70 years. The mean ejection fraction was 0.49. An intra-aortic balloon was present in 86% of patients. About three fourths of patients received IV nitroglycerin, and 12 had received thrombolytic therapy. The indication for surgery was postinfarction ischemia in 48% of cases and preinfarction unstable angina in 35%.

Four grafts per patient, on average, were placed. The hospital mortality was 0.8%, and there was one perioperative myocardial infarction. The actuarial survival at 45 months was 91%. The 117 long-term survivors had a mean New York Heart Association functional classification of 1.1. The mean follow-up of hospital survivors was 21 months. Three patients had nonfatal infarction during the follow-up interval. One patient required repeat revascularization.

Patients with unstable angina should be stabilized preoperatively with the intra-aortic balloon pump if necessary. Those with marked residual coronary obstruction following thrombosis should have some type of definitive revascularization. Patients with acute ischemic complications of angioplasty should have early balloon pump insertion and expeditious revascularization.

▶ This impressive series of 127 patients is another publication by Akins about the effectiveness of hypothermic fibrillatory arrest for performing coronary bypass. The results are impressive as there was only one hospital death and one perioperative infarction. As an accompanying editorial by Levitsky indicates, the criteria used for measure of infarction, that is, the appearance of a new Q wave, would miss subendocardial infarctions.

The series has an unusually high percentage of intra-aortic balloons, but the balloons were inserted simply to maintain myocardium if revascularization could not be done promptly, not because of hemodynamic instability. Nonetheless, the data clearly indicate the safety of this form of cardiac arrest, a reasonable alternative to cardioplegic arrest. Most surgeons would prefer the latter.—F.C. Spencer, M.D.

Determinants of Cardiac Failure After Coronary Bypass Surgery Within 30 Days of Acute Myocardial Infarction
Nevin M. Katz, Thomas E. Kubanick, Susan W. Ahmed, Curtis E. Green, David L. Pearle, Lowell F. Satler, Charles E. Rackley, and Robert B. Wallace (Georgetown Univ., Washington, D.C.)
Ann. Thorac. Surg. 42:658–663, December 1986   16–4

The proper time to perform coronary bypass surgery after acute myocardial infarction is uncertain, especially where myocardial function is impaired. Early grafting might lead to reperfusion injury and heart failure, but delay could risk a second ischemic event. The role of various preoperative factors in the development of postoperative heart failure was studied in a series of 145 patients having isolated coronary bypass within 4 weeks of acute infarction.

Heart failure developed in 26% of the patients, and all five postoperative deaths were in this group. Mean preoperative ejection fraction was 48.5% for patients with postoperative heart failure and 59% for those without heart failure. On multivariate analysis, the most important predictor of postoperative heart failure was preoperative failure, as defined by the need for catecholamine support. The next most prominent factor was an ejection fraction less than 45%, followed by the need for intravenous nitroglycerin preoperatively. The interval from infarction to surgery was not an important factor.

Preoperative heart failure, ischemia, and a low ejection fraction are independently predictive of heart failure after coronary bypass surgery, done within 1 month of acute infarction. If ischemia or threatening coronary anatomy is present early after infarction and the patient is not improving, immediate surgery should be strongly considered.

▶ Experiences with 145 patients undergoing coronary bypass within 4 weeks of acute myocardial infarction are described. There were five deaths. The data clearly show that the time elapsing since an infarction did not influence mortality, whereas ischemia or cardiac failure had an adverse effect. Hence, operation should not be automatically postponed simply for passage of time following an infarction if indications for bypass exist.—F.C. Spencer, M.D.

Emergency Coronary Bypass for Cardiogenic Shock
Robert A. Guyton, Joseph M. Arcidi, Jr., David A. Langford, Douglas C. Morris, Henry A. Liberman, and Charles R. Hatcher, Jr. (Emory Univ.)
Circulation 76 (Suppl. V):V-22–V-27, November 1987   16–5

Cardiogenic shock that is caused by myocardial ischemia is a therapeutic challenge. Emergency coronary artery bypass for this condition is associated with a high operative death rate. At one institution the approach to acute myocardial ischemia has been thrombolytic therapy and percutaneous transluminal coronary angioplasty of stenotic lesions. Emergency coronary artery bypass is done in patients with persistent ischemia after thrombolysis or angioplasty, or both, especially if ischemia is accompanied by a failure in left ventricular power.

In a retrospective review of the results of this approach the authors studied the data on 69 patients who underwent emergency coronary artery bypass from January 1983 through March 1986. Seventeen were in shock; 15 of them hypotension which required treatment. An intra-aortic balloon pump was used in ten, and catecholamines were used in six. The other two patients had a low cardiac index and a pulmonary capillary wedge pressure of more than 25 mm Hg. Among these patients nine presented with acute infarction, four had failed angioplasty, and four had uncontrollable angina. Four patients needed cardiopulmonary resuscitation.

After surgery 94% required catecholamine support, and 71% were treated with an intra-aortic balloon pump. Two patients died in the hospital. Median hospital stay after surgery for the survivors was 9 days. Forty-seven percent of patients suffered major complications. At a mean follow-up of 20.5 months, no further deaths were noted. At 3 years 88% were still alive. Six patients were in functional class I, seven were in class II, and two were in class III.

Of the 52 patients who underwent emergency coronary artery bypass and were not in shock one died in the hospital, 52% required catecholamines, and 12% required intra-aortic balloon pump after surgery. Median stay in the hospital after operation was 8 days. Thirteen percent suffered complications, and 91% were alive at 3 years. This retrospective review demonstrated that the coronary bypass approach to acute myocardial ischemia yielded excellent hospital survival (except in octogenarians) and short-term functional results, although emergency surgery in the presence of cardiogenic shock was associated with increased morbidity.

▶ This impressive report describes experiences with 17 emergency bypass procedures performed for patients in cardiogenic shock. Only two hospital deaths occurred. Mean follow-up analysis averaged 20 months. There were no late deaths. Clearly, prompt operation for cardiogenic shock that cannot be treated by thrombolytic therapy and percutaneous angioplasty is the therapy of choice.—F.C. Spencer, M.D.

Free (Aorta-Coronary) Internal Mammary Artery Graft: Late Results
Floyd D. Loop, Bruce W. Lytle, Delos M. Cosgrove, Leonard A.R. Golding, Paul C. Taylor, and Robert W. Stewart (Cleveland Clinic Found.)
J. Thorac. Cardiovasc. Surg. 92:827–831, November 1986   16–6

The authors placed free internal mammary artery (IMA) grafts in 156 patients from 1971 to 1985. Of 244 IMA grafts, 166 were free arterial grafts in the aorta-coronary position. The mean patient age was 54 years. Nearly half the patients were in New York Heart Association (NYHA) functional class III or IV preoperatively.

One hospital death was due to ischemia/infarction. Eight percent of patients required reoperation for persistent bleeding. Of 75 free IMA grafts reevaluated, 84% were patent, and the patency rate beyond 18 months was 91% (Fig 16–1). Sixty-two percent of 155 patients who survived initial hospitalization were in NYHA class I after a mean of 98 months. Another 28% of patients were in functional class II. Actuarial survival was 90% at 5 years and 73% at 10 years. Eight patients had later cardiac surgery.

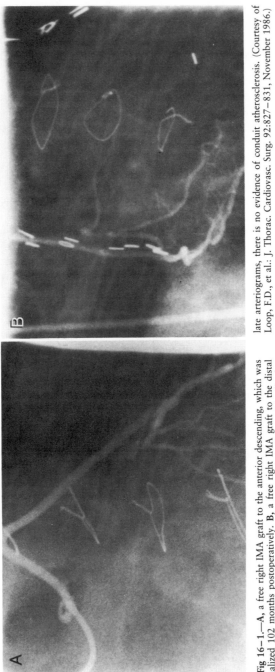

Fig 16–1.—A, a free right IMA graft to the anterior descending, which was visualized 102 months postoperatively. **B,** a free right IMA graft to the distal right coronary artery 132 months postoperatively. In these films and in all other late arteriograms, there is no evidence of conduit atherosclerosis. (Courtesy of Loop, F.D., et al.: J. Thorac. Cardiovasc. Surg. 92:827–831, November 1986.)

Use of the free IMA graft appears to be warranted because of good late patency rates, relief of angina, and good patient survival. The free IMA graft, like the in situ IMA graft, appears to be relatively immune to atherosclerotic change.

▶ This important report describes experiences with free internal mammary grafts in 156 patients, a method of grafting chosen because other problems prevented the use of standard techniques. Forty free grafts were restudied within 18 months, finding a patency rate of only 77 percent. This high rate of closure was attributed to technical problems occurring in the early experience. Quite significantly, however, 91% of 35 grafts studied about 8 years following operation were patent. Sequential catheterization studies found that 24 free grafts patent at 9 months remained patent at 80 months. Six of these were restudied at 93 months and again found to be uniformly patent.

It is unknown whether the remarkable high patency with internal mammary anastomoses is due to the internal mammary artery itself or due to its use as a pedicle graft. Data such as these support the inherent internal mammary hypothesis. The use of free grafts could significantly enlarge the applicability of bilateral internal mammary grafting in many patients.—F.C. Spencer, M.D.

Clinical and Angiographic Assessment of Complex Mammary Artery Bypass Grafting
J. Scott Rankin, Glenn E. Newman, Thomas M. Bashore, Lawrence H. Muhlbaier, George S. Tyson, Jr., T. Bruce Ferguson, Jr., J.G. Reves, and David C. Sabiston, Jr. (Duke Univ.)
J. Thorac. Cardiovasc. Surg. 92:832–846, November 1986   16–7

Sequential, bilateral, and free internal mammary artery (IMA) grafts are increasingly used in order to maximize the number of distal IMA

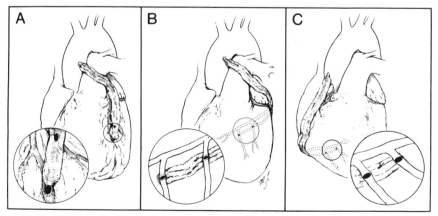

Fig 16–2.—Methods of free IMA grafting. (Courtesy of Rankin, J.S., et al.: J. Thorac. Cardiovasc. Surg. 92:832–846, November 1986.)

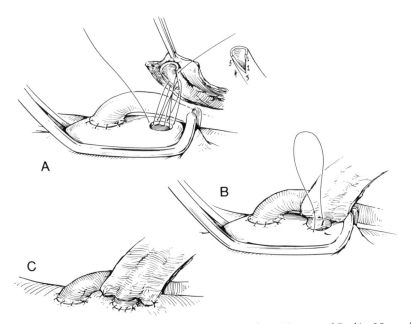

Fig 16–3.—Proximal aortic anastomosis for free IMA grafting. (Courtesy of Rankin, J.S., et al.: Thorac. Cardiovasc. Surg. 92:832–846, November 1986.)

anastomoses. The patency results were assessed in 207 patients having bypass graft angiography 1–32 weeks postoperatively in a 15-month period, representing a restudy rate of 85%. A total of 841 distal vessels had been grafted, averaging about four per patient. Patency was defined as complete filling of the graft and the distal bypassed vessel. The technique of free IMA grafting is shown in Figure 16–2, and the method of proximal aortic anastomosis, in Figure 16–3.

Overall graft patency was 94%. The rate for 503 distal saphenous vein graft anastomoses was 91%, and that for 338 IMA anastomses was 99%. Eighty-four percent of patients had all grafts patent. The patency rate for sequential IMA grafts was 99%, and all 15 free IMA grafts were patent. Three of 18 patent right IMA grafts to the circumflex marginal artery via the transverse sinus showed slow flow.

Attempts to increase the number of distal IMA anastomoses by complex grafting appear to be warranted. This is a most versatile approach to myocardial revascularization. Currently, multiple IMA grafting is done routinely, with the adjunctive use of vein grafts, in cases of multivessel ischemic heart disease.

▶ This important paper describes experiences with 207 patients operated on over a period of 15 months, 85% of whom were studied subsequently with angiograms. A total of 841 distal vessels were grafted. Patency rates were 91% for 503 venous anastomoses and 99% for 338 internal mammary grafts. Excellent patency rates were obtained with sequential grafts as well as with isolated grafts. It was quite significant, however, that five of 20 transverse sinus right internal mammary grafts were unsatisfactory, so this technique has been abandoned. These data fully support the mounting evidence about the usefulness of multiple internal mammary bypasses for revascularization.—F.C. Spencer, M.D.

17 Miscellaneous Cardiac Conditions and the Great Vessels

Results of Open Heart Surgery in Patients With Recent Cardiogenic Embolic Stroke and Central Nervous System Dysfunction
Zvi Zisbrod, Daniel M. Rose, Israel J. Jacobowitz, Marshall Kramer, Anthony J. Acinapura, and Joseph N. Cunningham, Jr. (Maimonides Med. Ctr. and Downstate Med. Ctr., Brooklyn, N.Y.; and St. Vincent's Hosp., New York)
Circulation 76 (Suppl. V):V-109–V-112, November 1987   17–1

Patients who undergo open heart surgery after a recent cardiogenic embolic stroke or have central nervous system dysfunction are difficult to treat. Cardiopulmonary bypass and heparinization may exacerbate the neurologic injury. There are no clear data to indicate what is a safe interval from the onset of neurologic symptoms to the time of surgery.

The authors describe experience with 15 patients with recent neurologic injury who had open heart surgery since 1982. All had sustained their injuries 2 to 28 days before surgery (mean, 12.7 days). Surgery was indicated by recurrent embolization, sepsis, and hemodynamic deterioration.

At the time of surgery three patients were comatose with no focal neurologic signs and 12 had focal neurologic deficits. Preoperative computed tomography scans were performed for all. Twelve patients had documented embolic cerebral infarctions, one had evidence of intracranial hemorrhage, and one had a subdural hematoma. Fourteen had native or prosthetic valvular endocarditis; one had a left atrial myxoma.

One patient died in the postoperative period from multisystem failure. At 6 months to 4 years all surviving patients showed improvement in neurologic symptoms. Eight patients had complete neurologic recovery.

These data suggest that although there is always a risk of infarct extension from hemorrhage, early surgery after recent cardiogenic embolic stroke can be done safely in a high percentage of patients. Patients with bacterial endocarditis and profound mental obtundation or coma may also recover completely after surgery. Most patients with focal neurologic deficits from cardiogenic emboli will partly or completely recover after operation. Early surgical intervention can also significantly improve hemodynamics, which may prevent further neurologic deterioration.

▶ The importance of this report is related to the important question of the safety of open heart surgery following an embolic stroke. The major question is whether heparinization may exacerbate the neurologic injury. This report describes experiences with 15 patients operated upon between 2 and 28 days following onset of neurologic injury. The results were most encouraging, for no exacerbation of neurologic injury was recognized.—F.C. Spencer, M.D.

Major Sternal Wound Infection After Open-Heart Surgery: A Multivariate Analysis of Risk Factors in 2,579 Consecutive Operative Procedures
Gianmaria Ottino, Ruggero De Paulis, Stefano Pansini, Giuseppe Rocca, Maria Vittoria Tallone, Chiara Comoglio, Paolo Costa, Fulvio Orzan, and Mario Morea (Univ. of Turin and S. Giovanni Battista Hosp., Turin, Italy)
Ann. Thorac. Surg. 44:173–179, August 1987   17–2

The incidence of major infections of sternal wounds after open heart surgery ranges from 0.4% to 5%, with a mortality of 7% to 80%. Complications in surviving patients can be long lasting. The influence of different predisposing factors to such infections has not been thoroughly investigated.

To identify significant risk factors, the authors conducted a retrospective analysis of major sternal wound infections which developed in 48 of 2,579 consecutive patients who were seen between 1979 and 1984. These patients underwent open heart procedures through a midline sternotomy and survived long enough for infection to develop.

Possible risk factors that were assessed by multivariate analysis included age, sex, hospital environment, interval between hospital admission and surgery, antibiotic prophylaxis, type of surgical procedure, reoperation, duration of surgical procedures, duration of cardiopulmonary bypass, amount of blood transfused, postoperative blood loss, chest reexploration, rewiring of a sterile sternal dehiscence, duration of mechanical ventilation, and number of days in intensive care.

After multiple stepwise logistic regression analysis, six variables emerged as significant: hospital environment, or the different locations of surgical facilities over the years; interval between admission and operation; reoperation; blood transfusions; early chest reexploration; and sternal rewiring. Age and sex were not significant factors. It was found that patient contamination can occur before, during, or after surgery and that any kind of reintervention may predispose to wound infection.

▶ This report from Italy found sternal wound infections in about 2% of more than 2,500 patients undergoing sternotomy. The frequency of wound infection is remarkably similar to different reports published in the United States. Factors of statistical significance associated with wound infection included the familiar ones of reoperation, sternal rewiring, blood transfusions, and reoperations. All of these, of course, are associated with both the increased likelihood of wound contamination as well as decreased vascularity in the sternal incision.—F.C. Spencer, M.D.

Delayed Sternal Closure After Cardiac Surgery
William J. Fanning, John S. Vasko, and James W. Kilman (Ohio State Univ.)
Ann. Thorac. Surg. 44:169–172, August 1987   17–3

After difficult cardiac operative procedures, sternal reapproximation may, although rarely, result in hemodynamically significant restriction to diastolic filling either from excessive cardiac edema and dilation or ongoing mediastinal hemorrhage. Clinically, it resembles cardiac tamponade. Wound closure without sternal reapproximation may alleviate cardiac compression, thus allowing ready access to the mediastinum when there is ongoing mediastinal hemorrhage.

The authors describe 57 who were managed with delayed sternal closure (DSC). The group included 11 female and 34 male patients aged 18–72 years and five girls and seven boys aged 10 weeks to 9 years. Delayed sternal closure ranged from 1 to 14 days after surgery. Thirty-eight patients survived and were able to leave the hospital.

Complications of DSC were seen in five patients and included superficial sternal wound infection, sternal osteomyelitis, and fatal infection in one patient. The cause of death in the remaining nonsurvivors included intracranial hemorrhage, pulmonary embolism, recurrent ventricular fibrillation, cardiogenic shock, and multiple-system organ failure. Of the 19 nonsurvivors nine had undergone DSC because of mediastinal hemorrhage and ten because of cardiac compression. Only one of the 19 deaths could be directly attributed to DSC.

The pediatric patients underwent DSC 1–8 days after repair of various complex congenital cardiac lesions. The need for DSC was indicated by cardiac compression in eight children and by mediastinal hemorrhage in four. Only one infectious complication occurred. One child died of cardiogenic shock and another died of intracranial hemorrhage. The ten surviving children were discharged in good condition with healing sternal wounds.

These data suggest that DSC may be beneficial in selected patients. The morbidity and mortality that were related to this technique in this high risk group were judged to be acceptable.

▶ This report describes experiences with 57 patients treated with delayed sternal closure for serious complications following a cardiac operation. This technique has emerged as a reasonably safe one in desperate circumstances when cardiac swelling is severe. As with other reports, the low frequency of sternal or mediastinal infection (2 of 57 patients in this report) is surprising.—F.C. Spencer, M.D.

Mediastinal Infection Following Open-Heart Surgery: Treatment With Retrosternal Irrigation
Kalervo Verkkala and Antero Järvinen (Helsinki Univ.)
Scand. J. Thorac. Cardiovasc. Surg. 20:203–207, 1986   17–4

Sternotomy infection with mediastinal involvement is a relatively rare but serious complication of open heart surgery. Mediastinitis developed in 15 of 1,083 consecutive open heart surgery patients in a 3-year period, or 1.4% of the total. The 13 men and two women had a mean age of 55 years. Most patients had coronary bypass surgery. Débridement of the sternal wound and anterior mediastinum was followed by sternal refixation and continuous retrosternal irrigation with antiseptic or antibiotic solution. Irrigation continued for nearly 2 weeks on average. Antibiotic solution was used in 13 cases, and povidone iodine was used in 2 cases.

Four patients were septic. *Staphylococcus aureus* was the most frequent isolate. Signs of infection were apparent a mean of 10 days after operation except in one patient who presented 3 weeks postoperatively. Patients requiring irrigation for longer than 10 days tended to have an unfavorable outcome. Three of seven such patients died, two of resistant infection. Three surviving patients required removal of the sternal wires, but the sternum remained stable in all of them.

Closed treatment of postoperative mediastinitis succeeded in 13 of 15 patients in this series. Use of β-lactam antibiotics is now preferred. Concentrations up to 1 gm per liter of irrigant may be used without causing local irritation.

▶ This report describes experiences with mediastinitis developing in 15 patients following 1,083 open heart operations. The technique of operative débridement, sternal closure and continuous mediastinal irrigation was successful in 13 of 15 patients. There were two deaths from persistent infection. Mediastinal irrigation was employed usually for about 12 days.

These data are quoted to support the use of operative débridement followed by sternal closure and mediastinal antibiotic irrigation in the majority of patients with mediastinitis, especially when an early diagnosis is made. This method of therapy remains successful in the majority of patients treated at New York University.

However, in the minority of patients not responding, usually because of delayed onset of treatment, the patient should be promptly treated by débridement and subsequent muscle flap closure, a more complicated but highly effective technique.—F.C. Spencer, M.D.

Transfusion of Predonated Autologous Blood in Elective Cardiac Surgery
Tim R. Love, William G. Hendren, Dennis D. O'Keefe, and Willard M. Daggett (Harvard Univ.)
Ann. Thorac. Surg. 43:508–512, May 1987   17–5

Substantial risks still are associated with homologous blood transfusion in cardiac surgery patients. Predonation of autologous blood reportedly can reduce the need for homologous blood, but routine implementation of predonation is poor. The efficacy of predonated autologous blood was studied in matched groups of 58 patients, one given homologous blood perioperatively, and the other, predonated autologous blood.

The study patients predonated an average of nearly 2 units of blood over 18 days. The whole blood hemoglobin level decreased by 2.2 gm/dl on average. No complications resulted from phlebotomy in these ambulatory patients. Transfusions of an average of 1.7 units of autologous blood lowered the volume of homologous transfusion by 46%, compared with the control group. Sixty-four percent of study patients and 38% of controls required no homologous transfusion. No complications resulted from autologous blood transfusion.

Homologous blood requirements can be significantly reduced by an autologous blood predonation program for patients having elective cardiac surgery. Patient acceptability is good, the risk is low, and there are no additional costs. The use of homologous blood can be avoided in up to 90% of cases.

▶ The data in this report are impressive. Two units of blood, on average, were predonated in one group of patients over a period of 18 days, decreasing the hemoglobin about 2 gm. At operation, however, this group required far less homologous blood than those who did not predonate. One third of the patients did not require any homologous blood. Clearly, the method is both effective and safe. Its more frequent use should be encouraged.—F.C. Spencer, M.D.

Hypothermia-Induced Reversible Platelet Dysfunction

C. Robert Valeri, George Cassidy, Shukri Khuri, Hollace Feingold, Gina Ragno, and Mark D. Altschule (Naval Blood Research Lab., Boston Univ., and Brockton-West Roxbury VA Med. Ctr., Boston)
Ann. Surg. 205:175–181, February 1987   17–6

Bleeding disorder may occur in association with hypothermia in patients having cardiopulmonary bypass. This possibility was examined in baboons, whose platelets and clotting proteins closely resemble those of humans.

Animals subjected to systemic hypothermia of 32 C had an arm skin temperature of 27.3 C and a bleeding time of 5.8 minutes. On local warming of the arm skin to 34 C, the bleeding time was lowered to 2.4 minutes. Normothermic animals with an arm skin temperature of 34.6 C had a bleeding time of 3.1 minutes, and local cooling to 27.6 C produced a bleeding time of 6.9 minutes. Increasing the local skin temperature reduced bleeding times in both normothermic and hypothermic baboons. Bleeding times correlated negatively with the thromboxane B2 level in blood taken at the template bleeding time site.

When a hypothermic patient bleeds without apparent surgical cause, the skin and wound temperatures should be returned to normal before blood products are administered. In this way expense is avoided, as is the risk of transmitting disease by blood product administration. Platelet thromboxane B2 production is temperature-dependent, and skin cooling leads to reversible platelet dysfunction.

▶ This experimental study in baboons clearly demonstrates the production of platelet dysfunction with hypothermia, fortunately reversed with rewarming. The frequent observation that hypothermia is associated with increased surgical bleeding is at least partly explained with these observations. Fortunately, in the experimental study the platelet abnormality disappeared with rewarming.—F.C. Spencer, M.D.

The Effect of Pericardial Insulation on Hypothermic Phrenic Nerve Injury During Open-Heart Surgery
Rick A. Esposito and Frank C. Spencer (New York Univ.)
Ann. Thorac. Surg. 43:303–308, March 1987   17–7

Fatal respiratory complications from phrenic nerve injury have followed the use of iced saline slush to produce local hypothermia at open heart surgery. The authors noted a marked increase in diaphragmatic paralysis and more perioperative respiratory morbidity shortly after a change from cold saline lavage to iced saline slush for topical hypothermia. A prospective study, therefore, was done in 133 consecutive adults having open heart surgery. Cardiopulmonary bypass was performed under moderate systemic hypothermia. Multidose cold blood cardioplegia was used, and topical hypothermia was produced with iced saline slush during the ischemic interval. In 63 cases, an insulation pad molded to fit the pericardial well was used to isolate the phrenic nerves from contact with ice. Both silastic and aluminum sheets were used.

Diaphragmatic palsy, usually affecting the left diaphragm, occurred in 73% of control cases and in 17% of patients in whom pericardial insulation was used. Two bilateral injuries occurred in the control group. Seven control patients and no study patients had serious respiratory morbidity. Both types of insulating pads were effective. Three control patients required tracheostomy in expectation of prolonged ventilatory assistance. Two patients had respiratory arrest postoperatively, requiring closed-chest cardiopulmonary resuscitation.

Phrenic nerve injury from iced saline slush may be avoided by using pericardial insulation. It remains uncertain that iced slush provides better protection from ischemic injury than cooled saline, and consideration should be given to abandoning the use of saline slush.

▶ This prospective study from the editor's institution clearly establishes the injurious effect of topical hypothermia with ice on the phrenic nerve, which occurred with a frequency of 73% unless protective measures were employed. A pericardial insulation pad decreased the frequency of injury to 17%.

The frequency of phrenic nerve injury seems to be much greater with ice than with simple cold electrolyte, perhaps because of the rapid caloric exchange that occurs when ice melts (640 calories/gram). The ice technique has been virtually abandoned at NYU since this time. The small advantages from the use of ice would seem to be far outweighed by the serious problems that can occur from phrenic nerve injury.—F.C. Spencer, M.D.

Clinical Temporary Ventricular Assist: Pathologic Findings and Their Implications in a Multi-Institutional Study of 41 Patients
Frederick J. Schoen, Diane C. Palmer, William F. Bernhard, D. Glenn Pennington, Christian C. Haudenschild, Norman B. Ratliff, Robert L. Berger, Leonard R. Golding, and John T. Watson (Harvard Univ., St. Louis Univ., Boston Univ., Cleveland Clinic Found., and Natl. Heart, Lung, and Blood Inst., Bethesda)
J. Thorac. Cardiovasc. Surg. 92:1071–1081, December 1986   17–8

The pathologic findings were reviewed in 41 patients having temporary ventricular assistance (TVA) at four centers in 1977–1983. Textured diaphragm pumps were used in 24 cases, and smooth-surfaced pumps were used in 17. Thirty-three patients had left, five had right, and three had bilateral TVA. The patients had postcardiotomy cardiogenic shock and could not be weaned from bypass or developed a refractory low-output state postoperatively.

Sixteen of the 41 patients gained a cardiac index of at least 2 L/minute/sq m without pump support. Five, however, died during TVA. Six patients were long-term survivors. The overall mean duration of TVA was 62 hours; the mean for patients having a favorable hemodynamic response was 127 hours. Acute myocardial necrosis was found in 88% of patients evaluated, including some with hemodynamic improvement on TVA. Prominent contraction bands, indicating severe myocardial ischemia, were noted in 11 cases. Pump-related complications included fatal aortic infection at the site of pump return and nonfatal pulmonary embolism.

Clinical TVA is relatively safe and effective in patients in cardiogenic shock or a low-output state after surgery. The presence of myocardial necrosis does not preclude a good hemodynamic response and, in surviving patients, functional myocardial recovery is frequent.

▶ This multi-institutional study among four centers describes experiences with 41 patients undergoing temporary cardiac support with a variety of pumps. Only six patients survived, a mortality of 85%. This grim mortality, considerably greater than that experienced at the editor's institution (NYU) over the past several years, strongly suggests that the mortality is related to irreversible ventricular injury, rather than the type of pump used. At the editor's institution the simple roller pump has been employed for several years.

Subendocardial edema can probably progress to irreversible necrosis within a short time, probably within a few hours in some patients. Almost surely the dismal results in this report resulted from either irreversible injury initially or excessive delay in starting circulatory support.—F.C. Spencer, M.D.

Mechanical Support of the Failing Heart
Sang B. Park, George A. Liebler, John A. Burkholder, Thomas D. Maher, Daniel H. Benckart, George J. Magovern, Jr., Ignacio Y. Christlieb, Race L. Kao, and George J. Magovern, Sr. (Allegheny Gen. Hosp., Pittsburgh)
Ann. Thorac. Surg. 42:627–631, December 1986   17–9

Although the efficacy and merit of mechanical assist for the failing heart following open heart procedure have been documented, a small group of patients develops pump failure refractory to these conventional supports. These patients require further mechanical assistance: mechanical ventricular assist device can provide adequate circulatory support while reducing the preload. Mechanical ventricular assist was investigated in 41 patients with postcardiotomy ventricular failure.

These patients underwent left ventricular, right ventricular, and biventricular assist. The patients were divided into three groups based on the outcome, including group 1, composed of 13 long-term survivors who were discharged from the hospital; group 2, eight patients who were weaned off ventricular assist but died within 30 days; and group 3, comprising 20 patients who could not be weaned from ventricular assist. Overall long-term survival was 32%, operative mortality was 49%, and short-term survival was 20%. The use of biventricular assist contributed to survival of two patients in whom initial left ventricular assist alone could not maintain satisfactory circulatory support. The longest survival was 5 years following operation: this patient is free from cardiac symptoms. Complications in the long-term survivors included severe congestive heart failure (three patients), renal failure requiring dialysis (one patient), cerebrovascular accident (one patient), and below-the-knee amputation (one patient). In all instances, the cause of death in the nonsurvivors was progressive deterioration of cardiac function associated with multiorgan failure.

It appears that severe ventricular dysfunction can unpredictably result from temporary ischemia; nevertheless, much of the damage may be reversible if adequate coronary flows are restored and circulatory support by means of ventricular assist is used. Unfortunately, it currently is difficult to predict which patients may have reversible ischemic damage, and it is not known whether all patients not easily weaned from cardiopulmonary bypass should receive ventricular assist.

▶ Experiences with cardiac support using a centrifugal pump were described for 41 patients. The use of the Bio-Medicus centrifugal pump is particularly significant because minimal amounts of heparin were required. Twenty-one of the patients were successfully weaned from ventricular support, 13 of whom were discharged from the hospital. Four of these 13 subsequently died. Intra-aortic balloon pumping was used in all of the patients as well. Hence, as with other reports of this technique for seriously ill patients, the chance of long-term salvage is small, primarily because of irreversible injury.

Pierce, in a discussion of the report, stated that the pump developed by his group in Hershey, Pennsylvania, has been used in 21 patients with a survival rate of more than 43%. The advantage of the Pierce pump is that it can be used for weeks, if necessary, usually as a bridge for cardiac transplantation.—F.C. Spencer, M.D.

Percutaneous Cardiopulmonary Bypass With a Synchronous Pulsatile Pump Combines Effective Unloading With Ease of Application

Howard I. Axelrod, Aubrey C. Galloway, Michael S. Murphy, John C. Laschinger, F. Gregory Baumann, Eugene A. Grossi, Ephraim Glassman, and Frank C. Spencer (New York Univ.)
J. Thorac. Cardiovasc. Surg. 93:358–365, March 1987   17–10

Percutaneous total cardiopulmonary bypass is a rapid, simple approach avoiding thoracic incision that can be used for both left and right ventricular failure as well as for pulmonary insufficiency. Roller pump bypass has, however, been only partly successful because of incomplete unloading of the left ventricle. The authors evaluated synchronous pulsatile pumping in a normal canine model to determine whether such pumping, synchronized with the ECG, can effectively unload the left ventricle and reduce myocardial energy demands.

Fourteen dogs were placed on percutaneous bypass for 1 hour, half with a roller pump and half with a synchronous pulsatile pump having an ECG triggering mechanism. The tension-time index decreased 56% in the pulsatile pump group and 19% in the control group. Myocardial oxygen consumption decreased 46% and 2%, respectively. The endocardial/epicardial blood flow ratio increased 28% in the pulsatile pump group and decreased 6.5% in the roller pump group. A large increase in overall coronary sinus flow occurred with both pumping systems.

The addition of diastolic counterpulsation to percutaneous cardiopulmonary bypass solves many problems. This type of percutaneous bypass may be a more practical approach than percutaneous left heart bypass in patients with potentially reversible lesions who require temporary hemodynamic stabilization. It may be especially useful as an adjunct to prompt reperfusion of acute myocardial infarction.

▶ This significant laboratory study from the editor's institution demonstrates that a synchronized pulsatile cardiopulmonary bypass effectively decreases left ventricular oxygen consumption whereas a nonsynchronized bypass does not. All currently used cardiac assist pumps require a thoracotomy to drain blood directly from the left atrium. This method indicates that a synchronized peripheral bypass is equally effective, although an oxygenator is required.—F.C. Spencer, M.D.

The Value of Computed Tomography in Postoperative Pneumothorax Following Open-Heart Surgery

Rick A. Esposito, Arthur Boyd, and Frank C. Spencer (New York Univ.)
Ann. Thorac. Surg. 42:699–701, December 1986   17–11

Serial chest radiographs were misleading in two patients with pneumothorax following open heart surgery. In both cases, persistent air leakage occurred despite intercostal tube drainage. Computed tomography demonstrated pleural air pockets and malpositioning of the intercostal tube, and the indicated changes in treatment avoided prolonged tube drainage.

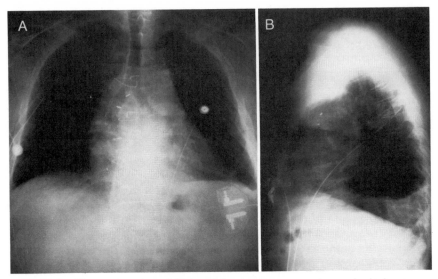

Fig 17–1.—(A) posteroanterior and (B) lateral chest roentgenograms taken on the third postoperative day following reoperative coronary artery grafting. Although a small air leak persisted, the lung appeared to be fully expanded. (Courtesy of Esposito, R.A., et al.: Ann. Thorac. Surg. 42:699–701, December 1986.)

Man, 59, an asthmatic who smoked heavily, underwent reoperative coronary bypass grafting. A 100% right pneumothorax was present the day after surgery, although the right pleural space had not been entered at initial operation. Apparent full expansion of the lung (Fig 17–1) followed placement of an intercostal tube, but an air leak persisted. Computed tomography demonstrated an unsuspected residual anterior air pocket and a posteriorly located intercostal tube (Fig

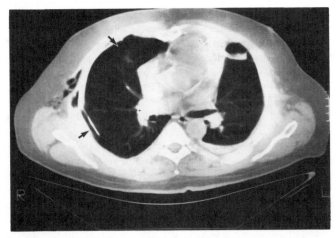

Fig 17–2.—Computed tomographic scan done on the third day postoperation shows a residual anterior pneumothorax on the right *(top arrow)* and an intercostal tube positioned posteriorly *(bottom arrow)*. (Courtesy of Esposito, R.A., et al.: Ann. Thorac. Surg. 42:699–701, December 1986.)

17–2). A second anterior chest tube was placed and the posterior tube was removed, and air leakage ceased within 24 hours. The anterior tube was removed 2 days later.

Persistent air leakage after open heart surgery usually is an indication for thoracotomy for bronchopleural fistula. Computed tomography may, however, demonstrate an occult air leak not seen on conventional radiographs. If a roentgenogram shows complete lung expansion but an air leak persists, a computed tomography scan should be promptly obtained.

▶ This short report from the editor's institution illustrates the value of computed tomography in the troublesome problem of continuing air leakage following thoracotomy despite multiple chest tube insertions. The basic principle with such patients, of course, is the precise insertion of a chest tube that will enable the lung to expand and adhere to the pleural surfaces. A persisting residual pneumothorax inevitably leads to empyema.—F.C. Spencer, M.D.

Dire Consequences of the Indiscriminate Use of Teflon Felt Pledgets
H.G. Borst (Hannover Med. School, Hannover, West Germany)
J. Thorac. Cardiovasc. Surg. 94:442–443, September 1987   17–12

A recent report described the successful use of resorbable material to control bleeding. However, the indiscriminate use of Teflon felt pledgets and strips when infection occurs have dire consequences. Four such cases are described.

CASE 1.—Man, 55, underwent surgery initially for a cardiac lipoma. One month later multiple sternal and parasternal fistulas were noted. After 8 months of multiple attempts to eradicate the sinus tracts by local procedures, radical resection of the sternum was done, and infected pledgets at the site of aortic cannulation were removed. A total of 37 weeks of hospitalization and seven reoperations had been required. The patient is free of infection at 4½ years.

CASE 2.—Man, 24, had undergone aortic valve repair for congenital aortic stenosis at age 8 years and valve replacement at age 20 years. After 2½ years of intermittent sepsis, he was reoperated on for a large infected retrosternal false aneurysm of the ascending aorta. This aneurysm orignated at the site of aortotomy, which had been secured with Teflon felt pledgets. Additional Teflon strips were used in this first attempted repair. Finally, a large segment of the anterior wall of the ascending aorta, including the original site of aortotomy and its infected Teflon strips, was removed. Although the patient survived this extensive procedure, he died 12 days later of continuing sepsis and pneumonia.

CASE 3.—Man, 36, had left ventricular aneurysmectomy and endocardial resection and implantation of a nonfunctional myocardial pacemaker electrode. Five months later the pacemaker lead was found to be infected where it traversed the Teflon strips that secured the original ventriculotomy. The strips were removed with some difficulty, and the patient has remained infection free for 4½ years.

CASE 4.—Woman, 53, had undergone combined aortic and mitral valve replacement. Infection from a large pack of Teflon felt resulted in four hospitalizations comprising 29 weeks and 6 reoperations. This patient was successfully treated and has been infection free for 6 years.

Placement of Teflon felt pledgets and strips outside the heart and aorta for bleeding control or to reinforce friable tissue should be avoided. The same results can almost always be achieved with pericardial pledgets or strips.

▶ This short report from Germany sharply cautions against the casual use of Teflon pledgets, describing serious or fatal complications in four patients. At the editor's institution, the use of Teflon felt has gradually decreased over recent years to where it is now very rarely used. As the author indicates, if pledgets are necessary, autogenous pericardium or autogenous vein is simpler and safer.—F.C. Spencer, M.D.

Left Ventricular Aneurysm With Predominating Congestive Heart Failure: A Comparative Study of Medical and Surgical Treatment
Yves Louagie, Taoufik Alouini, Jacques Lespérance, and L. Conrad Pelletier (Montreal Heart Inst. and Université de Montréal)
J. Thorac. Cardiovasc. Surg. 94:571–581, October 1987   17–13

When a left ventricular aneurysm leads to congestive heart failure, surgery is associated with high operative mortality and the long-term outlook is poor. A review was made of experience with 109 patients treated between 1979 and 1985 for congestive failure secondary to postinfarction left ventricular aneurysm. Of these, 73% were in New York Heart Association functional class III or IV at the time of diagnosis. The total ejection fraction averaged 30%, and the mean telediastolic volume of the aneurysm was 76 ml.

Aneurysmectomy was performed in 49 patients and 60 clinically similar patients were managed medically. The patients treated surgically had more extensive coronary disease. Survival was similar in the two groups after an average follow-up of 4 years. Surgically treated patients, however, had significantly fewer complications. Surgery independently lowered the risks of both cardiac complications and death, as did a shorter interval between initial infarction and the diagnosis of aneurysm, and the absence of right ventricular failure. Functional improvement was directly related to surgical treatment.

Aneurysmectomy improves the quality of life in patients with left ventricular aneurysm who present with predominant congestive failure. Patients who have a proximal left anterior descending artery lesion and a contractile segment ejection fraction of at least 41% have an excellent long-term outlook after surgical treatment.

▶ A major important question is the expected benefit with aneurysmectomy in patients with congestive heart failure and a left ventricular aneurysm. This report analyzed 109 patients with congestive heart failure and a left ventricular aneurysm; left ventricular end-diastolic pressure was near 24 mm and ejection fraction, 30%. Aneurysmectomy was performed in 49 patients. With an average follow-up of 2 years, 5-year actuarial survival curves were similar in surgical and medical groups: 70% vs. 64%. The 5-year complication free rate, however, was significantly better among surgical patients, 52% vs. 31%. An unanswerable question is whether a longer period of follow-up would demonstrate an improvement in survival with surgical resection.—F.C. Spencer, M.D.

Cryoablative Techniques in the Treatment of Cardiac Tachyarrhythmias
David A. Ott, Arthur Garson, Jr., Denton A. Cooley, Richard T. Smith, and Jeffrey Moak (Texas Heart Inst., Houston; Texas Children's Hosp., Houston; and St. Luke's Episcopal Hosp., Houston)
Ann. Thorac. Surg. 43:138–143, February 1987   17–14

For drug-resistant, incessant, or life-threatening cardiac tachyarrhythmias, surgery is recommended in selected patients. Recently, cryoablative techniques have been demonstrated to be effective in eliminating foci or pathways causing tachycardia when used alone or in conjunction with surgery.

Of 175 patients treated surgically for cardiac tachyarrhythmias, 53 underwent confirmatory operative mapping and definitive operation using cryoablative procedures. Sixteen patients had supraventricular tachycardia caused by Kent's bundle in the right anterior or posterior paraseptal location; six patients had permanent junctional reciprocating tachycardia; and 19 had atrial ectopic tachycardia. Of 19 infants with critical ventricular tachycardia, 13 were treated with cryoablation at the site of the ectopic focus, either alone or combined with excision of the area.

In patients with Kent's bundle, cryoablation was successful in eliminating tachycardia in 15 of 16 patients. Cryoablation was successful in all patients with permanent junctional reciprocating tachycardia and in all infants with critical ventricular tachycardia. The success rate was 83.3% in patients having atrial ectopic tachycardia but 100% in patients having a single focus. Results indicate that cryoablative techniques have a high rate of cure when used either alone or in combination with other treatments in selected cases of tachyarrhythmias.

▶ This report describes the use of cryoablative techniques in 53 of 175 patients treated surgically for cardiac arrhythmias. The cryoablative techniques have many attractive features that will undoubtedly increase their popularity. Such techniques avoid extensive dissection and permit destruction of electrical activity without destroying the fibrous matrix of the heart.—F.C. Spencer, M.D.

Closed-Heart Technique for Wolff-Parkinson-White Syndrome: Further Experience and Potential Limitations
Gerard M. Guiraudon, George J. Klein, Arjun D. Sharma, Simon Milstein, and Douglas G. McLellan (Univ. of Western Ontario, London, Ontario, Canada)
Ann. Thorac, Surg. 42:651–657, December 1986   17–15

The endocardial approach to Wolff-Parkinson-White (WPW) syndrome necessitates cold cardioplegic arrest, and surgical mortality has not lessened significantly. The authors evaluated the epicardial approach in 105 consecutive cases of WPW syndrome treated in 1982–1985. The mean age was 33 years. Three patients had multiple accessory pathways. There were 74 left ventricular free wall accessory pathways, 23 in the posterior septal region, and 11 right ventricular free wall paths. Twenty-one of the patients had "concealed" WPW syndrome. The most frequent indication for surgery was refractory reciprocating supraventricular tachycardia or potentially life-threatening atrial fibrillation.

Normothermic cardiopulmonary bypass usually was not used in patients with right ventricular free wall accessory pathways. Electrophysiologic mapping was carried out using a hand-held exploring electrode. The atrioventricular (AV) junction was cryoablated. No deaths occurred, and none of the patients had temporary or permanent AV block. Five patients required more than one operation. All but one of the AV accessory paths were successfully ablated. No patient had recurrence after a mean follow-up of 18 months.

The epicardial approach to ablation of accessory pathways in WPW syndrome is associated with low morbidity and mortality and is effective. If subendocardial AV pathways are present, an alternative approach may be necessary. Ablation of accessory pathways in the closed heart without cardioplegic arrest allows concomitant procedures to be done without augmenting arrest time.

▶ This report describes experiences with 105 patients treated with a closed heart technique and cryoablation. A successful result was achieved in all but one patient: there were no deaths and no heart block. These data would indicate that the closed technique may be preferable to the more complicated open heart technique developed by several groups. Further experiences will be particularly significant.—F.C. Spencer, M.D.

Surgical Treatment of Endomyocardial Fibrosis
M.S. Valiathan, K.G. Balakrishnan, R. Sankarkumar, and C.C. Kartha (Trivandrum, India)
Ann. Thorac. Surg. 43:68–73, January 1987   17–16

Dubost introduced endocardial resection and valve replacement for advanced endomyocardial fibrosis. The authors reviewed 46 patients having endomyocardial fibrosis (Fig 17–3) who underwent endocardiectomy and tricuspid or mitral valve replacement, or both, in 1981–1984. The disorder is relatively frequent in Kerala State, India. The mean age at operation was 24 years. Surgery was performed under bypass with moderate systemic hypothermia and cold potassium cardioplegia. Local pericardial cooling also was used. In cases of left ventricular involvement,

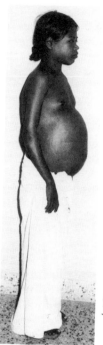

Fig 17–3.—Patient with biventricular endomyocardial fibrosis. (Courtesy of Valiathan, M.S., et al.: Ann. Thorac. Surg. 43:68–73, January 1987.)

tricuspid annuloplasty frequently was carried out. Five patients with advanced biventricular disease required biventricular endocardiectomy and mitral and tricuspid valve replacement.

The operative mortality was 22%. The postoperative period generally was difficult. Two of four deaths that followed readmission to hospital were a result of prosthetic valve thrombosis. Six of 30 survivors, followed for a mean of 26 months, had nonfatal thromboembolic complications. Twelve patients were in New York Heart Association functional class I postoperatively. Thirteen other patients improved to class II, and four were reclassified from class IV to class III. The life table estimate for survivors, including operative mortality, was 67% at 2 years.

In 16 more recent cases, there were five early deaths but no late deaths. Endocardiectomy and atrioventricular valve replacement are the best approaches to advanced endomyocardial fibrosis. Earlier operation may lower operative mortality and improve the hemodynamic results in surviving patients.

▶ This short report describes experiences with 46 patients treated by endocardiectomy and replacement of different cardiac valves in a hospital in India where there is a high frequency of this disease. Operative mortality was near 22%; late mortality, about 13%. The degree of disability with the condition is most impressive. Although the disease is fortunately geographically limited to different sections of the world, the effectiveness of the operation merits emphasis.—F.C. Spencer, M.D.

Primary Repair of Traumatic Aortic Disruption

Lawrence R. McBride, Stephen Tidik, Joseph C. Stothert, Hendrick B. Barner, George C. Kaiser, Vallee L. Willman, and D. Glenn Pennington (St. Louis Univ.) Ann. Thorac. Surg. 43:65–67, January 1987   17–17

Prompt surgical repair is vital in traumatic disruption of the thoracic aorta. The majority of repairs are made by prosthetic graft; only 4% of recent cases were repaired by primary anastomosis. A retrospective study was undertaken to evaluate 22 patients who underwent repair of acute traumatic rupture of the aorta by prosthetic graft or by primary anastomosis.

All patients had suffered deceleration injuries as a result of motor vehicle accidents. The operative procedure was determined by the surgeon: in 64% of patients, a modified Gott shunt was selected. Primary anastomosis was performed in 68% of patients. Wherever possible, intercostal arteries were preserved. Ligation of no more than one pair of intercostal arteries was usually required for sufficient mobilization, although additional branches were sometimes temporarily occluded. Sufficient mobilization permitted the transected end to be approximated with gentle traction.

The overall survival rate was 82%: in the shunt group, technical problems related to the shunt contributed to the deaths of 3 patients. One patient died intraoperatively; postoperative morbidity usually stemmed from associated injuries. Aortic cross-clamp time averaged 37 minutes for primary anastomosis and 58 minutes for insertion of a prosthetic graft.

Primary repair of aortic tears has several advantages, including shorter aortic cross-clamp time, reduced risk of infection, and reduced risk of pseudoaneurysm formation from suture dehiscence. Although primary anastomosis is more technically demanding, successful application of this technique is feasible in most patients, if adequate mobilization of the proximal and distal aorta can be obtained. Preservation of the intercostal arteries is important for the success of this procedure.

▶ This report indicates that a primary repair can be done in a significant percentage of patients with traumatic rupture. Mobilization of the injured aorta for a short distance provides enough mobility for anastomosis. In this series of 22 patients, primary repair was performed in 15, including the last ten consecutive patients.

Details regarding shunting are not given. A Gott shunt was used in about two thirds of the patients. Neurologic injury occurred in two of this group; one of the "no shunt" group after a cross-clamp time of 35 minutes.

At the editor's institution, a femoral artery–femoral vein bypass with a pump oxygenator is routinely used to maintain distal perfusion, with a blood pressure above 60 mm. This is by far the most effective method for protection from paraplegia. The Gott shunt was a valuable contribution in its time but is now inferior to other techniques and should be rarely, if ever, used.—F.C. Spencer, M.D.

Hypothermic Circulatory Arrest in the Treatment of Thoracic Aortic Lesions

J. Thomas Crepps, Jr., Philip Allmendinger, Lee Ellison, Chester Humphrey, Paul Preissler, and Henry Low (Hartford Hosp./Univ. of Connecticut)
Ann. Thorac. Surg. 43:644–647, June 1987   17–18

Treatment of arteriosclerotic and dissecting aneurysms that involve the ascending aorta and aortic arch is one of the most technically difficult procedures in cardiovascular surgery. Hypothermic circulatory arrest has been used to treat aortic arch lesions.

The authors describe three women and seven men aged 23 to 77 years who had this type of circulatory arrest during treatment of thoracic aortic lesions. Seven had dissecting aneurysms of the ascending aorta with extension into the aortic arch, one had a mycotic aneurysm of the arch, and two had arteriosclerotic aneurysms of the ascending aorta and entire aortic arch.

The patients were supported and cooled with cardiopulmonary bypass. Hypothermic circulatory arrest lasted from 21 to 63 minutes, with an average of 35.7 minutes. Total bypass time averaged 169 minutes. All patients survived the surgery; nine remained neurologically intact. An average of 2.9 units of blood was given during operation. Blood loss in the first 24 hours after surgery averaged 683 ml. In all patients renal function returned to baseline.

The hemorrhagic cerebrovascular accident that occurred in one patient was not considered to be a result of the hypothermic circulatory arrest. Three additional patients experienced transient somnolence, lethargy, or dizziness after operation, which resolved within 2 weeks in each case. At an average of 21 months after surgery, nine patients were alive. One had died of transfusion hepatitis at 6 months.

From this experience it was concluded that hypothermic circulatory arrest facilitates the surgical approach to thoracic aortic lesions. The technique appears to be the safest method of preserving vital organs.

▶ This short report, describing surgical experiences with ten patients with large aneurysms of the ascending and transverse aortic arch, is a refreshing example of the increasing use of hypothermic circulatory arrest for complex aortic lesions. If the brain is properly cooled to near 15 C, published data continue to support the premise that circulatory arrest for at least 30–45 minutes is neurologically safe. In this report, all ten patients survived, nine of whom were free of neurologic problems.—F.C. Spencer, M.D.

Aortic Dissection

Roman W. DeSanctis, Robert M. Doroghazi, W. Gerald Austen, and Mortimer J. Buckley (Massachusetts Gen. Hosp., Boston, Harvard Univ., and Boone Clinic, Columbia, Mo.)
N. Engl. J. Med. 317:1060–1067, Oct. 22, 1987   17–19

Dramatic advances in the management of aortic dissection have occurred in the past 30 years. The authors review old and new concepts in the diagnosis and treatment of this lethal disease.

In aortic dissection a tear in the aortic intima allows blood to surge into the aortic media, separating the intima from the adventitia. Usually, dissections propagate from the intimal tear distally in the aorta, but proximal extension can occur. Controversy continues as to whether the initial event is the intimal tear or hemorrhage into a diseased aortic media with secondary rupture of the overlying intima. In a recent study of 158 postmortem specimens, an intimal tear was found in every case. Usually, dissection begins in the ascending aorta, within a few centimeters of the aortic valve.

Type I dissection extends beyond the ascending aorta; type II is confined to it. Type III dissections originate in the descending thoracic aorta. Another classification system designates all dissections that involve the ascending aorta as type A, regardless of the site of the primary intimal tear. All other dissections are called type B. Dissections are "acute" if presentation occurs within 2 weeks of onset; 65%–75% of patients with untreated dissection die within the first 2 weeks after onset.

The classic assumption that aortic dissection is associated with degenerative changes in the elastic tissue and smooth muscle of the aorta has been challenged. The most important predisposing factor is hypertension. Others include congenital disorders of connective tissue, particularly Marfan's syndrome and Ehlers-Danlos syndrome. Dissections predominate in men. Half the dissections in women younger than age 40 years occur during pregnancy. The etiologic role of arteriosclerosis, which commonly coexists with aortic dissection, is unclear. Iatrogenic dissections can originate at the sites of suturing of saphenous veins to the aorta for coronary artery bypass.

Clinical findings include severe chest pain, which is present in 90% of patients. Its intensity is maximal at inception. The three chief neurologic complaints of dissection are stroke, ischemic peripheral neuropathy, and paraparesis or paraplegia. Patients often appear cool, clammy, and vasoconstricted, although blood pressure is increased in many cases. For confirming diagnosis, aortic angiography has a 95%–99% accuracy.

Early short-term treatment usually involves intravenous injection of sodium nitroprusside, 25–50 μg/minute, and propranolol, 0.05–0.15 mg/kg every 4–6 hours. Acute proximal dissections should be treated surgically. For acute distal dissections definitive therapy is more controversial.

Long-term follow-up should include routine chest films every 3 months for the first year and at least twice a year thereafter. Long-term survival of patients with this disease has improved, with overall actuarial 10-year survival now at about 40%.

▶ This review article well summarizes current knowledge about dissecting aneurysms. Surgical therapy has improved remarkably in recent years to where routine excision of acute dissections in the ascending aorta, the preferred approach, can be performed with an operative risk near 15%. The importance of permanent long-term follow-up is emphasized by all reports, for nearly 30% of late deaths result from development and rupture of another aneurysm.—F.C. Spencer, M.D.

Techniques of Aortic Arch Replacement: Profound Hypothermia Versus Moderate Hypothermia With Innominate Artery Perfusion
Michael J. Janusz and Frank O. Tyers (Vancouver Gen. Hosp., Vancouver, B.C.)
Am. J. Surg. 153 511–514, May 1987   17–20

The chief difficulties in resecting an aortic arch aneurysm are due to surgical exposure, bleeding, and possible ischemic neurologic injury from interrupting circulation to the aortic arch vessels. Of the many approaches to these problems, the use of profound hypothermia and circulatory arrest has met with the most consistent success. However, coagulopathy that is associated with profound hypothermia has been a problem.

To reduce the time and potential difficulties of cooling and rewarming, a technique of moderate hypothermia and low-flow, pressure-monitored innominate artery perfusion has been developed as an alternative. From January 1985 until July 1986, eight patients had resection of an aortic arch aneurysm. Profound hypothermia, 12–17 C, and circulatory arrest were used in six patients (group 1). Moderate hypothermia, 20 C, with a low flow of 200 ml/minute and pressure-monitored innominate artery perfusion by means of a 14-gauge cannula were used in two patients (group 2).

The arch was repaired by patch graft in two patients and by tube graft in six. Concomitant ascending aortic replacement was done in five patients, aortic valve replacement was performed in four, and coronary bypass was used in two. Circulatory arrest lasted 15–71 minutes in group 1 and 15 and 35 minutes in the 2 patients in group 2. All patients survived surgery. One patient in group 1 suffered a minor residual neurologic deficit after postoperative cardiac arrest was brought on by rapidly progressing hypoxia.

The technique of low-flow, pressure-monitored innominate artery perfusion was found to be simple and expedient. Cooling and rewarming for a nasopharyngeal temperature of 20 C was quicker and simpler than cooling to between 12 C and 15 C. Coagulopathy has not been a serious problem with this new technique.

▶ Surgery of the aortic arch is one of the frontiers of cardiovascular surgery in which vast progress has been made in the past few years. This report describes experiences with eight patients, six of whom were operated upon with hypothermia and circulatory arrest for 15–71 minutes, and two with hypothermia and low flow cerebral perfusion. All patients recovered, though one with the hypothermic arrest technique had a moderate neurologic injury. Though the data are few, the authors quite properly emphasize that the techniques of low flow cerebral perfusion remain an alternate method of treatment and may be considered with complicated lesions for which longer periods of circulatory arrest would be required.—F.C. Spencer, M.D.

Operative Management of Acute Aortic Arch Dissection Using Profound Hypothermia and Circulatory Arrest
Joseph M. Graham and D. Mitchell Stinnett (St. John's Regional Med. Ctr., Joplin, Mo.)
Ann. Thorac. Surg. 44:192–198, August 1987   17–21

Acute aortic dissection that involves the transverse aortic arch poses special technical problems. The authors report that profound hypothermia and circulatory arrest have proved to be valuable adjuncts in treating acute aortic dissection with extension into the transverse aortic arch. They describe six consecutive patients who had acute aortic dissection that involved the transverse aortic arch and underwent surgery with the use of profound hypothermia and circulatory arrest. The five men and one woman were aged 32 to 78 years.

Complete aortic dissection and aortic valvular insufficiency occurred in

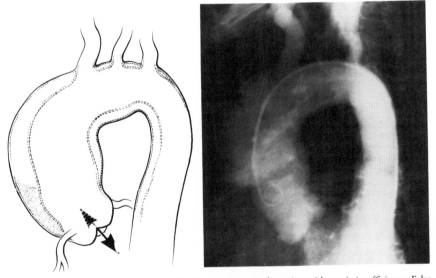

Fig 17–4.—Preoperative aortogram showing type 1 aortic dissection with aortic insufficiency. False lumen was present to middescending thoracic aorta, and intimal tears were noted in ascending and midtransverse arch. (Courtesy of Graham, J.M., and Stinnett, D.M.: Ann. Thorac. Surg. 44:192–198, August 1987.)

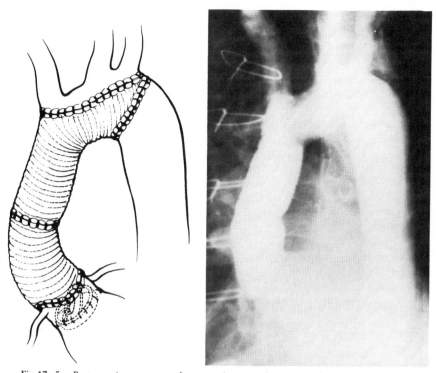

Fig 17–5.—Postoperative aortogram demonstrating operative repair with aortic valve replacement and total ascending and transverse arch replacement. No residual false lumen was noted then or by computed tomography during subsequent 4 years. (Courtesy of Graham, J.M., and Stinnett, D.M.: Ann. Thorac. Surg. 44:192–198, August 1987.)

each patient. Dissection was spontaneous in four and iatrogenic in two. All underwent surgery emergently.

Body temperatures were reduced to 14–18 C. The aortic arch was drained of blood and inspected after pump perfusion was stopped and the brachiocephalic vessels were clamped. In 4 patients complete or partial replacement of the arch was done with reimplantation of the aortic arch vessels (Figs 17–4 and 17–5) or with their incorporation into a beveled distal anastomosis.

Total circulatory arrest in all patients lasted 16–42 minutes. Ischemic cardiac arrest lasted 56–85 minutes, and total perfusion lasted 132–241 minutes. All patients recovered without neurologic deficit. Pulmonary insufficiency occurred in two patients and was the most noteworthy complication. In all cases postoperative angiographic assessment showed complete resection or obliteration of patent false lumen in the aortic arch and ascending aorta. Five patients were alive and well 8–49 months after surgery.

The use of profound hypothermia and circulatory arrest in the operative management of aortic arch dissection allowed bloodless inspection and repair of extensive intimal tears, complete intimal adventitial reapproximation or resection, avoidance of injury by a clamp to fragile dissected aortic tissue, and assurance of patent arch-cerebral revascularization.

▶ This short report from Joplin, Missouri, is quite significant in that it does not come from a large tertiary medical center with a long history of experience with operations for thoracic aneurysms. Six patients with acute aortic dissection involving the transverse aortic arch were successfully operated upon with the technique of profound hypothermia and circulatory arrest. The length of cerebral circulatory arrest varied from 16 to 42 minutes. All patients recovered without neurologic defect. Hence, this report is an excellent example of both the safety of the hypothermic circulatory arrest technique and its applicability by experienced vascular surgeons in smaller medical centers.—F.C. Spencer, M.D.

Budd-Chiari Syndrome Resulting From a Membranous Web of the Inferior Vena Cava: Operative Repair Using Profound Hypothermia and Circulatory Arrest
J. Peter Murphy, Jr., Igor Gregoric, and Denton A. Cooley (Texas Heart Inst., Houston)
Ann. Thorac. Surg. 43:212–214, February 1987   17–22

The present patient had Budd-Chiari syndrome due to a subdiaphragmatic inferior caval web, with associated caval and hepatic venous thrombosis. Repair was successfully performed under cardiopulmonary bypass with profound hypothermia and circulatory arrest.

Man, 47, presented with right upper quadrant abdominal pain, hepatomegaly, and ascites. Lower limb edema had been present sporadically for 8 years. The liver was diffusely enlarged. Inferior cavography showed a suprahepatic membrane with proximal caval dilation. The inferior cava was controlled from within the pericardium at operation. Cardiopulmonary perfusion was stopped when the core temperature was 24 C, allowing incision of the cava and removal of a large amount of thrombus from both the cava and hepatic veins. Patch angioplasty then was done using autologous pericardium. A postoperative study showed unobstructed caval flow and normal opacification of the hepatic veins.

Profound hypothermia and circulatory arrest allowed precise resection of the caval membrane and complete thrombectomy in this case, as well as repair of the vena cava. If inadequate flow is established after caval and hepatic venous thrombectomy, a mesocaval or mesoatrial shunt could be created, depending on the flow status of the inferior vena cava.

▶ This impressive case report describes the application of the hypothermic circulatory arrest technique for removal of a web obstructing the vena cava and producing the Budd-Chiari syndrome. The amount of thrombus removed was impressive. The authors state that a 1970 report from Japan found 74 cases of vena caval occlusion by caval webs. Hopefully, this report will stimulate others to try this direct approach for relief of the caval obstruction in this serious problem.—F.C. Spencer, M.D.

Intracardiac Extension of Wilms' Tumor: A Report of the National Wilms' Tumor Study
Don K. Nakayama, Alfred A. deLorimier, James A. O'Neill, Jr., Patricia Norkool, and Giulio J. D'Angio (Children's Hosp. of Philadelphia and American Academy of Pediatrics, Elk Grove Village, Ill.)
Ann. Surg. 204:693–697, December 1986   17–23

Tumor thrombus from Wilms' tumor sometimes extends through the vena cava into the heart, presenting a difficult challenge. Excision without embolization may necessitate cardiopulmonary bypass. Intracardiac extension was present in 15 (0.7%) of 2,280 patients enrolled in the first three National Wilms' Tumor Studies. The mean age was 3½ years. Only one patient had cardiac symptoms at the outset. Preoperative studies demonstrated intracardiac extension of tumor in six patients.

All patients but one, with clear-cell sarcoma, had favorable histologic findings. Cardiopulmonary bypass was used in ten cases. Nearly three fourths had operative complications, most frequently major intraoperative bleeding. Only three of the six preoperatively diagnosed patients had such complications. Two patients had embolization. Eighty-six percent of the patients with favorable histology lived 2 years without sequelae. The patient with clear-cell sarcoma died.

Intracardiac Wilms' tumor should be suspected in patients with extensive caval thrombosis, hypotension, or heart failure. Aggressive multidrug chemotherapy and radiotherapy, in addition to surgical removal of tumor, may improve the outlook.

▶ This remarkable paper describes experiences with 15 patients enrolled in three consecutive National Wilms' Tumor Studies who had intracardiac tumor extension. Cardiopulmonary bypass was used in ten of the patients. Fortunately, there were no operative deaths, and embolization occurred in only two patients. Eleven of 14 patients survived, with an actuarial 2-year survival of 86%. Hence, these data indicate both the safety and effectiveness of an aggressive approach for this unusual form of malignancy.—F.C. Spencer, M.D.

18 The Arteries

Use and Limitations of Thrombolytic Therapy in the Treatment of Peripheral Arterial Ischemia: Results of a Multi-Institutional Questionnaire
John J. Ricotta, Richard M. Green, and James A. DeWeese (Univ. of Rochester)
J. Vasc. Surg. 6:45–50, July 1987

18 – 1

Vascular thrombosis is frequently treated by infusion of thrombolytic drugs. To determine the effectiveness of this therapy for peripheral arterial ischemia, the results of a questionnaire answered by 45 vascular surgeons who have experience with thrombolytic infusion in 623 patients were analyzed.

A successful outcome was obtained in 50.2% of cases. Complications included hemorrhage requiring transfusion or operation in 20.1% of cases and amputation, which was required in 16.5% of cases. There were nine strokes in this series. Six of these strokes were fatal. The total mortality rate was 2.5%. There was no significant correlation between experience and outcome.

The use of thrombolytic infusion should be limited in the treatment of peripheral ischemia due to high morbidity and mortality rates. Thrombolytic infusion therapy should be compared to surgical intervention in prospective randomized trials before becoming accepted treatment for arterial thrombosis.

▶ Koltun et al. (*Arch. Surg.* 122:901, 1987) reviewed an experience with 64 consecutive episodes of limb-threatening graft or native vessel occlusion. The overall success rate of thrombolytic therapy in their hands was 59%, with a complication rate or mortality rate of 28%. Thrombolytic therapy in patients with occluded vascular grafts required identification of the causative lesion and subsequent management in 64% of the cases. By contrast, 70% of native vessel occlusions maintained their patency. Patients who failed thrombolytic therapy had a 38% amputation rate, while patients with reconstructable occlusions had a 64% salvage rate at 6 months. These authors emphasized that graft occlusion successfully treated with thrombolysis requires correction of precipitating lesions for long-term limb salvage.—S.I. Schwartz, M.D.

Intra-Arterial Thrombolysis for Acute Limb Ischemia: A Three-Year Experience
Patrick M. Battey, J. Timothy Fulenwider, Robert B. Smith III, Louis G. Martin, Mark T. Stewart, and Garland D. Perdue (Emory Univ. and VA Med. Ctr., Atlanta)
South. Med. J. 80:479–482, April 1987

18–2

In acute limb ischemia following arterial grafts, percutaneous intra-arterial thrombolysis (IAT) has been used alone or as an adjunct to balloon catheter embolectomy and arterial graft revision. Incomplete thrombolysis, peripheral thromboembolic migration, hypersensitivity reactions, and high costs are significant disadvantages of IAT. This article reviews a retrospective study designed to determine which patients would most benefit from IAT.

The charts of 28 patients who underwent IAT procedures for native arterial thromboembolism in 15 limbs and arterial graft thrombosis in 17 limbs were reviewed. Half of the limbs were painful at rest, while the other half were painful upon walking. Baseline segmental Doppler limb pressures—and, in some cases, plethysmographic hemodynamic measurements—were conducted on the patients. Angiography was performed before IAT to locate the acute arterial obstruction and 1, 6, 12, and 24 hours after IAT to monitor thrombolysis. Streptokinase alone or in conjunction with urokinase was injected through a no. 5 French end-hole polyethylene catheter into the proximal end of the thrombus. The initial bolus was 10,000 units of streptokinase followed by 5,000 units of streptokinase or urokinase hourly. A low-dose heparin drip was used in most cases. If necessary, drug infusion was decreased to maintain the fibrinogen level above 100 mg/dl. The IAT lasted an average of 28 hours, and it was stopped if progression of ischemic symptoms, lack of effective thrombolysis, or hemorrhaging was found.

Of 32 involved extremities, 27 were salvaged. Of the 17 limbs operated on for arterial graft thrombosis, five required a smaller operation than predicted or none at all following IAT. The IAT alone cleared the thrombi from four of six limbs with native arterial embolism. Major complications in 8 patients required abandonment of IAT; overall mortality was 6%.

The IAT technique is most successful in patients whose acute limb ischemia results from arterial embolus, in those whose ischemic condition would tolerate a 1-day IAT trial, and in patients whose femoropopliteal or tibial runoff is unlikely to require remedial operation.

▶ The role of intra-arterial thrombolysis for acute limb ischemia has not been defined. Hurley et al. (*Am. J. Surg.* 148:830, 1984) reported an experience with intra-arterial fibrinolytic therapy applied to 34 patients with severe peripheral ischemia. Fifty-six percent required surgical intervention; 71% of patients were significantly improved. Complications occurred in almost two thirds of their patients, and many of these were major. Sicard et al. (*J. Vasc. Surg.* 2:65, 1985) examined the efficacy of this mode of therapy in 40 patients. Forty-five percent of patients with native artery occlusion had improvement and did not need further surgical intervention. Only 21% of graft occlusions were successfully managed.—S.I. Schwartz, M.D.

Comparison Between the Transabdominal and Retroperitoneal Approach for Reconstruction of the Infrarenal Abdominal Aorta

Gregorio A. Sicard, Michael B. Freeman, John C. VanderWoude, and Charles B. Anderson (Washington Univ.)
J. Vasc. Surg. 5:19–27, January 1987   18–3

Infrarenal abdominal aortic occlusive or aneurysmal lesions have traditionally been repaired through a transperitoneal route. Nevertheless, the retroperitoneal approach has been suggested as an alternative in patients with multiple intra-abdominal operations or when previous transperitoneal aortic surgery has been carried out. The research reported in this article compared the transperitoneal (TP) and the retroperitoneal (RP) approaches with regard to multiple intraoperative and postoperative parameters in the elective reconstruction of the infrarenal abdominal aorta.

The study population consisted of 104 consecutive patients who under-

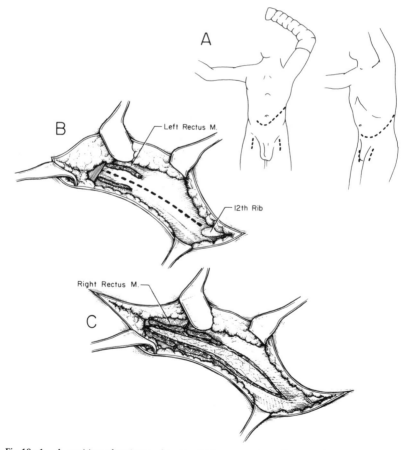

Fig 18–1.—**A,** position of patient and incision(s) for retroperitoneal approach to aortoiliac system. **B,** division of left rectus muscle and exposure of twelfth rib. **C,** division of both recti and abdominal wall muscles. (Courtesy of Sicard, G.A., et al.: J. Vasc. Surg. 5:19–27, January 1987.)

went elective reconstruction of the infrarenal abdominal aorta. Fifty patients underwent aortoiliac reconstruction through the TP approach, and 54 patients underwent operation through the RP approach. Both groups were observed to have similar revascularization procedures, associated diseases, and preoperative cardiac and pulmonary function parameters. The TP approach was noted to be associated with larger intraoperative blood loss when compared to the RP approach (Fig 18–1). The intraoperative crystalloid requirements were higher for the TP approach when compared to the RP approach. Furthermore, the intraoperative blood requirements were higher for the TP approach than for the RP approach. Both groups were shown to have similar operative times, but the nasogastric intubation and initiation of oral feeding were markedly prolonged in the TP group relative to the RP group. Postoperative hospitalization was substantially prolonged in the TP group when compared to the RP group. It is concluded that the RP approach is a preferable alternative to the TP route in elective aortoiliac reconstruction.

▶ This paper is important because it gives objective proof that the retroperitoneal approach may be superior to the transperitoneal approach in many aortic reconstructions. As the discussants point out, exposure to the distal right renal artery is a drawback of the procedure. While the proximal right renal artery can be controlled by this approach, if distal control is necessary, the peritoneum has to be entered. Having the opportunity to watch Dr. Charles Rob, who introduced this approach to Rochester, I can attest to its effectiveness and advantages.—S.I. Schwartz, M.D.

Supraceliac Aortofemoral Bypass
Clifford S. Canepa, Peter J. Schubart, Lloyd M. Taylor, Jr., and John M. Porter (Oregon Health Sciences Univ., Portland)
Surgery 101:323–328, March 1987   18–4

There are occasionally patients who have anatomical situations that preclude or render the standard arterial repair hazardous, including retroperitoneal scar formation that results from multiple previous failed attempts at infrarenal reconstruction, disease extending to or above renal artery origins, retroperitoneal sepsis, primary retroperitoneal fibrosis, and extensive infrarenal arterial calcification, which precludes the use of this vessel for arterial inflow. This report details experience with seven patients with limb threatening ischemia of the lower extremity who had prosthetic bypass from the supraceliac aorta to the femoral arteries.

In four patients, the aorta was exposed through a left thoracoabdominal incision, which divided the diaphragm radially and divided the costal margin with reflection of the stomach, pancreas, spleen, and left colon to the right and anastomosis of the bypass graft to the lateral aspect of the supraceliac aorta as described by Elkins et al. In the two most recent patients the aortic exposure provided by a left posterolateral incision from the upper border of the eleventh rib to the edge of the rectus muscle with the patient in the semilateral position was used. The dissection is both extrathoracic and extraperitoneal with this exposure, and the aorta is exposed by reflecting the left kidney forward and dividing the diaphragm crus fibers to anastomose the bypass graft to the posterolateral aspect of the aorta, as described by O'Mara and Williams. To prevent excessive myocardial afterload strain, aortic clamping is performed with pharmacologic control of blood pressure. The aortic clamps are removed after the anastomosis is complete, and the graft is occluded with a soft jawed clamp.

The authors' current preferred graft configuration consists of a single 8- or 10-mm aorta to the left femoral tube graft with an 8-mm left-to-right femorofemoral crossover subcutaneous graft. There were no deaths from surgery. A graft infection related to passage of the right limb of a retroperitoneally placed bifurcation graft developed through the incisional scar of a previous hysterectomy in one patient, who was treated by graft removal and axillofemoral grafting, and she recovered. The current follow-up ranged from 6 months to 6 years (mean, 3½ years). Two years after surgery one patient died of a myocardial infarction. No other deaths have occurred. There have been no late graft occlusions. At 3½ years' mean follow-up, there was one graft limb occlusion that resulted in amputation for an overall graft limb patency rate and overall limb salvage rate of 93% each.

The authors' experience led to their current preference for a single graft to the left femoral artery with a separate femorofemoral component. They believe that bypass from the supraceliac aorta to the femoral arteries performed through a left flank incision with extraperitoneal extrathoracic exposure of the aorta is well tolerated with excellent long-term patency.

▶ As the authors point out, with an increasing number of patients with failed prior infrarenal aortic reconstructions, this procedure will have an increased role. The excellent limb salvage rate reported is better than that achieved by axillary-bifemoral bypassing. In the poor risk patient the axilla-bifemoral procedure represents a lesser insult and despite its decreased patency rate may remain the procedure of choice in that subset of patients.—S.I. Schwartz, M.D.

The Management of Aortoduodenal Fistula by In Situ Replacement of the Infected Abdominal Aortic Graft
William E. Walker, Denton A. Cooley, J. Michael Duncan, Grady L. Hallman, Jr., David A. Ott, and George J. Reul (Univ. of Texas and Texas Heart Inst., Houston)
Ann. Surg. 205:727–732, June 1987   18–5

Standard treatment of an infected abdominal aortic graft involves complete removal followed by oversewing. Blood flow is restored by an extra-anatomic bypass graft. Because of the association of this method with a high complication rate, mortality, infection, and loss of limb, 20

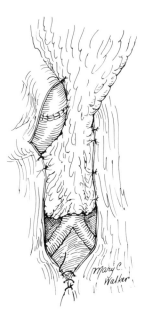

Fig 18–2.—The greater omentum is passed down between the duodenum, *upper left,* and aorta-graft, anchored securely to the tissues between the aorta and vena cava and sutured to the edges of the retroperitoneal incision, separating effectively the graft from the small bowel. A similar technique is applicable when the jejunum is involved rather than the duodenum. (Courtesy of Walker, W.E., et al.: Ann. Surg. 205:727–732, June 1987.)

such patients with secondary aortoduodenal fistula were treated with a more conservative approach: the graft was simply excised and replaced. Three patients with aortic graft erosion in the jejunum were treated in the same way and were followed for an average of 5.2 years. The results are reported in this article.

Fourteen patients had interposition of the greater omentum as a barrier between the new aortic graft and small bowel (Fig 18–2). Nine had closure of the retroperitoneal incision. Eighteen patients survived the repair process. Three had recurrent rupture or false aneurysm of the proximal aortic anastomosis. Two died. The remaining 15 had no problems or complications. There was no loss of limb.

Conservative operative management appears to be the optimal treatment for the majority of such patients; it avoids the complications and morbidity of more radical techniques.

▶ This is certainly an iconoclastic report because most authors indicate a preference for removal of the infected graft and for performing a remote bypass. In the discussion of this paper Rich indicated that eight patients were treated in this fashion with no operative mortality and no morbidity. There is evidence to suggest that the omental interposition represents a critical step in the avoidance of future problems. The entire subject of arterioenteric fistulas was reviewed recently by Bergqvist (*Acta Chir Scand* 153:81, 1987), and was originally described in 1825 by Astley Cooper, whose review uncovered 631 cases. Reconstructive vascular surgery was the etiologic agent in 95% of these cases. When lifetime analysis was performed, the long-term prospects were dismal.—S.I. Schwartz, M.D.

Secondary Aorto-Enteric Fistulae: Towards a More Conservative Approach

W.E.G. Thomas and R.N. Baird (Bristol Royal Infirmary, England)
Br. J. Surg. 73:875–878, November 1986

18–6

Although aortoenteric fistulae rarely occur, they can be devastating in their outcome. Primary fistulae almost always result from erosion of an aortic aneurysm into the duodenum, although they can occur with trauma or malignancy. Secondary fistulae usually follow the insertion of a Dacron or other aortic prosthesis. There currently is no consensus on how secondary fistulae should be managed. Although most U.S. researchers advocate mandatory graft excision, this carries a high incidence of

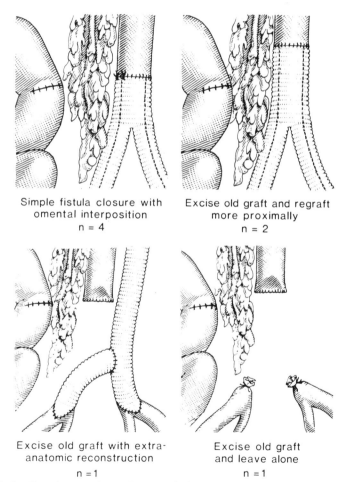

Simple fistula closure with
omental interposition
n = 4

Excise old graft and regraft
more proximally
n = 2

Excise old graft with extra-
anatomic reconstruction
n = 1

Excise old graft
and leave alone
n = 1

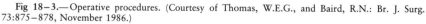

Fig 18–3.—Operative procedures. (Courtesy of Thomas, W.E.G., and Baird, R.N.: Br. J. Surg. 73:875–878, November 1986.)

CLINICAL DETAILS OF PATIENTS WITH SECONDARY AORTOENTERIC FISTULAE

Case no.	Age	Sex	Time from surgery	Reason for surgery	Findings	Procedure	Outcome
1	66	F	2 years	Ischaemia	Simple fistula	Direct suture	Well at 1 year
2	54	M	5 years	Ischaemia	False aneurysm	Regraft	Well at 5 years
3	58	M	4 years	Ischaemia	Simple fistula	Direct suture	Recurred at 2 months. Well at 3 years
4	59	M	2 years	Ischaemia	Simple fistula	Direct suture	Well at 3 years
5	14	F	9 months	Aneurysm	Infected graft	Graft excised	Died at 9 months (aortic stump rupture)
6	63	M	5 years	Ischaemia	Infected graft	Regraft	Femoral false aneurysm. Well at 1·5 years
7	58	F	10 years	Ischaemia	Infected graft	Graft excised. Axillobifemoral graft	Died of sepsis at 1 month
8	81	M	6 years	Aneurysm	Simple fistula	Direct suture	Well at 2 years

(Courtesy of Thomas, W.E.G., and Baird, R.N.: Br. J. Surg. 73:875–878, November 1986.)

aortic stump disruption. This article reviews experience with a more conservative approach for management of secondary aortoenteric fistulae.

The study population consisted of eight patients with secondary aortoenteric fistulae; all had previously undergone aortic Dacron grafting a median of 5 years previously (table). Procedures fell into four groups (Fig 18–3). Four patients had a simple fistula between the anastomosis and the adherent duodenum, three patients had clinically infected grafts, and one patient had a false aneurysm that had ruptured into the bowel. The four patients with a simple fistula had direct suture repair of the defect; one developed a recurrent fistula at 1 month but was successfully repaired again by direct suture. All four of these patients remain well at a follow-up of 1–5 years. The remaining four patients had their grafts excised, and two of them underwent local regrafting. Both patients who had local regrafting remain well at follow-up. One of the patients whose graft was excised had an axillobifemoral graft but died at 30 days of overwhelming sepsis. The final patient, who had diffuse aneurysmal disease, underwent oversewing of the aortic stump but had no reconstruction. This individual died at 9 months of aortic stump disruption. These results lead the authors to recommend a more conservative approach to the operative corrective surgery of secondary fistulae wherever possible.

▶ As the authors point out, most American authors feel that graft excision accompanied by extra-anatomical vascularization is mandatory. Removal of the graft is a high risk procedure, particularly if infection is present. Martin-Paredero et al. (*Am. J. Surg.* 146:194, 1983) reviewed 18 patients who required removal of an aortofemoral graft. Sixteen grafts were removed because of infection and two for thrombosis. The overall mortality was 39%, and the incidence of amputation was 28%. Champion et al. (*Ann. Surg.* 195:314, 1982) reported an overall mortality of 77% for 22 patients considered. The encouraging results achieved in the present article may lead to a more conservative approach.—S.I. Schwartz, M.D.

Carotid Artery Occlusion: Natural History
Stephen C. Nicholls, Ted R. Kohler, Robert O. Bergelin, Jean F. Primozich, Ramona L. Lawrence, and D.E. Strandness, Jr. (Univ. of Washington, Seattle)
J. Vasc. Surg. 4:479–485, November 1986   18–7

A retrospective study was performed among patients with carotid occlusion to determine the incidence rate of subsequent stroke or death.

The study covered a 5-year period during which 212 patients, 170 men, aged 42 to 90 years, and 42 women, aged 41 to 88 years, were diagnosed with internal carotid artery (ICA) occlusion by means of duplex scanning. Arteriograms of 89 patients (40%) available for comparison showed a 94% agreement with duplex scanning results. The average follow-up period was 24.9 months.

There were 40 deaths, for a cumulative 5-year survival rate of 62%, including 7 from stroke (17%) and 22 of cardiac origin (55%). The cumulative 5-year stroke-free survival rate was 75%. Of 31 strokes that occurred, 18 (64%) were ipsilateral. The overall cumulative survival rate for patients who had no transient ischemic attacks (TIAs) was 82%, and for those with ipsilateral TIAs, it was 92%. There was no statistically significant difference between male and female patients for either death or stroke, nor was there any correlation between age and stroke during follow-up. Diabetes and hypertension both increased the risk of stroke, however. Aspirin consumption did not modify the risk of stroke. Although endarterectomy of the opposite carotid artery did not significantly affect the natural history of stroke, it lowered the incidence of stroke in the hemisphere ipsilateral to the operated artery.

Of 111 patients treated for stroke, 22 (20%) suffered another stroke, and 21 patients (19%) died. Of 42 patients treated for TIA, only 2 (5%) suffered a stroke, and none died. Of 23 patients with TIAs during follow-up, 3 (13%) eventually had a stroke.

It appears that the occurrence of TIA is not helpful in predicting which patients are at increased risk for stroke following carotid occlusion.

▶ The authors' concluding statement that TIA is of limited value in predicting stroke and a higher mortality rate related to stroke in this group of patients is an important consideration. Prescribing therapy has broad implications. Hertzer et al. (*Ann. Surg.* 204:154, 1986) indicated that carotid endarterectomy appears to be most useful in preventing stroke in patients with unilateral carotid stenosis of more than 70% or in patients with bilateral stenosis more than 50%. In the other groups of patients there was no definite advantage related to endarterectomy as a method of preventing neurologic complications. There is an increasing number of reports that carotid endarterectomy may not be superior to nonoperative management for the prevention of stroke (Bardin et al.: *Arch. Surg.* 117:1401, 1982).—S.I. Schwartz, M.D.

The Role of External Carotid Endarterectomy in the Treatment of Ipsilateral Internal Carotid Occlusion: Collective Review
Jonathan P. Gertler and Richard P. Cambria (Yale Univ., and Massachusetts Gen. Hosp., Boston)
J. Vasc. Surg. 6:158–167, August 1987   18–8

Several studies indicate that external carotid artery (ECA) reconstruction improves cerebral perfusion in cases of ipsilateral internal carotid artery (ICA) occlusion. More than two thirds of such patients will have significant intracerebral collateral circulation via the ECA through the ophthalmic artery. Review was made of 195 EC endarterectomies and 23 ECA bypasses, accumulated from 23 series and case reports. Both subclavian-ECA and common carotid-ECA bypass graft procedures were included.

Eighty-three percent of patients had no neurologic events after surgery. Another 7% of patients improved but had rare residual transient ischemic attacks. External carotid artery reconstruction was more effective

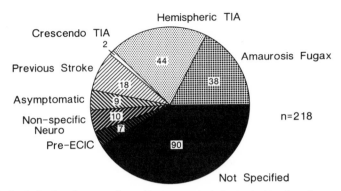

Fig 18–4.—Indications for external carotid artery revascularization in 23 collected series. *TIA,* transient ischemic attack; *ECIC,* extracranial- intracranial. (Courtesy of Gertler, J.P., and Cambria, R.P.: J. Vasc. Surg. 6:158–167, August 1987.)

in patients with specific retinal and hemispheric events (Fig 18–4) than in those with nonspecific neurologic symptoms. Perioperative mortality was 3%. No patient had late stroke ipsilateral to the ECA repair. Four of 19 patients having contralateral ICA occlusion had a poor neurologic outcome after the ECA procedure.

Symptomatic patients with ICA occlusion have a poor outlook, if managed conservatively; an attempt to increase flow through a stenotic ECA is warranted in these cases. External carotid reconstruction is a useful approach to ipsilateral internal carotid occlusion in symptomatic patients. The best results are obtained when specific hemispheric or retinal symptoms are present.

▶ McIntyre et al. (*Am. J. Surg.* 150:58, 1985) reported patients with transient neurologic deficits and an internal carotid artery occlusion on the side referrable to symptoms who had reconstruction of external artery. External carotid endarterectomy was carried out; all patients were relieved of their symptoms. Countee and Vijayanathan (*Stroke* 10:450, 1979) reported that external carotid endarterectomy was of no value if substantial intracranial flow could not be demonstrated on a preoperative angiogram. Friedman et al. (*J. Vasc. Surg.* 5:715, 1987) demonstrated that external carotid artery revascularization may be effective therapy for patients with bilateral internal carotid artery occlusion.—S.I. Schwartz, M.D.

Symptomatic Internal Carotid Thrombosis After Carotid Endarterectomy
Thomas A. Painter, Norman R. Hertzer, Patrick J. O'Hara, Leonard P. Krajewski, and Edwin G. Beven (The Cleveland Clinic Found.)
J. Vasc. Surg. 5:445–451, March 1987   18–9

The major cause of delayed neurologic deficits, occuring after carotid endarterectomy, is cortical ischemia caused by cerebral embolization or internal carotid artery (ICA) occlusion. In the period from 1977 to 1984,

298 / Surgery

RESULTS OF EARLY REOPERATION FOR SYMPTOMATIC POSTOPERATIVE THROMBOSIS AFTER CAROTID ENDARTERECTOMY IN COLLECTED SERIES

Series	Year	No.	Neurologic deficit					
			Improved		Unchanged		Deaths	
			No.	%	No.	%	No.	%
Najafi et al.	1971	7	3	42	2	29	2	29
Kwaan et al.	1979	3	3	100	0	—	0	—
Lindberg	1980	4	1	25	2	50	1	25
Treiman et al.	1981	7	3	42	2	29	2	29
Novick et al.	1985	4	4	100	0	—	0	—
Meyer et al.	1986	5	3	60	1	20	1	20
Present series	1986	11	8	73	2	18	1	9
Total		41	25	61	9	22	7	17

(Courtesy of Painter, T.A., et al.: J. Vasc. Surg. 5:445—451, March 1987.)

11 of 2,651 Cleveland Clinic patients who underwent carotid endarterectomy required emergency reoperation because of thrombosis of the ICA. The outcomes of these 11 patients are discussed in this paper and compared to those reported in the literature.

Neurologic deficits usually occurred after lucid intervals following recovery from general anesthesia. Two patients underwent thrombectomy, eight patients underwent thrombectomy and vein patch angioplasty, and one patient underwent thrombectomy of the external carotid artery with ligation of the ICA. Six patients had nearly complete recovery, and two more had substantial recovery from the neurologic symptoms. One patient had a fatal hemorrhagic cerebral infarction. Prompt surgical treatment of thrombosis was associated with clinical improvement in 61% of patients gleaned from a literature search (table).

Surgical treatment for thrombosis occurring after endarterectomy allows for improvement of neurologic symptoms, without an increase in mortality. Therefore, this approach is recommended for this serious complication of carotid endarterectomy.

▶ The results of thrombectomy in the postendarterectomy patient probably depend upon the extent of ischemia and the promptness of the restoration of circulation. Operative intervention has been considered contraindicated in patients with progressing and acute completed strokes because of delayed intracranial hemorrhage in some patients with successful revascularization (Gonzalez and Lewis: *Surg. Gynecol. Obstet.* 122:773, 1966; Bland et al.: *Ann. Surg.* 171:459, 1970). Beebe and Rob (*Complications of Vascular Surgery.* Philadelphia, JB Lippincott Co, 1973, p. 162) state that unless a stroke is diagnosed in the recovery room, it is rarely possible for an operation to improve the situation.—S.I. Schwartz, M.D.

Recurrent Carotid Stenosis: Incidence and Management
Sara J. Shumway, William H. Edwards, Judith M. Jenkins, Joseph L. Mulherin, Jr., and William H. Edwards, Jr. (Vanderbilt Univ. and St. Thomas Hosp., Nashville, Tenn.)
Ann. Surg. 53:61–65, February 1987   18–10

A retrospective study was done of 54 patients who underwent at least one second carotid endarterectomy or reconstructive procedure. Five of them required a third procedure. Dacron patch angioplasty, either preclotted sauvage or knitted, was done for most of the patients in this study at their second operation. For a third procedure most underwent carotid bifurcation resection and vein graft replacement.

In recurrent carotid stenosis, risk factors involved are the same as those for patients who have carotid occlusive disease for the first time. Hypertension and smoking were the two most common risk factors. Any recurrence of the original carotid endarterectomy within 4 years was defined as early recurrence, and after 8 years was defined as late recurrence. Myointimal hyperplasia was seen primarily in early recurrence, while atherosclerosis was dominant after 4 years. No difference in Dacron patch versus vein patch angioplasty was found. The use of antiplatelet drugs minimized thrombosis.

In six patients who underwent a total of 66 procedures, complications occurred for an overall incidence of 9%. After resection of the carotid bifurcation and vein graft replacement were performed as a second procedure in one patient with bilateral disease, graft thrombosis occurred. Follow-up ranged from 1 to 84 months. Nine patients (16.7%) died between 1 and 33 months after their operations; five (9.2%) were lost to follow-up, and 36 (66.7%) are asymptomatic.

▶ Rapp et al. (*Surgery* 101:277, 1987) presented data to suggest that hypercholesterolemia has a strong association with early restenosis after carotid endarterectomy, but not with late recurrent disease, and that hypertension, even when treated, may be associated with both early and late recurrence stenosis. Stewart and associates (*Arch. Surg.* 122:364, 1987) presented data to suggest that vein-patch angioplasty would have a positive effect. Although the venous patching in dogs did not influence early patency, after endarterectomy vein-patch angioplasty increased the vessel diameter and prevented the development of circumferential intimal thickening.—S.I. Schwartz, M.D.

A Comparison of In Situ and Reversed Saphenous Vein Grafts for Infrainguinal Reconstruction

Martin A. Fogle, Anthony D. Whittemore, Nathan P. Couch, and John A. Mannick (Brigham and Women's Hosp., Boston)
J. Vasc. Surg. 5:46–52, January 1987   18–11

Many series have suggested the superiority of in situ to reversed saphenous vein for infrainguinal arterial reconstruction, recently disputed in one report. A review of 675 infrainguinal vein grafts done during 1976–1986 was undertaken. Over the 10-year period, there was no substantial modification in the technique used for 535 reversed vein grafts, and the 140 in situ vein grafts during the last 3 years were carried out with the leather valvulotome used to incise the venous valves. Of the 140 in situ bypasses, 15% were anastomosed to vessels at the ankle or foot level, but none of the reversed bypasses were carried that far distally.

When analyzed for 3 years, bypasses to the popliteal level demonstrated no significant advantages on the basis of the surgical technique employed (P = .059). The patency rate for reversed vein bypasses declined from 81% at 1 year to 73% at 3 years and 63% at 5 years, while for in situ popliteal bypasses the cumulative patency rate of 84.7% at 1 year remained stable for 3 years. When compared with the patency rate of 61.7% for reversed vein graft (p = .002) at 3 years, however, in situ bypasses to the infrapopliteal vessels retained a significantly higher pa-

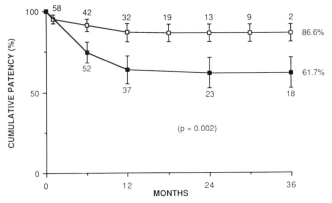

Fig 18–5.—Life-table comparison of cumulative patencies of femoroinfrapopliteal bypasses: in situ versus reversed vein techniques. *Open squares* = in situ vein group (n=65); *closed squares* = reversed vein group (n=86). (Courtesy of Fogle, M.A., et al.: J. Vasc. Surg. 5:46–52, January 1987.)

tency rate, 86.6% (Fig 18–5). During the first 6-month interval this difference became apparent, and it persisted throughout the next 3 years.

In the in situ vein group, seven patients (5%) complained of recurrent symptoms or had diminished blood pressure in routine follow-up. Patent reconstruction with localized lesions, including one arterial fistula, and six stenotic segments were demonstrated by subsequent arteriography. From 1 day to 13 months after operation, stenoses became manifest and were repaired locally with vein patch angioplasty or valve excision, and in one case, by lysis of an adventitial band. For the duration of follow-up, all seven of the grafts have remained patent. Of the 535 reversed vein bypasses, 32 (6%) had stenoses without graft thrombosis and underwent similar repair with vein patch or percutaneous transluminal angioplasty. Among the in situ grafts, 17 occlusions occurred (12%).

The contention that in situ use of the greater saphenous vein for infrapopliteal bypass provides significantly better cumulative patency rates is supported in this series. It is particularly applicable to distal infrapopliteal reconstruction and those patients with vein of limited quality or caliber. Reversed vein grafts no longer are used in the authors' institution when ipsilateral saphenous vein is available.

▶ Two recent articles have addressed this same issue. Bandyk et al. (*J. Vasc. Surg.* 5:256, 1987) reported on 192 in situ saphenous vein bypasses. The primary patency rate at 36 months was only 48% for femoral popliteal bypass and 58% for femorotibial bypasses. In contrast, the secondary patency rate, i.e., patency maintained by thrombectomy, thrombolysis, or revision, at 36 months was 89% and 80%, respectively. Problems unique to the in situ technique, i.e., incomplete valve incision, residual AV fistula, and graft torsion and entrapment accounted for over half the early and half the late revisions. The authors suggest the use of Doppler spectral analysis at operation and duplex scanning to locate unsuspected technical errors. Harris et al. (*Br. J. Surg.* 74:252, 1987) conducted a prospectively randomized trial to compare in situ and reversed saphenous vein grafts for femoropopliteal bypass. The results indicated that the reversed and in situ veins were equally effective in this region.—S.I. Schwartz, M.D.

The Reoperative Potential of Infrainguinal Bypass: Long-Term Limb and Patient Survival
Stephen T. Bartlett, Andrew J. Olinde, William R. Flinn, Walter J. McCarthy III, Victora A. Fahey, John J. Bergan, and James S.T. Yao (Northwestern Univ. and Northwestern Mem. Hosp., Chicago)
J. Vasc. Surg. 5:170–179, January 1987   18–12

A return of the severe lower limb ischemia that necessitated the primary procedure is usually experienced in patients with femorodistal graft failure. With recurrence of limb jeopardy, further surgical intervention must be considered. The fate of 202 patients during a 10-year period with failed distal bypass grafts undergoing reoperation after the failure is reviewed.

The patients had 389 infrainguinal reoperative procedures, an average of 1.9 reoperations per patient. In 101 patients a secondary bypass was performed: 51 had a tertiary procedure; 30, a fourth bypass; and in 20 patients, more than four operations were required. In 377 (97%) of 389 cases, reoperation was performed to treat severe ischemia, rest pain, ulceration, or gangrene. In 21 cases (7.4%) repetitive bypasses were performed with autogenous vein; for 16 patients (5.6%) composite grafts were made; and polytetrafluoroethylene was used in 247 cases (87%). The remaining 105 reoperations included 77 thrombectomy, 20 thrombectomy plus distal angioplasty, and 8 profundaplasty. In 14% the distal anastomosis was to the popliteal artery, and in 59%, to the tibial or peroneal artery.

There were four operative deaths (within fewer than 30 days) in the 389 reoperative procedures (1.0%) and 35 late deaths. The cumulative life-table 5-year survival rate for all patients was 80%. The operative morbidity rate was 12.3%, including wound infection in 3.1% and hematoma in 6.4%. Graft patency was 80% at 1 year and 37% at 5 years in this study (Fig 18–6). Limb salvage rates were 87% at 1 year and 59% at 5 years.

This current series seems to contradict the belief that late mortality rates are always high among these patients, with its most striking observation being that 80% of the patients lived for 5 years or more from the time of initial entry into the study. These data seem to make clear the patients' ischemic symptoms, and threatened limbs cannot be ignored on the basis of a compromised longevity. Better control of hypertension and more aggressive evaluation and treatment of associated carotid and coronary disease in these patients may be reflected in the low late mortality rate in this series. They were treated with an aggressive policy of reoperation, resulting in acceptable long-term graft patency and limb salvage rates, low operative mortality rates, and no significant compromise of subsequent amputation level.

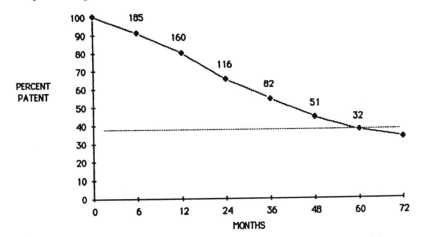

Fig 18–6.—Life-table curve of cumulative graft patency shows that at 5 years 37% of the patients have patent grafts. Number at risk for each interval is shown above the curve. (Courtesy of Bartlett, S.T., et al.: J. Vasc. Surg. 5:170–179, January 1987.)

► It is important to emphasize that these patients require continuous attention. Veith et al. (*J. Vasc. Surg.* 3:104, 1986) demonstrated that it is possible to detect lesions that will cause graft failure before thrombosis occurs. This is predominantly progression of atherosclerosis by detecting the failing state. Reintervention by angioplasty or simple operation may be effective. The same group (Ascer et al.: *J. Vasc. Surg.* 5:298, 1987) reported their reoperation for polytetrafluoroethylene (PTFE) bypass failure. Femoral above-knee prostheses reported on had 3-year patency rates from the time of first operation of 52%, whereas it was only 13% for below-knee prostheses. This slow rate may relate to the fact that PTFE was used liberally in the below-knee and infrapopliteal positions.—S.I. Schwartz, M.D.

Nonoperative Management of Selected Popliteal Aneurysms

Jon Schellack, Robert B. Smith III, and Garland D. Perdue (Emory Univ. and VA Med. Ctr., Decatur, Ga.)
Arch. Surg 122:372–375, March 1987   18–13

Popliteal arterial aneurysms (PAAs) are well known for their propensity to develop limb-threatening complications; consequently, most surgeons advocate prophylactic repair of even small asymptomatic ones as soon as they are discovered. The management of 95 PAAs was reviewed for a period from 1965 to 1985. In 90% of the operations surgical therapy was initially successful, and in 6% major limb amputation was required.

In 62 PAAs reconstructive surgery was performed; exclusion of the aneurysm with bypass grafting was the most common technique employed. In 2 limbs restoration of arterial continuity was accomplished by primary end-to-end anastomosis, and in 60 it was accomplished with bypass grafting. In 32 extremities autogenous saphenous vein (ASV) grafts were used, and nonautogenous grafts were used in 28. If ASV was used, and if reconstruction was performed before development of complications, durability of surgical reconstruction was improved.

In six symptomatic PAAs, conservative management was initially used; three had evidence of distal embolization, but because of poor tibial runoff, reconstruction was not performed. In one of these three aneurysms, total thrombosis developed later but did not require surgical repair. The

COMPARISON OF PATENCY RATES

Category	No.	Five-Year Cumulative Patency Rate, %	
		Primary	Secondary
Autogenous saphenous vein grafts	32	89	92
Nonautogenous grafts	28	29	55
Complicated aneurysms	42	53	66
Noncomplicated aneurysms	20	77	93
All reconstructions	62	61	75

(Courtesy of Schellack, J., et al.: Arch. Surg. 122:372–375, March 1987.)

other 2 ruptured; surgical reconstruction was attempted, but early graft failures made major amputations eventually necessary. There was no follow-up available for a fourth patient, and the last two with thrombosed PAAs continued to describe stable claudication.

Of 46 asymptomatic PAAs, 26 were initially managed without operation, and 20 were subjected to elective surgical repair. Only 2 cases of 26 (8%) had significant complications as a result of the conservative management. Of the remaining 24, none have described symptoms that could be attributed to their PAAs. The small size of the aneurysm (13 cases); surgical risk factors believed to be prohibitive (7 cases); and patients refusing recommended surgical therapy (4 cases) were the most common reasons for choosing conservative management. The 20 asymptomatic PAAs had a 5-year secondary cumulative patency rate of 93% (table).

Based on the demonstrated effectiveness of surgical therapy for asymptomatic PAAs, surgical correction of all definitively diagnosed popliteal aneurysms is recommended unless specific contraindications exist. It appears that, when faced with a high risk patient with a small asymptomatic popliteal aneurysm, taking a conservative nonoperative approach is reasonably safe.

▶ Most surgeons feel that a popliteal aneurysm is a foreboding lesion, related to its being an etiologic factor in limb ischemia. Vermillion et al. (*Surgery* 90:1009, 1981) reviewed 147 cases and made a plea for aggressive therapy. Nonsurgical management of aneurysms was considered a dangerous practice, but the current report suggests that there is a group of high risk patients in whom a nonoperative approach is safe. Szilagyi et al. (*Arch. Surg.* 116:724, 1981) reviewed 87 popliteal aneurysms in 62 patients of which 50 were treated surgically. They recommended surgical treatment not only in all symptomatic but in all asymptomatic aneurysms larger than 2 cm. Like the present authors, they felt that an autogenous saphenous vein graft provided the best conduit.—S.I. Schwartz, M.D.

Sympathectomy for Causalgia: Patient Selection and Long-Term Results
Mary B. Mockus, Robert B. Rutherford, Camilo Rosales, and William H. Pearce (Univ. of Colorado, Denver)
Arch. Surg. 122:668–672, June 1987   18–14

Sympathectomy for the management of arterial occlusive disease has largely been replaced by arterial reconstruction. Nevertheless, causalgic pain or reflex sympathetic dystrophy is still a valid indication for the use of sympathectomy because of the immediate and dramatic relief the technique often provides. The long-term efficacy of sympathectomy for causalgia is not well documented; a 15-year experience with this procedure for causalgia is described.

All cases of sympathectomy done for causalgic pain from 1970 to 1985 at one institution were reviewed. Potential relief of pain was assessed preoperatively by one or more regional sympathetic blocks using local anesthetic agents. A retroperitoneal approach to lumbar sympathectomy through an oblique anterolateral abdominal incision was used. Three ganglia were removed. Dorsal sympathectomy was always done through a transaxillary incision. Thirty-four sympathectomies were done. Overt extremity trauma was found to be the precipitating event in 26%. In 48%, nerve compression necessitating surgical relief preceded the onset of pain; 37% had lumbar disk surgery. In the remaining 26%, miscellaneous vascular conditions contributed. Satisfactory immediate relief was achieved in 97%; 61% were initially completely relieved of pain. There were no deaths. Wound complications of hematoma and infection occurred in 10%, and there was one instance of Horner's syndrome. Postsympathectomy neuralgia occurred in almost 40% of the patients and lasted for slightly more than 1 month on average; it did not persist in any patient for more than 10 weeks. In extended follow-up, only one patient did not sustain satisfactory relief, and 84% continued to enjoy the same degree of pain relief as they had immediately after surgery. Surgical sympathectomy offers high frequency, high degree, and long duration of benefit for causalgic pain. Moreover, causalgic pain is one of the best indications for sympathectomy.

▶ The results reported in this series are extremely encouraging. A word of caution, however, is introduced by Dr. Poulos (discussion). He points out that sympathectomy for full-blown clinical causalgia is normally beneficial, but in a second group selected by pain and relief by sympathetic block, results were disappointing because most patients got temporary relief only. The results have been so bad in that group of patients with so-called mimocausalgia that they do not recommend the procedure. One third of male patients become impotent after low lumbar sympathectomy: this should be mentioned in the informed consent.—S.I. Schwartz, M.D.

Limb Sparing Operations for Sarcomas of the Extremities Involving Critical Arterial Circulation
David L. Steed, Andrew B. Peitzman, Marshall W. Webster, Jr., Sai S. Ramasastry, and Mark A. Goodman (Univ. of Pittsburgh)
Surg. Gynecol. Obstet. 164:493–498, June 1987   18–15

Therapeutic operations for sarcomas of the extremities involve either amputation or wide local excision, based on tumor grade, location, and the presence of neural or vascular involvement. Vascular displacement by the pseudocapsule implies an extracompartmental lesion. When a major vessel is involved, wide local resection with limb sparing surgery may be precluded. An experience with seven patients who underwent resection of a sarcoma of the extremity requiring excision of a vital artery and revascularization is discussed.

From 1980 through 1986, 350 patients with sarcomas of the extremity were seen at one institution. One third underwent amputation, and two thirds underwent local excision. Seven patients (2%) had resection of the

LIMB SPARING OPERATIONS

Patient No.	Age, yrs., Sex	Tumor and location	Vessel involved	Comment
1	21 M	Low grade chrondosarcoma in osteochondroma of tibia	Popliteal artery	Contralateral saphenous vein interposition graft; well and disease-free at six years
2	57 F	Recurrent myxoid liposarcoma of the thigh	Superficial femoral artery and vein	Previous tumor excised 20 years ago; contralateral saphenous vein interposition graft to both artery and vein; wound closed with omental pedical graft; died of myocardial infarction three months later
3	47 M	Moderately-well differentiated osteosarcoma of the pubis	External iliac artery and vein	6 mm. Polyetrafluoroethylene graft to external iliac artery; wound closed with contralateral rectus pedicle flap; died eight months later of metastatic disease
4	33 F	High grade osteosarcoma of distal femur	Superficial femoral and popliteal arteries	Amputation refused, 6 mm. polytetrafluoroethylene graft to superficial femoral artery; margins involved, amputation still refused; well at 16 months
5	48 M	Recurrent low grade liposarcoma of popliteal space	Popliteal artery	Previous tumor resected two years ago; contralateral saphenous vein interposition graft; well at eight months
6	21 M	Alveolar rhabdomyosarcoma of the thenaremminence	Radial artery	Cephalic vein interposition graft; well at one year
7	68 F	Undifferentiated sarcoma of thigh	Superficial femoral artery	Contralateral saphenous vein interposition graft; well at six months

(Courtesy of Steed, D.L., et al.: Surg. Gynecol. Obstet. 164:493–498, June 1987.)

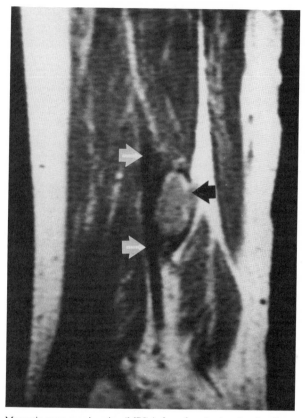

Fig 18–7.—Magnetic resonance imaging (MRI) in lateral projection showing the tumor of the thigh *(black arrow)* adjacent to the superficial femoral artery *(white arrows)*. Note the fine anatomical detail seen with MRI. (Courtesy of Steed, D.L. et al.: Surg. Gynecol. Obstet. 164:493–498, June 1987.)

tumor with limb-sparing operation with vascular reconstruction. The seven patients had osteosarcoma of the pubis, osteosarcoma of the distal femur, undifferentiated sarcoma of the thigh (Fig 18–7), liposarcoma of the thigh, liposarcoma of the popliteal space, chondrosarcoma of the proximal tibia, or rhabdomyosarcoma of the thumb (table). Surgery involved excision of the iliac artery in one case, the femoral artery in three, the popliteal artery in two, and the radial artery in one. Autogenous vein from the contralateral extremity was the arterial conduit, if available. Wide local resection, including revascularization, was done when the tumor was low-grade malignant, could be resected with the artery, and could be separated from the nerve or when the patient refused amputation for a high-grade malignant disease. Tumor margins were adequate in five patients. Coverage of the soft tissue and vascular grafts was achieved in two patients with a distant pedicle flap. Amputation was avoided; all patients remained ambulatory. Five patients remained disease-free with patent grafts at 6 months to 6 years of follow-up. The sixth patient died of late myocardial infarction; the seventh, who underwent palliative re-section, died of metastatic disease 8 months later.

Five of seven patients undergoing limb sparing operations for sarcomas of the extremities involving critical arterial circulation remained disease free up to 6 years after surgery. It is concluded that involvement of the major arterial circulation does not preclude adequate resection of sarco-mas of the extremity with limb salvage.

▶ In recent years the principles of management of soft tissue sarcomas have undergone major changes, and there is an increasing emphasis on limb sparing operations. Karakousis reported on nine consecutive patients with soft tissue sarcomas, only three of whom required amputation. The 5-year survival has in-creased to 63% from 45% reported in the previous decade (*Cancer* 57:484, 1986). Shiu (*Cancer* 57:1632, 1986) also stressed the feasibility of limb preser-vation and tumor control in treatment of popliteal and antecubital soft tissue sarcomas combining surgical excision and radiation. Nambisan and Karakousis recently reported on ten patients with soft tissue sarcoma of the lower extrem-ity and involvement of the blood vessels that were resected along with the sur-rounding tumor. Resection involved the iliac vessels in three patients, the fem-oral vessels in six, and the posterior tibial vessels in one. Ten arterial and six venous grafts were used. Of the eight patients who underwent curative resec-tion and arterial reconstruction, none has relapsed locally for a mean of 24 months (*Surgery* 101:668, 1987).—S.I. Schwartz, M.D.

19 The Veins and the Lymphatics

The Early Fate of Venous Repair After Civilian Vascular Trauma: A Clinical, Hemodynamic, and Venographic Assessment
Joseph Meyer, James Walsh, James Schuler, John Barrett, Joseph Durham, Jens Eldrup-Jorgensen, Thomas Schwarcz, and D. Preston Flanigan (Cook County Hosp. and Univ. of Illinois, Chicago)
Ann. Surg. 206:458–464, October 1987   19–1

It is proposed that major venous injuries in the extremities be repaired to improve limb salvage and prevent sequelae of venous interruption. Nevertheless, the contribution of vein repair to the surgical outcome is uncertain. Early venous patency was related to surgical outcome in a series of 36 patients with major venous injuries in the upper or lower extremity who underwent venous reconstruction. Gunshot wounds were most frequent. The lower extremity was involved in 78% of cases. All patients but two had major arterial injuries.

Systemic heparin was routinely used. Distal venous thrombus was extracted by catheter thrombectomy. Vein repairs were done with interrupted or running monofilament sutures. Fasciotomy was necessary in 11 cases. There were no perioperative deaths, and all limbs were salvaged. Fourteen venous repairs had thrombosed a week postoperatively. The rate of thrombosis was 21% for local venous repairs and 59% for interposition vein grafting. Two patients with thrombosis had persistent but

ACCURACY OF CLINICAL AND NONINVASIVE EVALUATION
IN DETERMINING PATENCY OF VEIN REPAIR

	N
Clinical evaluation*	
True (+)	6
True (−)	18
False (+)	4
False (−)	8
Noninvasive testing†	
True (+)	6
True (−)	13
False (+)	9
False (−)	8

*Accuracy = 0.666, positive predictive value = 0.60, negative predictive value = 0.69.
†Accuracy = 0.527, positive predictive value = 0.4, negative predictive value = 0.62.
(Courtesy of Meyer, J., et al.: Ann. Surg. 206:458–464, October 1987.)

mild lower limb edema at 3 months. Clinical evaluation was 67% accurate in assessing patency compared with contrast venography. Noninvasive venous evaluation was only 53% accurate (table).

Maintenance of venous outflow from the extremity via the main conduit is not necessary for limb salvage. Local repair, as by lateral venorrhaphy or limited vein patching, has an acceptable early patency rate. Vein grafting, however, may not be warranted since it does not appear to enhance limb salvage.

▶ The results of this study, indicating that limb salvage was not adversely influenced by venous thrombosis, disagrees with the findings of Rich, who noted that lower extremity venous ligation led to amputations in some patients and emphasized that patients in whom veins were ligated developed sequelae of postphlebitic syndrome (*Surgery* 91:492, 1982). Most authors feel that simple, primary venous repair is almost always indicated if it is feasible. Complicated venous repair is indicated only when it does not compromise the overall management. In general, venous thrombosis has a minimal effect on the patency of the associated arterial repair. As Bergan points out in the discussion, pulmonary embolus after failed venous repair does not represent a threat. Dr. Webb substantiated the authors' findings related to the absence of limb loss in patients who underwent ligation of the vein.—S.I. Schwartz, M.D.

Results of Surgical Treatment for Iliofemoral Venous Thrombosis
J. Swedenborg, R. Hägglöf, H. Jacobsson, J. Johansson, H. Johnsson, S. Larsson, E. Nilsson and S. Zetterquist (Karolinska Hosp., Stockholm, and Danderyd Hosp., Sweden)
Br. J. Surg. 73:871–874, November 1986   19–2

The goal of treatment for venous thrombosis is to prevent primary embolism and the development of the postthrombotic syndrome. Anticoagulation, thrombolysis, and surgery can all be used, but the optimal treatment has not been determined. A group of 19 patients was treated for iliofemoral venous thrombosis by thrombectomy and a temporary arteriovenous fistula. Patency was assessed with isotope phlebography, and venous function was studied with plethysmographic and foot volumetric methods at follow-up of 13–75 months.

The operation was successful in 17 of the 19 patients. The remaining 2 patients had chronic iliac vein occlusions. Three months later, at closure of the arteriovenous fistula, the iliac vein was patent in 14 patients. At follow-up, eight patients had a completely patent vein, eight had partial patency, and three had an occluded iliac vein. Impaired venous emptying was detected in the patients with occluded veins.

Good long-term results can be achieved by venous thrombectomy with a temporary arteriovenous fistula. Impaired emptying is rare after successful thrombectomy.

▶ The Swedes have been the prime proponent of this approach to iliofemoral venous thrombosis. This represents the first long-term follow-up of patients treated with thrombectomy and temporary arterial venous fistula, and the results are excellent. Roder et al. (*Acta Chir Scand.* 150:31, 1984) reported on the effects of venous thrombectomy alone for iliofemoral thrombosis. Controlled phlebography on the fifth postoperative day showed a patent iliofemoral segment in 26 of the 46 patients undergoing thrombectomy. Of 30 patients alive after 10 years, 40% were asymptomatic, and 33% had signs of severe venous insufficiency. Correlation of the late clinical results with the postoperative phlebographic findings showed that patients with unsuccessful recannulization generally had venous insufficiency; those with good results had patent veins at phlebography. There is growing evidence that the addition of the arteriovenous fistula provides significant improvement in the results.—S.I. Schwartz, M.D.

Modifications of Techniques and Early Results of Pulmonary Thromboendarterectomy for Chronic Pulmonary Embolism
Pat O. Daily, Walter P. Dembitsky, Kirk L. Peterson, and Kenneth M. Moser (Univ. of California, San Diego)
J. Thorac. Cardiovasc. Surg. 93:221–233, February 1987   19–3

Pulmonary embolism rarely leads to chronic pulmonary hypertension. It is not known whether the chronic disease results from failure of resolution of a massive embolus, repeated embolic episodes, or both. Nevertheless, patients in whom chronic pulmonary hypertension does develop have a poor prognosis. In 1980, the authors described bilateral pulmonary thromboendarterectomy with median sternotomy, cardiopulmonary bypass, deep hypothermia, and circulatory arrest for the relief of pulmonary hypertension caused by chronic pulmonary embolism. Their subsequent experience with the technique in 41 patients is described.

Three groups of patients were characterized by differences of intraoperative management. In group A (n = 16), myocardial protection included a single-dose crystalloid cardioplegia, followed by pericardial irrigation with cold saline; extrapericardial dissection of the pulmonary arteries was carried out. In group B (n = 7), treatment was the same, except for the substitution of saline slush contained in a laparotomy pad for iced saline. In group C (n = 18), myocardial protection involved single-dose blood cardioplegia, followed by the application of a specially designed cooling jacket to the right and left ventricles. Another change was that of intrapericardial dissection of the pulmonary arteries with extension of the dissection into the hilar tissues without entrance to the pleural spaces. The hospital mortalities of groups A, B, and C were 18.7%, 14.3%, and 5.5%, respectively. Other differences between groups included phrenic nerve paresis, which occurred in five of seven patients in group B (71%) but not in groups A or C. Group B patients required ventilatory support for 32.2 days, compared with 8.4 days for group A and 6.2 days for group C. Time in the intensive care unit was 36 days for group B patients, versus 13 days for group A patients and 10.3 days for group C patients. Pulmonary vascular resistance dropped 59% intraoperatively in 13 patients in group C.

Simultaneous bilateral pulmonary thromboendarterectomy with median sternotomy, cardiopulmonary bypass, deep hypothermia with circulatory arrest, and the modified methods of myocardial preservation and dissection represent current optimal surgical management of this problem.

▶ This remarkable report describes experiences with 41 patients with chronic pulmonary embolism treated by thromboendarterectomy. I imagine this is the largest such series in the world.

The operative technique is a complex one requiring periods of circulatory arrest to prevent massive bleeding from bronchial arteries. Among 40 patients the arrest periods varied from 7 to 41 minutes, with as many as seven separate periods of arrest in one person. Individual periods of arrest were limited to 20 minutes. It is remarkable that neurologic injury did not occur.

The paper should be studied in detail because the accomplishments in some patients are most impressive.—F.C. Spencer, M.D.

20 The Esophagus

Surgical Treatment of the Gastroesophageal Reflux Syndrome in Infants and Children

Eric W. Fonkalsrud, William Berquist, Jorge Vargas, Marvin E. Ament, and Robert P. Foglia (Univ. of California, Los Angeles)

Am. J. Surg. 154:11–18, July 1987

20–1

Gastroesophageal reflux is associated with abnormally low pressure in the lower esophageal sphincters in infants and children. Delayed gastric emptying is a frequent finding in symptomatic patients. Esophageal motility is also frequently impaired. Review was made of 352 infants and children with symptomatic gastroesophageal reflux, including 340 who underwent gastroesophageal fundoplication in 1969–1987. Some patients with predominant gastric dysmotility had pyloroplasty alone. Reflux was demonstrated by thin barium esophagography, and gastric emptying was demonstrated by a technetium-99m (^{99m}Tc)-sulfur colloid study. All patients younger than 3 years of age and many older patients underwent tube gastrostomy.

There were three perioperative deaths. Eight posterior paraesophageal hernias developed, necessitating reoperation. Vomiting was consistently relieved by surgery. Recurrent pulmonary problems nearly always were less marked or absent postoperatively. No patient required reoperation for recurrent reflux in the absence of paraesophageal hernia.

Gastroesophageal fundoplication plus pyloroplasty is indicated when gastric emptying is delayed, the lower esophageal sphincter (LES) pressure is reduced, and esophageal pH monitoring gives abnormal results. If the esophageal pH is mildly abnormal, the LES pressure is high-normal, and gastric emptying is markedly delayed, pyloroplasty alone is indicated. Both approaches are effective in properly selected infants and children having symptomatic gastroesophageal reflux.

▶ The selected application of pyloroplasty based on preoperative assessment is of interest. Delayed gastric emptying occurs more commonly in the neurologically impaired group. St. Cyr et al. (*J. Thorac. Cardiovasc. Surg.* 92:661, 1986) reported improvement in the great majority of patients operated on for recurrent aspiration, and improved function in all patients with bronchopleural dysplasia. Randolph (*Ann. Surg.* 198:579, 1983) reported excellent results in 61 of 72 infants with gastroesophageal reflux undergoing Nissen fundoplication. —S.I. Schwartz, M.D.

Complications and Reoperation After Nissen Fundoplication in Childhood

Gregory K. Dedinsky, Dennis W. Vane, C. Thomas Black, Mary K. Turner, Karen W. West, and Jay L. Grosfeld (Indiana Univ. and James Whitcomb Riley Hosp. for Children, Indianapolis)
Am. J. Surg. 153:177–183, February 1987   20–2

In pediatric patients with gastroesophageal reflux, a considerable percentage of them also have severe neurologic impairment. Complications and the need for reoperation after a Nissen fundoplication procedure in 429 infants and children treated at a single pediatric facility were evaluated. In 297 children (69%), some degree of neurologic impairment was present. Ages ranged from 1 month to 18 years (mean, 65 months).

In 69 patients (16%) postoperative complications occurred. The most common was herniation or breakdown of the fundic wrap, which occurred in 29 patients (6.7%). In 14 children, there were 18 instances of postoperative intestinal obstruction (4.2%). In 28 patients, esophageal dilations were required postoperatively (6.5%). Other postoperative complications included stricture in ten, intra-abdominal abscess and enterocutaneous fistula in three each, and wound infection, wound dehiscence, and inadvertent splenectomy in two each. Before 30 days after operation, there were four deaths (0.9%), caused by underlying pulmonary disease in two and by sepsis or a severe, uncorrectable, congenital metabolic disorder in one each; all had severe neurologic impairment.

Indications for a second antireflux procedure included recurrence of gastroesophageal reflux symptoms, vomiting, and aspiration pneumonia, among others. Herniation or breakdown of the wrap occurred in 28 of the children, stricture occurred in six, and four had a radiologically intact wrap but remained symptomatic.

Over a follow-up period ranging from 6 months to 10 years, fundoplication successfully controlled symptoms of gastroesophageal reflux in 395 children (92%). A second antireflux operation was required because of recurrent symptoms in 38 patients (8.8%). There was severe neurologic impairment in 29 patients: five of these had associated congenital malformations, and three had significant pulmonary problems.

▶ This is a somewhat unusual group because 69% had some degree of neurologic impairment. Those patients did not have demonstrable gastroesophageal reflux. The majority of the literature is related to Nissen fundoplication for gastroesophageal reflux in infants. Recently, Randolph (*Ann. Surg.* 198:579, 1983) reviewed 72 patients who underwent the procedure. Ninety-four percent had good results. In five of these patients reoperation was required because of recurrence before a long-term good result was effected. Rather than approximating the hiatus, most people suture the fundus to the diaphragm.—S.I. Schwartz, M.D.

Gastric Transposition for Esophageal Replacement in Children

Lewis Spitz, Edward Kiely, Tony Sparnon (Hosp. for Sick Children, London)
Ann. Surg. 206:69–73, July 1987   20–3

Technical problems and the possibility of major postoperative complications make the decision to perform esophageal reconstructive surgery on children difficult. Various methods of esophageal substitution have been attempted. The use of stomach to restore continuity to the alimentary tract has been successful in adults. Esophageal replacement by total gastric transposition through either the posterior mediastinum or posterior thorax was done on 34 infants in a 5.5-year period at one institution.

Thirty-two infants had esophageal atresia; 18 had associated tracheoesophageal fistulas as well. Nine of the 27 infants with long gap esophageal atresia had undergone previous attempts at delayed anastomosis. In 16 infants, the operative procedure consisted of a transhiatal gastric transposition through the posterior mediastinum without a thoracotomy (Fig 20–1). In 18 children, thoracoabdominal gastric transposition through the posterior thorax was done. A thoracotomy was also considered necessary in children with extensive esophageal strictures and some of the failed primary anastomoses where extensive scarring from the leak necessitated careful dissection to remove the esophagus. All but one infant underwent gastric outlet drainage procedures; 20 had pyloroplasties and 13 had pyloromyotomies. In each child, a 12-gauge nasogastric tube was inserted to prevent postoperative gastric distention. A fine-bore jejunal feeding tube was placed to provide enteral nutrition before oral feeding was established. Three children (9%) died, two in the early postoperative period, and the third 1 year after surgery from persistent chronic respiratory problems. Fourteen children had a totally uncomplicated course and have not required further hospitalization. Thirteen had early

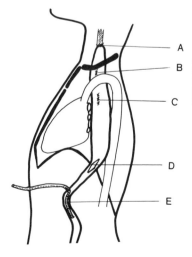

Fig 20–1.—Posterior mediastinal gastric transposition. *A,* anastomosis of cervical esophagus to fundus of stomach. *B,* oversewn junction of lower esophageal stump with stomach. *C,* oversewn gastrostomy site. *D,* pyloroplasty. *E,* jejunal feeding tube. (Courtesy of Spitz, L., et al.: Ann. Surg. 206:69–73, July 1987.)

COMPARISON OF TWO METHODS OF ESOPHAGEAL REPLACEMENT

	Colon Interposition 1952–1981	Gastric Transposition 1981–1986
Number	112	34
Mortality	13%	9%
Graft failure	14%	0%
Cervical anastomotic		
Leakage	48%	6%
Stricture	30%	12%
Outcome of survivors		
Excellent	56%	81%
Good	35%	13%
Fair	9%	6%

(Courtesy of Spitz, L., et al.: Ann. Surg. 206:69–73, July 1987.)

postoperative complications: six had delayed gastric emptying, four had anastomotic strictures requiring dilatation, and two had radiologic anastomotic leaks. Late complications included two adhesion intestinal obstructions, a perforation related to a jejunal feeding tube, and subsequent malabsorption. Twenty-five children are entirely asymptomatic and manage a normal diet. Of the 23 children followed up for at least 1 year after surgery, six remain below the third percentile for height and weight.

The results of this procedure compare favorably with extensive previous experience in colon interposition (table). Although the follow-up period in this study was short, 70% of the children treated with the gastric transposition procedure who are at least 1 year postsurgery are thriving, with heights and weights within normal range.

▶ Esophageal replacement generally has been accomplished with colon and has achieved excellent results. Stone et al. (*Ann. Surg.* 203:346, 1986) reported that 86% of 36 children who were subjected to colon interposition as a method of esophageal replacement remained asymptomatic. The results achieved in the present series are most attractive, particularly the reduction in cervical anastomotic leak and stricture formation.—S.I. Schwartz, M.D.

Colon Interposition for Benign Esophageal Disease
Myriam J. Curet-Scott, Mark K. Ferguson, Alex G. Little, and David B. Skinner (Univ. of Chicago)
Surg. 102:568–574, October 1987   20–4

This report describes the recent experience of the University of Chicago Medical Center with esophageal resection followed by colon interposition as a treatment for benign disease in 53 patients. The purpose of this review was to assess operative morbidity and long-term function.

In this series of patients, 32 had gastroesophageal reflux, eight had advanced motility disorders, six had esophageal perforation, and seven had strictures not related to reflux. The operative death rate was 3.8%. Major complications, which included graft infarcts, graft perforations, and anastomotic leaks, occurred in 26.4% of patients. During follow-up averaging 5 years, eight patients required dilations and 15 underwent reoperation. A gastric emptying procedure was required in 25% of the cases that did not have pyloroplasty initially. Despite symptoms of postprandial fullness in 78% and dysphagia in 42%, 75% of patients felt the results were good to excellent. The surgeons rated 72% of the results as good to excellent.

Colon interposition for benign esophageal disease has a 30% major complication rate and a 37% reoperation rate. However, it can be performed with a low mortality rate and has a high patient satisfaction rate. Therefore, it is recommended for the reconstruction of benign esophageal disease.

▶ The colon also provides an excellent conduit in children requiring esophageal replacement. Stone et al. (*Ann. Surg.* 203:346, 1986) reported that 31 of 36 patients survived and were asymptomatic. Only four patients had mild dysphagia. All patients had normal growth curves. Satisfactory long-term results were also reported by Hendren and Hendren (*J. Pediatr. Surg.* 20:829, 1985) who used the colon to bridge an esophageal defect. The authors stress that the operations are performed only in patients who are very symptomatic, and indicate they perform gastric emptying procedures in all patients having esophagectomies.—S.I. Schwartz, M.D.

Jejunal Interposition for Benign Esophageal Disease: Technical Considerations and Long-Term Results
C. Wright and A. Cuschieri (Univ. of Dundee, Scotland)
Ann. Surg. 205:54–60, January 1987   20–5

Jejunal interposition has had criticism directed at it because of the limited length that can be achieved, its inadequate blood supply, its technical difficulty, overall safety of the operation in terms of anastomotic leakage, necrosis, and postoperative mortality rates. However, the authors believe excellent long-term results can be obtained from this procedure. Benign intractable or complicated esophageal disease in 30 patients was treated with esophageal resection and isoperistaltic jejunal interposition in this study.

Distal anastomosis is performed with the anterior wall of the stomach a few centimeters distal to the closed cardiac end, previous mobilization of which greatly facilitates this step. At the distal end of the interposed loop any excess length is trimmed, and the adjacent stomach wall is incised to fashion an appropriate size stoma. Anastomosis is done in a single-layer technique with a running nonabsorbable 3 = 0 suture for the posterior wall and interrupted sutures anteriorly. The completed anastomosis is buried in the stomach wall by 2–3 seromuscular gastric sutures, which results in a fundal wrap around the anastomosis to prevent reflux of gastric contents into the interposed jejunal segment.

There were three anastomotic leaks, all occurred at the proximal anastomosis. One of the patients died 35 days after operation for persistent sepsis, the only death in this study. The remaining two patients had minor radiologic leaks that were managed conservatively. Pyloroplasty or pyloromyotomy was not performed during the interposition because of frequent sequelae of dumping and bile vomiting. Of the 30 patients, 19 still survive, eight dying of unrelated disease, and all but one patient was free of dysphagia until death. Long-term follow-up results in all but one patient who had scleroderma were favorable.

No evidence of inflammation in the interposed segment in any patients was shown by late endoscopy 12 months beyond the operation. Retention of normal villous pattern showed in the endoscopic biopsies. Histologic changes seen in late biopsies included hyperplasia of the Paneth cells together with an infiltrate of eosinophils and plasma cells, but no evidence of metaplasia. Radionuclide transit studies showed total transit time after jejunal interposition averaged 3.6 ± 0.4 minutes compared to a control group that averaged 10.4 ± 2.6 seconds.

Using the jejunum as an esophageal substitute has the advantages of a size similar to the esophagus, relative freedom from intrinsic disease, and ease of preoperative preparation. Its contents are usually sterile, and after interposition the jejunum retains peristaltic activity. The transit studies showed that contractions are predominantly segmental and for this reason overall transit time is significantly slower than normal.

▶ This article is selected because it provides description of the technical considerations. The jejunum represents an excellent conduit in replacement of the esophagus. Free grafts of jejunum have been placed, using microvascular anastomosis; this is now considered the method of choice for reconstructing the cervical esophagus (Jurkiewicz: *J. Thorac. Cardiovasc. Surg.* 88:893, 1984).—S.I. Schwartz, M.D.

Management of Esophageal Gunshot Wounds
Lawrence J. Pass, Leroy A. LeNarz, J. Tracy Schreiber, and Aaron S. Estrera (Univ. of Texas, Dallas)
Ann. Thorac. Surg. 44:253–256, September 1987   20–6

Gunshot wounds of the esophagus constitute a relatively small percentage of injuries that are caused by penetrating chest trauma; however, mortality from such injury ranges from 7% to 21% and morbidity can be as high as 23%. Patients often have major concomitant injuries that obscure an esophageal perforation. Unless specifically sought, such perforations can be overlooked.

The authors examined the records of 20 patients with esophageal gunshot wounds who were treated from 1973 to 1985. Nine perforations were cervical, ten were thoracic, and one was abdominal. Diagnosis was made by esophagoscopy in nine patients, esophagography in four, and surgical exploration in seven.

Mean time from hospital admission to surgery was 3.8 hours. Associated injuries were common. Eighteen patients were managed by primary closure and wide drainage; the remaining two were treated by esophageal exclusion. Two patients died at operation from associated aortic injuries. One late death brought overall mortality to 15%. Fourteen complications occurred in ten patients, but only one sustained an esophageal leak. No leaks were noted in any of the patients with thoracic repair.

Because physical findings and plain radiographs lack specificity, a high index of suspicion that is based on the bullet path is needed for early diagnosis of esophageal gunshot wounds. Such injury should be suspected particularly when the bullet wound is transcervical or transmediastinal. Primary repair can be safely accomplished with prompt diagnosis and surgery. When sepsis from esophageal leak is avoided, mortality and major morbidity are associated with other injuries.

▶ This report presents important diagnostic considerations with esophageal gunshot wounds describing experiences with 20 patients. A high index of suspicion with any missile that traverses the mediastinum is crucial because symptoms are nonspecific. This fact is the basis of the fundamental rule that bullet wounds that traverse the mediastinum should be routinely explored surgically, regardless of the presence of gross abnormalities.—F.C. Spencer, M.D.

Surgical Management of Esophageal Perforation
Jonathan C. Nesbitt and John L. Sawyers (Vanderbilt Univ.)
Am. Surg. 53:183–191, April 1987   20–7

In terms of both diagnosis and management, esophageal perforation remains a difficult problem. Improved adjunctive modalities have increased overall survival, but morbidity and mortality remain high. Nonmalignant esophageal perforation was reviewed in a total of 115 consecutive cases treated from 1935 to 1984. Of these, 69 were thoracic, 27 were cervical, and 19 were abdominal perforations (table).

In 65 patients, the etiology of the perforations was iatrogenic; in 28 it was traumatic, and in 22 it was spontaneous. Seventy one percent had pain; 51% had fever; 24%, dyspnea; and 22%, crepitus. In 78 patients contrast roentgenography was used and demonstrated the perforation in all but two of them. Ninety-five of the 115 patients had surgery.

Overall delay in treatment beyond 24 hours occurred in 29.4%. For those patients treated within 24 hours, the mortality rate was 11.4% versus 26.6% for those treated beyond 24 hours, for an overall mortality of 15.7%. No substantial worsening of prognosis was found until treatment delay reached the 48-hour mark; there were no deaths in the patients treated between 24 and 48 hours, but in those treated after 48 hours, mortality was 40%.

For the 51 patients treated from 1975 to 1984, there were no deaths in those who sustained cervical esophageal perforations, 11 of whom

TREATMENT AND RESULTS IN 115 PATIENTS WITH ESOPHAGEAL PERFORATIONS

	1935–1974			1975–1984		
Location	Number of Patients	Deaths	Mortality (%)	Number of Patients	Deaths	Mortality (%)
Cervical	10			17		
N †	1	1	100	4	0	
D ‡	2	0	0	1	0	
C						
CD§	7	0	0	11	0	
DD‖				1	0	
Thoracoabdominal	51*			34		
N †	9	6	100	2	1	50
D ‡	8	4	50	4	3	75
C	4	2	50			
CD§	30	7	23	20	3	15
DD‖				8	1	12.5

*Three patients deleted from this study.
†N, nonoperative (conservative).
‡D, conservative treatment with drainage only.
§CD, closure with drainage.
‖DD, diversion or exclusion with drainage.
(Courtesy of Nesbitt, J.C., and Sawyers, J.L.: Am. Surg. 53:183–191, April 1987.)

received closure and drainage and four of whom were treated nonoperatively. Patients with sustained thoracic or abdominal perforations who were treated early had a 19% mortality rate; with treatment delay, the rate rose to 30%, and if the delay was beyond 48 hours, the rate was 44%. There were no deaths in the patients who had traumatic esophageal perforations. Mortality was zero when spontaneous perforations were treated within 24 hours. With treatment delayed for 28–48 hours or longer, mortality was 29% and 40%, respectively.

The authors' choice for treating esophageal perforations is primary closure with drainage, regardless of the duration of the perforation, and their mortality rate is lower than that mentioned in the literature. It is also recognized that, in selected patients who have cervical esophageal perforation, nonoperative therapy has a role.

▶ The results of this series provide evidence for the authors' conclusion that the treatment of choice is primary closure, but that in selected patients with cervical esophageal perforation, nonoperative management has a role. The need for an individualized approach has been reported by Ajalat and Mulder (*Arch. Surg.* 119:1318, 1984). Deaths occurred in patients with thoracic perforations, but no death occurred in the group of patients treated within 24 hours of perforation. An operative delay of more than 24 hours was associated with a mortality of 33%. Nine patients with small well-contained instrumental injuries were successfully managed nonoperatively. There is little question that most spontaneous, traumatic, and larger instrumental perforations require early operative intervention.—S.I. Schwartz, M.D.

Early Blunt Esophagectomy in Severe Caustic Burns of the Upper Digestive Tract: Report of 29 Cases

D. Gossot, E. Sarfati, and M. Celerier (Hôpital Saint-Louis, Paris)
J. Thorac. Cardiovasc. Surg. 94:188–191, August 1987 20–8

High mortality from transthoracic esophagectomy in cases of caustic burn injury has prompted a trial of transhiatal blunt dissection and stripping to remove necrotic esophagus. This procedure was performed in 29 patients who had total esophageal necrosis from attempted suicide. A strong base was ingested by 18 patients and a strong acid, by seven patients. The average age was 38 years.

A bilateral subcostal incision and a cervical incision along the anterior sternomastoid muscle are made. Total gastrectomy is done if necessary. The cervical esophagus than is mobilized by blunt dissection, and a silicone tube is introduced into the lumen (Fig 20–2) and sutured to the esophagus. Dissection begins using the fingers through the hiatal orifice, producing intussusception of the organ along with stripping from the mediastinum. A cervical esophagostomy and a feeding lateral jejunostomy complete the procedure (Fig 20–3).

Nine of 11 deaths resulted from tracheobronchial stenosis. No patient died during operation. Only two patients lost excessive blood. Only one of nine patients operated on within 6 hours of injury died, as did two of six treated 6–12 hours after ingestion. Digestive continuity was restored after 2–4 months by retrosternal esophagoplasty, usually using the right ileocolon.

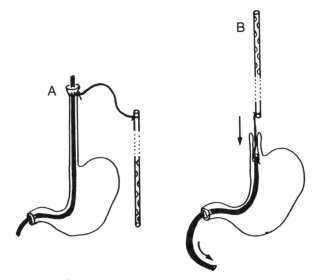

Fig 20–2.—**A**, insertion of the nasogastric tube. **B**, traction on the tube provides esophageal intussusception. Placement of the mediastinal drainage tube follows the specimen. (Courtesy of Gossot, D., et al.: J. Thorac. Cardiovasc. Surg. 94:188–191, August 1987.)

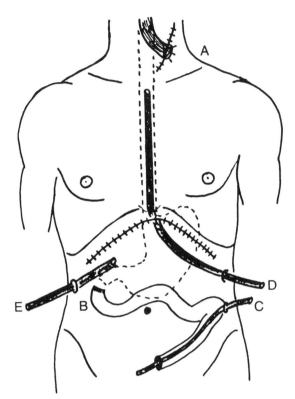

Fig 20–3.—Postoperative diagram. A, esophagostomy; B, duodenal closure; C, feeding jejunostomy; D, mediastinal drainage; E, drainage under the liver. (Courtesy of Gossot, D., et al.: J. Thorac. Cardiovasc. Surg. 94:188–191, August 1987.)

Transhiatal blunt esophagectomy with stripping is a simple and rapid procedure. Hemorrhage is minimal because of thrombosis of the periesophageal vessels. Avoidance of thoracotomy may prevent tracheobronchial lesions associated with mediastinal necrosis and sepsis. Viable muscle flap transplants might lower mortality from localized tracheobronchial perforation.

▶ In most patients with corrosive burns of the esophagus or stomach, initial management consists of esophagoscopy, steroids, antibiotics, and dilatation. Estrera et al. (*Ann. Thorac. Surg.* 41:276, 1986) suggested that early surgery, consisting of radicoresection, achieved better results. The use of blunt esophagectomy in that circumstance is certainly appropriate and the authors' technical trick facilitates the procedure.—S.I. Schwartz, M.D.

Esophageal Carcinoma: Improved Quality of Survival With Resection
Michael K. Bluett, John L. Sawyers, and Dean Healy (Vanderbilt Univ.)
Am. Surg. 53:126–132, March 1987   20–9

Experience with carcinoma of the esophagus was reported 20 years ago in 263 patients, with 2% overall 5-year survival. Esophagectomy was possible in 89 patients (34%) and was associated with a 32% mortality. To update that study, 311 patients seen from 1966 to 1985 were reviewed. Esophageal resection was accomplished in 104 patients with a 10% operative mortality and 41% complication rate. Overall 5-year survival increased to 6%.

Following esophageal resection, actuarial survival rates were 51% at 1 year, 21% at 2 years, and 13% at 5 years. These survival rates were not influenced by adjuvant radiotherapy. In 83 patients, radiation therapy was used for attempted cure, and actuarial survival rates were 29% at 1 year, 15% at 2 years, and 4% at 5 years, significantly lower than survival rates following esophagectomy ($P < .0001$). Survival rates following esophagectomy were not affected significantly with the use of adjuvant radiotherapy ($P > .05$) but tumor stage at time of resection significantly affected the survival rates ($P < .05$; Fig 20–4). Tumor site for patients undergoing esophagectomy had no statistically significant effect on survival ($P > .05$). The effect of adjuvant therapy is difficult to determine, but there was no significant improvement in survival statistically ($P > .05$). The overall operative, 30-day mortality was 10% and was not affected by the adjuvant use of preoperative radiation therapy. Preoperative radiation therapy did not significantly affect the postoperative complication rate ($P > .05$). The use of hyperalimentation did not influence overall survival ($P > .05$).

Although not as effective as surgical resection, radiation therapy in curative doses significantly improved survival when compared to no treatment ($P < .01$). Palliative esophageal bypass using the stomach was done in seven patients or colon in one patient and was associated with a 13% operative mortality, mean survival being 6 months. The quality of palliation was considered poor in two patients and fair or good in five. A poor quality of life in approximately 90% of the patients was associated

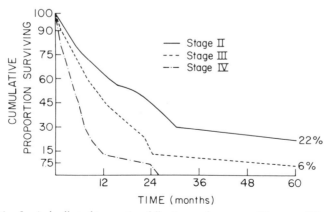

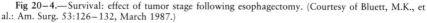

Fig 20–4.—Survival: effect of tumor stage following esophagectomy. (Courtesy of Bluett, M.K., et al.: Am. Surg. 53:126–132, March 1987.)

with palliative operations such as gastrostomy and jejunostomy without surgical resection or radiation therapy for the tumor. Following treatment, quality of life was good or fair in 83% of patients undergoing esophagectomy and in 64% of patients receiving "curative" doses of radiation.

This retrospective study supports growing optimism clinicians have toward esophageal carcinoma, with results similar to those reported by others. Five-year survival rates have improved from 6.7% to 14% at the authors' institution. The authors believe that using the Lewis operation or transhiatal esophagectomy can provide an acceptable operative mortality, result in prolonged survival, and improve quality of life.

Survival After Resection for Carcinoma of the Oesophagus

M. Eeftinck Schattenkerk, H. Obertop, H.J. Mud, W.M.H. Eijkenboom, J.G. van Andel, and H. van Houten (Dijkzigt Univ. Hosp., Erasmus Univ., and Rotterdam Radiotherapeutic Inst., Rotterdam, the Netherlands)
Br. J. Surg. 74:165–168, March 1987   20–10

The outcomes for 276 patients with cancer of the esophagus or gastroesophageal junction, selected after preoperative radiotherapy during the period 1978–1984, were assessed. During operation, 52 (19%) were found to be incurable, and in 224 patients (81%), resection of the involved esophagus was carried out. As a rule patients were selected and operated on 4 weeks after radiotherapy (40 Gy/4 weeks). For 154 patients (69%), the stomach or part of it was used for reconstruction; in 47 patients (21%), a colonic segment was used; in 15 patients (7%), a free ileal graft; and in 8 patients (3%), an esophagojejunostomy Roux-en-Y was performed. Mortality was higher when the colon was used rather than the stomach.

There were 82 patients (16%) who had stages I and II tumors, and in 141 (27%) the resection was for stage III tumors. The estimated 3-year survival for all patients with adenocarcinoma was 31%; for all patients with squamous cell carcinoma, it was 33%; for stage I and II tumors, 52%; and for stage III tumors, 21%. The difference was statistically significant ($P < .001$). Patients with stage I and II adenocarcinoma had a significantly longer survival than for stage III: 52% vs. 18% ($P < .001$) at 3 years. For patients with stage I or II squamous cell carcinoma, survival was significantly longer than for those with stage III: 48% vs. 25% ($P < .001$) at 3 years. The 3-year estimated survival for female patients was 42%, and for males, 28%.

It seems unlikely that lymph node dissection, as carried out by Skinner et al. or radiotherapy, as in this study, contribute much to survival in patients with esophageal cancer, nor is there evidence that adjuvant chemotherapy is effective to date. Proper selection of patients in good condition with curable disease, optimal patient care during the various phases of treatment, good surgical technique, and postoperative care are of utmost importance.

► The Chinese have an extraordinary experience. Lu et al. (*Ann. Thorac. Surg.* 43:176, 1987) reported on resection for carcinoma of the esophagus and esophagogastric junction in 1,025 patients between 1953 and 1973. Among the carcinomas of the esophagus, metastasis was present in 41% whereas it was present in 61% of patients with esophagogastric carcinoma. The rate of resectability was 81% for esophageal carcinoma and 74% for cancer of the esophagogastric junction. The five-year survival after complete resection for carcinoma of the esophagus was 28% and 16% for complete resection for carcinoma of the esophagogastric junction. The 5-year survival for patients with cancer of the lower third of the esophagus was 33%, and it was 64% for patients with a localized lesion and negative nodes in this subgroup.—S.I. Schwartz, M.D.

Ivor Lewis Esophagogastrectomy for Carcinoma of the Esophagus: Early and Late Functional Results
R. Michael King, Peter C. Pairolero, Victor F. Trastek, W. Spencer Payne, and Philip E. Bernatz (Mayo Clinic and Found., Rochester, Minn.)
Ann. Thorac. Surg. 44:119–122, August 1987   20–11

Early functional results from the Ivor Lewis esophagogastrectomy, involving separate laparotomy and right thoracotomy incisions, have been favorable, but the long-term results are uncertain. One hundred adults (mean age, 61 years) had this operation for documented esophageal cancer in 1980–1982. Seven patients were classed in stage I after operation, 11 in stage II, and 82 in stage III.

Three patients died postoperatively. Nine patients had mediastinal or pleural leakage from the esophagogastric anastomosis. Ten reoperations were necessary in nine patients. Follow-up of 95 operative survivors for a mean of 2.3 years revealed recurrent tumor in 60 cases. Forty-three patients had further cancer treatment. Dysphagia resulted

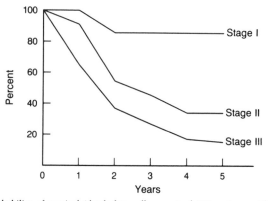

Fig 20–5.—Probability of survival (death from all causes) of 100 patients with carcinoma of the esophagus by postsurgical TNM classification. Zero time on abscissa represents day of operation. (Courtesy of King, R.M., et al.: Ann. Thorac. Surg. 44:119–122, August 1987.)

from benign stenosis in 35 patients and from recurrent cancer in five others. Twenty-two patients presently are living, three with known recurrence. Overall actuarial 5-year survival, including operative mortality, was 23%. Survival varied substantially with the stage of disease (Fig 20–5).

The Ivor Lewis esophagogastrectomy has acceptable operative mortality, and it provides good palliation without prejudicing care. A thorough assessment of node status and local spread is possible.

▶ Skinner et al. (*Ann. Surg.* 204:391, 1986) suggest the use of end-block esophagectomy, a more extensive procedure than standard esophagectomy for patients who have potential for long-term survival. They propose a new staging system based on wall penetration lymph nodes with systemic metastases. The results of treatment of this lesion are usually poor. McKeown (*J. R. Coll. Surg. Edinb.* 30:1, 1985) reported an overall cure of 15%. Orringer reported similar results using transhiatal esophagectomy (Ann Surg 200:282, 1984). By contrast, Nishihira et al. (*World J. Surg.* 8:778, 1984) reported 5-year survivals of 31%. Perhaps the most encouraging recent report is that of Wolfe et al. (*Ann. Surg.* 205:563, 1987. See Abstract 20–13).—S.I. Schwartz, M.D.

Abdominal and Right Thoracotomy Approach as Standard Procedure for Esophagogastrectomy With Low Morbidity
Robert L. Mitchell (Cardiovascular Inst. and El Camino Hosp., Mountain View, Calif.)
J. Thorac. Cardiovasc. Surg. 93:205–211, February 1987   20–12

Perioperative morbidity was assessed in a series of forty esophagogastrectomies for tumor done in 1978–1985. The standard approach has comprised en bloc resection through an upper abdominal incision and a limited right thoracotomy, the modified Lewis procedure. Removal of adjacent tissues and nodes and adequate control of tumor-free margins are possible using this approach. A limited thoracotomy minimizes chest trauma. Use of a double-lumen endotracheal tube provides excellent exposure of the thoracic esophagus.

Tumor penetrated the outer esophageal wall in 30 of 39 cases, and abnormal nodes were present in 25 patients. Estimated blood loss averaged 580 ml; only four patients required transfusion. There were no hospital deaths, and no patient had evidence of anastomotic leakage. Respiratory failure also did not occur. Two patients required reoperation. Three required esophageal dilatation for anastomotic dysfunction in the first year after surgery. Ten of the 11 surviving patients are free of disease, two longer than 5 years postoperatively.

En bloc esophagogastric resection via an abdominal and right thoracic approach has low morbidity and mortality. Lung injury is limited by a relatively small thoracic incision and the use of self-retaining retraction on the lung. Whether the particular type of resection used influences survival remains to be determined. The options include transhiatal esophagectomy, standard transthoracic esophagectomy, and radical en bloc resection.

▶ This impressive report was selected because of the frequent enthusiastic statements that blunt esophagectomy through cervical and abdominal incisions provides exceptive palliation with a low mortality and morbidity. This author reports 40 consecutive operations performed in a small community hospital with extremely good results. There was neither operative mortality nor anastomotic leaks. Only four of the 40 patients required blood transfusions. Certainly, these are impressive data. The surgeon is to be congratulated.—F.C. Spencer, M.D.

Early Results With Combined Modality Therapy for Carcinoma of the Esophagus
Walter G. Wolfe, Gary V. Burton, Hilliard F. Seigler, Ian R. Crocker, Anna L. Vaughn (Duke Univ.)
Ann. Surg. 205:563–571, May 1987   20–13

The prognosis for patients with carcinoma of the esophagus has continued to be poor over the past 10 years. The overall 5-year survival rate has been about 15%, regardless of the type of surgery used. In 1984, one institution initiated a combined modality protocol of multidrug chemotherapy and radiation followed by surgery. Patients undergoing this treatment were evaluated.

The 74 patients treated were 61 men and 13 women, aged 43 to 76 years. Fifty-two patients had squamous cell carcinoma, and 22 had adenocarcinoma. Sixty-three had preoperative chemotherapy and radiation, consisting of cisplatinum 5-fluorouracil (5-FU) and VP-16 for patients with squamous cell carcinoma and cisplatinum 5-FU for patients with adenocarcinoma combined with 4,500 to 6,000 rad. Thirty-four patients were staged as inoperable at the completion of the 4-month treatment

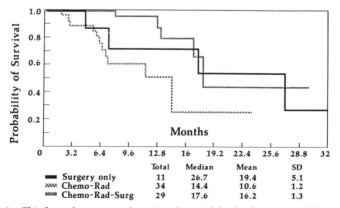

	Total	Median	Mean	SD
■ Surgery only	11	26.7	19.4	5.1
▧ Chemo-Rad	34	14.4	10.6	1.2
▨ Chemo-Rad-Surg	29	17.6	16.2	1.3

Fig 20–6.—This figure demonstrates the projected survival for the three groups. These curves were derived using the method of Kaplan-Meier (Kaplan, E.L., and Meier, P.: J. Am. Stat. Assoc. 53:456–481, 1958. Courtesy of Wolfe, W.G., et al.: Ann. Surg. 205:563–571, May 1987.)

regimen. Eleven patients had surgery alone. The surgical procedure included esophagectomy and esophagogastrostomy. All of the patients who received chemotherapy and radiation therapy had improved swallowing and a dramatic reduction of tumor mass early in the treatment course and were able to maintain oral nutrition without other support in the post-treatment period. Of the 34 patients who received chemotherapy and radiation therapy as palliation, 16 died within 2 to 16 months of therapy. One died of complications from chemotherapy, 1 died from myocardial infarction 9 months after therapy, and the remainder died from their disease. Of the 29 patients who had chemotherapy, radiation, and surgery, two died of their disease within 4 months; one died of a stroke at 9 months; one died of the disease at 11 months; and one died at 16 months, probably of the disease. (The longest survival in this group is 30 months.) Ten patients completing integrated therapy had no evidence of residual tumor in the specimen, and only microscopic foci were found in an additional five. Of the 11 patients who had surgery alone, two are dead—one of disease at 17 months, and one of unknown causes at 26 months. The longest survival in this group is 32 months (Fig 20–6).

These early results of combined modality therapy for patients with carcinoma of the esophagus should encourage investigators to continue the multidisciplinary approach to this disease.

▶ These are among the most encouraging results reported. In our institution we have had several patients who showed no evidence of residual tumor in the specimen after preoperative radiation, but all have died subsequently of the disease. In general, the results have been dismal. Galandiuk et al. (*Ann. Surg.* 203:101, 1986) reported 238 patients with esophageal carcinoma, 73% of whom were treated surgically. Only 5.5% survived: overall survival time was about 18 months, and the 5-year survival was 6%. The issue of preoperative radiation therapy has not been resolved. Wilson et al. (*Am. J. Surg.* 150:114, 1985) reported data to suggest that preoperative radiation therapy improved 2- and 3-year survival rates. It would be interesting to follow these patients 5 years and determine whether the mortality improves the 5-year survival statistics.—S.I. Schwartz, M.D.

21 The Stomach and the Duodenum

Association of *Campylobacter Pylori* on the Gastric Mucosa With Antral Gastritis in Children
Brendan Drumm, Philip Sherman, Ernest Cutz, and Mohamed Karmali (The Hosp. for Sick Children, Toronto, and Univ. of Toronto, Canada)
N. Engl. J. Med. 316:1557–1561, June 18, 1987   21–1

In a prospective study of 71 children with gastrointestinal (GI) symptoms who were undergoing upper GI tract endoscopy and gastric biopsies, the presence of *Campylobacter pyloris* was examined using silver staining, culture, and urease production.

Antral gastritis was diagnosed in 18 patients. *Campylobacter pyloris* was identified by culture and silver stain in 7 of 10 children with unexplained primary gastritis. It was not identified in any of the patients with gastritis secondary to other causes; *C. pyloris* was identified only in cases of antral gastritis. The urease test was positive in only half of the cases with positive cultures. Duodenal ulcers were detected in 5 children, and these patients had *C. pyloris* on the antral mucosa.

The presence of *C. pyloris* on the antral mucosa is associated with primary antral gastritis in children. It may also be associated with duodenal ulcers.

▶ Ever since the rediscovery of curved bacilli (now known as *Campylobacter pyloridis)* in the gastric epithelium of patients with chronic gastritis (*Lancet* [letter] 1:1273–1275, 1983), there has been a whirlwind of speculation regarding the relationships among the organism, antral gastritis, and peptic ulcer disease (reviewed by Rathbone, B. J.: *Gut* 27:635–641, 1986). There appears to be at least two kinds of gastritis. One is associated with chemical injury due to alkaline bile reflux, and the other appears to be associated with *C. pyloris*. This article confirms the presence of the condition in children and again confirms its absence in gastritis due to other causes. Five of the 7 children with the organism had duodenal ulcer, a startlingly high correlation. Are we going to have to relearn a whole new concept of the pathogenesis of duodenal ulcer? The answer is not clear yet, but all ulcer mavens are suddenly looking into that disquieting possibility.—J.C. Thompson, M.D.

Effect of Duodenal Ulcer Surgery and Enterogastric Reflux on *Campylobacter pyloridis*

H.J. O'Connor, M.F. Dixon, J.I. Wyatt, A.T.R. Axon, D.C. Ward, E.P. Dewar, and D. Johnston (General Infirmary at Leeds, Leeds, England)
Lancet 2:1178–1181, Nov. 22, 1986   21–2

There is a strong relationship between peptic ulcer disease, especially duodenal ulcer (DU), and the presence of *Campylobacter pyloridis* on gastric mucosal biopsy. This study evaluated the effect of gastric surgery on the presence of this organism.

Thirty-five patients had active duodenal ulcers, and 54 had previously undergone highly selective vagotomy (HSV), Billroth I partial gastrectomy (BIPG), Billroth II partial gastrectomy (BIIPG), or truncal vagotomy and gastroenterostomy (TVGE) for treatment of duodenal ulcer. After an overnight fast, two or more gastric mucosal biopsy specimens were obtained from each patient. Total bile acid concentrations were measured in 71 (80%) patients. The biopsy sections were evaluated blind for the presence of *C. pyloridis* and for severity of reflux gastritis using a histologic grading system.

There was no statistically significant difference in the proportion of patients positive for *C. pyloridis* between the untreated group and the HSV group. In comparison, significantly fewer patients had biopsy specimens positive for *C. pyloridis* in the BIPG, BIIPG, and TVGE groups. Both mean reflux scores and bile acid concentrations were significantly higher in *C. pyloridis*-negative patients than in *C. pyloridis*-positive patients and were significantly higher in patients who had undergone BIPG, BIIPG, and TVGE, compared with the untreated or HSV groups. A significant relationship was also found between presence of severe reflux gastritis and high bile acid concentration.

These results indicate that reflux of bile acids may produce disruption of the gastric mucous barrier. This results in a decrease of pH at the cell surface and a microenvironment preventing growth of *C. pyloridis*. Injury of the gastric mucosa may also be the cause of a reflux-specific gastritis, which may predispose to stump cancer. Since operations that destroy or bypass the pylorus appear to be associated with more enterogastric reflux, HSV may be the preferred technique to avoid adverse changes in the gastric mucosa.

▶ This paper must be read carefully. One might get the mistaken idea that, if *Campylobacter pyloridis* is bad for you, enterogastric reflux might be good for you. What it means to say, in my opinion, is that all operations for duodenal ulcer except highly selective vagotomy are associated with enterogastric reflux, and that this reflux is sufficiently severe to make the antrum mucosa inhospitable to the organism. Noting these findings and noting the conclusion of the authors, it is fascinating to speculate on just what their hypothesis was when they began the study. They may have been smart enough to have anticipated this finding and this interpretation, but I would not have been.—J.C. Thompson, M.D.

Life Events Stress and Psychosocial Factors in Men With Peptic Ulcer Disease: A Multidimensional Case-Controlled Study

Mark Feldman, Pamela Walker, Janet L. Green, and Kathy Weingarden (Univ. of Texas, Dallas, and Dallas VA Med. Ctr.)
Gastroenterology 91:1370–1379, December 1986   21–3

A case-controlled study of peptic ulcer disease (PUD) was performed, examining both personality attributes and environmental factors. The subjects were given a series of tests: a demographic questionnaire, a life experiences survey, the Minnesota Multiphasic Personality Inventory (MMPI), the Profile of Adaption to Life–Holistic Scale, and the Crisis Support Questionnaire. The study included 49 men with PUD, 32 with renal stones or gallstones, and 20 healthy controls.

The three groups did not differ significantly in age, race, marital status, or education. Nevertheless, PUD patients had more unemployment and lower-status occupations. All groups experienced similar amounts of potentially stressful life events; however, ulcer patients perceived these events significantly more negatively. Ulcer patients had significantly lower ego strength (Fig 21–1) and significantly more personality disturbances (Fig 21–2). Ulcer patients felt there were fewer people they could rely on in a crisis and exhibited significantly more depression and anxiety.

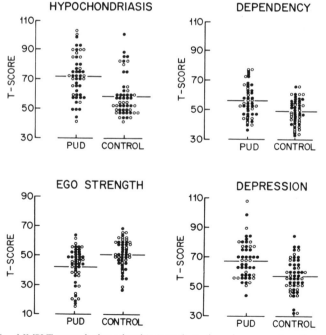

Fig 21–1.—MMPI T-scores for hypochondriasis (scale 1), dependency, ego strength, and depression (scale 2) in 49 patients with peptic ulcer disease (PUD) and in 52 controls. Inpatients with PUD and stone patients are shown as *closed circles;* PUD outpatients and healthy subjects are shown as *open circles*. Mean values are shown as *horizontal lines*. Differences between PUD patients and both control groups were significant for each variable examined. (Courtesy of Feldman, M., et al.: Gastroenterology 91:1370–1379, December 1986.)

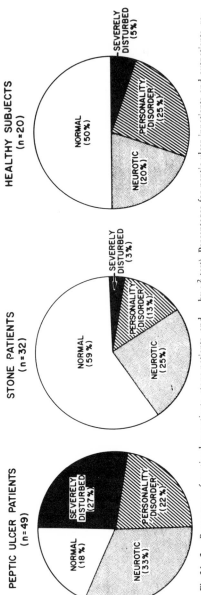

Fig 21–2.— Percentage of peptic ulcer patients, stone patients, and healthy subjects blindly classified into four general psychologic categories based on their overall MMPI profiles. Fewer normal profiles and a greater percentage of severely disturbed profiles were found in ulcer patients than in controls ($P < .001$, ulcer patients vs. combined controls by χ^2 test). Percentages for peptic ulcer inpatients and outpatients, respectively, were 16% and 24% (normal); 34% and 29% (neurotic); 31% and 6% (personality disorder); and 19% and 41% (severely disturbed). (Courtesy of Feldman, M., et al.: Gastroenterology 91:1370–1379, December 1986.)

Hypochondriasis, negative perception of life events, dependency, and low ego strength are the four variables that best separated ulcer patients and controls. This study indicates an association between stressful life events, psychosocial factors, and PUD. Future research should encompass both environmental factors and psychosocial variables.

▶ Although our grandmothers were clear about the role of stress in development of ulcers, most recent studies (*Gut* 22:1011–1017, 1981, for example) have concluded that ulcer patients have not been subjected to greater stress than their normal colleagues, and therefore most students of ulcer disease have concluded that emotional factors are not important in the pathogenesis of peptic ulcer. This article presents a series of meticulous arguments that ulcer patients are not as well equipped to handle the normal problems of life as are nonulcer patients. The point is that everyone has stressful occurrences during their lives, but that ulcer patients do not respond as well to stress as do others. What about patients who have had their ulcers cured by surgery? Do they continue to have this same set of personality disorders? The question could be answered only by a similarly detailed study, but I would be surprised if the scores did not improve. Perhaps we could interest Dr. Feldman and colleagues in attacking that problem.—J.C. Thompson, M.D.

Should It Be Parietal Cell Vagotomy or Selective Vagotomy-Antrectomy for Treatment of Duodenal Ulcer?
Paul H. Jordan, Jr., and John Thornby (Baylor College of Medicine and VA Med. Ctr., Houston)
Ann. Surg. 205:572–590, May 1987   21–4

In a prospective, randomized study 200 consecutive patients were treated electively by either parietal cell vagotomy (PCV) or selective vagotomy and antrectomy (SV-A). Both groups were similar with respect to duration of their ulcer symptoms, number of previous complications, acid secretory rates, and the degree of inflammatory response, and both had pyloric, prepyloric, or duodenal ulcers.

No operative deaths occurred, and in the 10-year follow-up period, 32 subsequent operations that could possibly be attributed to the initial operation were performed without mortality—72 in the SV-A group and 15 in the PCV group. For patients in the PCV group, diarrhea was never a significant problem, although there was no significant difference between the two groups. At all follow-up periods, dumping occurred significantly more frequently after SV-A than after PCV (Fig 21–3). In all but the 8th and 10th years the percentage of patients who lost weight was significantly greater after SV-A than after PCV.

There were nine recurrent ulcers after PCV and two after SV-A, for accumulated recurrence rates of 10.1% at 10 years by life-table analysis for the PCV patients and 2.2% for the SV-A patients; the recurrence curves were also significantly different (Fig 21–4). If pyloric and prepyloric ul-

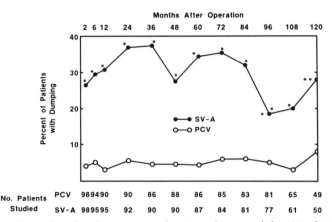

Months After Operation

No. Patients Studied

	PCV			90	86	88	86	85	83	81	65	49
	SV-A			92	90	90	87	84	81	77	61	50

Fig 21–3.—The graphs reflect the percentage of patients who reported dumping after PCV and SV-A. The frequency of dumping after PCV was significantly less (P <.005) than after SV-A for each period indicated by a single asterisk. The significance at 8 and 10 years was P <.01 and P <.03, respectively. (Courtesy of Jordon, P.H., Jr., and Thornby, J.: Ann. Surg. 205:572–590, May 1987.)

cers were deleted, there was no significant difference in the recurrent ulcer rate between the two groups. Of the 9 patients in the PCV group who had recurrent ulcers, 3 had an inadequate vagotomy, and 4 had a pyloric or prepyloric ulcer before operation. Three were successfully treated with antrectomy; 5 were treated by medical therapy and remained healed for long periods without recurrence; and 1 had five recurrences.

Five patients in the SV-A group and 1 in the PCV group required gastroenterostomy because of poor gastric emptying. There were signifi-

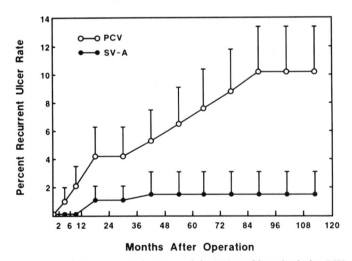

Months After Operation

Fig 21–4.—The cumulative recurrent ulcer rate and the 95% confidence level after PCV and SV-A were calculated using the Lee-Desu life table analysis. (Courtesy of Lee, E., et al.: Comput. Programs Biomed. 2:315–321, 1972.) The PCV recurrence curve was significantly higher (P <.033) than the SV-A curve. The monthly average recurrence was 0.018% after SV-A and 0.088% after PCV. (Courtesy of Jordon, P.H., Jr., and Thornby, J.: Ann. Surg. 205:572–590, May 1987.)

cantly more patients in the Visick I category after PCV than after SV-A. There is considerable controversy regarding some aspects of PCV. Nevertheless, in this study, except for a 10% risk for development of a recurrent ulcer, there were virtually no specific, serious, long-term sequelae associated with this procedure, and even this was significantly less if only patients with duodenal ulcers were considered. Thus, effective treatment is available for this complication, whereas effective treatment of severe sequelae from the destruction of pyloric function is not always possible. Even though results obtained with SV-A were good, the results obtained with PCV make this the operation of choice for the elective surgical treatment of duodenal ulcers.

▶ This is the largest personal series of prospectively randomized operative procedures for duodenal ulcer, followed for the longest time, that has ever been achieved in this country. It is clearly comparable, and in some ways perhaps superior, to the other great ongoing series in England and in Denmark. On first appraisal, it appears strange that Dr. Jordan concludes that PCV, with a 10-year recurrence rate of 10%, is superior to SV-A, with a recurrence rate of 2%. His point is that all other complications are significantly greater with resection and that these complications ultimately are more serious than recurrence. In my opinion, this is a landmark paper that shows that, in spite of a high rate of ulcer recurrence, selective proximal vagotomy (called parietal cell vagotomy in this paper) is the likely procedure of choice for the surgical treatment of duodenal ulcer.—J.C. Thompson, M.D.

Laser Photocoagulation for the Treatment of Acute Peptic-Ulcer Bleeding: A Randomized Controlled Clinical Trial
Guenter J. Krejs, Katherine H. Little, Henrik Westergaard, J. Kent Hamilton, David K. Spady, and Daniel E. Polter (Univ. of Texas, Dallas; Southwestern Med. School, Dallas; and Baylor Univ., Dallas)
N. Engl. J. Med. 316:1618–1621, June 25, 1987   21–5

Peptic ulcers cause upper gastrointestinal (GI) tract bleeding. To determine whether therapeutic endoscopy with neodymium:yttrium–aluminum–garnet (Nd:YAG) laser photocoagulation benefits patients with active peptic ulcer bleeding, 174 patients with active bleeding or signs of recent bleeding from peptic ulcers were randomly assigned during endoscopy to laser photocoagulation or therapy without photocoagulation.

In the laser-treated group bleeding was seen in 22%, and in the control group bleeding was seen in 20% of cases. Emergency surgery was required in 16% of those treated with laser and in 17% of the control group. Laser patients stayed in intensive care an average of 41 hours, and controls spent an average of 32 hours in intensive care. The laser patients stayed in the hospital an average of 12 days, and the control group stayed in the hospital an average of 11 days. There were no deaths in either group.

There were no significant differences in these parameters between the two groups. When the patients with active bleeding were analyzed separately, there was no significant difference in outcome. Nd:YAG laser photocoagulation does not significantly improve the outcome of patients with acute upper GI bleeding from peptic ulcer.

▶ Tremendous effort and great resources have been expended in attempts to answer the question of whether massive hemorrhage from duodenal ulcer can be controlled without operation. For some endoscopists, the answer is their Holy Grail. The authors conclude that it is not possible to achieve control by photocoagulation with the Nd:YAG laser. They quote four studies that reached the opposite conclusion (another appeared in the same issue of the same journal as this one: Laine, L.: *N. Engl. J. Med.* 316:1613–1617, June 25, 1987). I chose to include this paper because its results are not surprising to surgeons who have difficulty envisioning selective control of massive hemorrhage without the threat of irreparable damage and perforation. The evidence is strong that any effort to control massive hemorrhage should be labeled experimental and should be confined to teaching centers. The great hazard is that in their zeal to protect their patients from the real and perceived hazards of surgery, some physicians may delay appropriate surgical treatment or cause harm in attempts at photocoagulation of ulcer hemorrhage. Since the results of different studies are disparate, any student of this problem will want to read the other references cited, as well as the editorial by D. Fromm in the same issue (*N. Engl. J. Med.* 316:1652–1654, 1987). One aspect of the problem must be clearly understood. Surgeons and gastroenterologists look upon an operative approach to bleeding ulcer from vastly different viewpoints. The gastroenterologist often regards the need to send his patient to "the surgeons" as a personal failure and anticipates the operation with fear. To the surgeon it is part of coming to work in the morning. We must be aware of the hazards of the procedure, but we are familiar with them and believe that in the vast majority of cases we know how to handle them. Only by realizing the two different viewpoints, however, can we mutually consider the problem and arrive at the best decision for our patient's welfare.—J.C. Thompson, M.D.

Risk Stratification in Perforated Duodenal Ulcers: A Prospective Validation of Predictive Factors
John Boey, Samuel K.Y. Choi, T.T. Alagaratnam, and A. Poon (Univ. of Hong Kong and Queen Mary Hosp., Hong Kong)
Ann. Surg. 205:22–26, January 1987   21–6

The authors prospectively evaluated the value of three risk factors, i.e., concurrent medical illnesses, preoperative shock, and a long-standing perforation (more than 24 hours), in guiding surgical management of perforated duodenal ulcer patients. A total of 259 consecutive patients (mean age, 51.3 ± 17.8 years) with simple closure or definitive operation for perforated duodenal ulcers were studied.

Fourteen (6.2%) of 16 hospital deaths occurred after simple closure. Nine patients died of chest infections and respiratory failure. The overall morbidity rate was 14.3% with respiratory problems predominating. Many patients died after prolonged mechanical ventilation. Intraabdominal sepsis occurred in 8, and 7 patients had superficial wound infections in spite of prophylactic antibiotic therapy. The three risk factors, evaluated correctly, predicted the outcome in 93.8% of patients. The 16 postoperative deaths were identified with no false negative error. With increasing numbers of risk factors, the mortality rate increased progressively: 0%, 10%, 45.5%, and 100% in patients with no, one, two, and three risk factors, respectively.

Patients must be grouped into different risk categories before surgical results can be meaningfully compared. The value of the three independent variables in identifying high-risk patients with perforated ulcers was reaffirmed by this study. Clinical assessment can readily determine these variables and act as a guide in surgical management. The importance and feasibility of patient selection is attested by the fact that no patient whose case was defined as a good risk died after surgery. For patients with uncomplicated perforations, simple closure is preferable when any risk factor is present. If bleeding or stenosis coexists, truncal vagotomy and drainage may be required. Because of the poor postoperative outcome of patients with all three risk factors, nonoperative treatment should be considered.

▶ The message is clear. If you operate on patients with perforated ulcers who have all three risk factors (major medical illness, preoperative shock, and perforation of more than 24 hours), you can expect a devastating mortality rate (100% in this study). If there was ever an argument for nonoperative management, it would seem that Dr. Boey and his colleagues have offered one. His suggestion that definitive surgery is safe in patients with no risk factors and that simple closure is preferable if risk factors are present appears tenable, if we limit definitive surgery to those who have previous history of ulcer problems. Bleeding or stenosis is rarely concomitant with perforation of an ulcer, but if present, either requires definitive treatment, and I would agree with the authors' suggestion of truncal vagotomy and drainage. I would prefer gastroenterostomy for drainage.—J.C. Thompson, M.D.

Perforated Duodenal Ulcer Managed by Simple Closure Versus Closure and Proximal Gastric Vagotomy

J. Christiansen, O.B. Andersen, T. Bonnesen, and N. Baekgaard (Univ. of Copenhagen, Glostrup, Denmark)
Br. J. Surg. 74:286–287, April 1987   21–7

The authors compared the outcome of simple closure and closure combined with proximal gastric vagotomy without drainage (PGV) for perforated duodenal ulcer in 50 patients seen consecutively. Patients were studied regardless of the length of ulcer history. The 23 males and 27 females had a median age of 48 years (range, 12–63 years). By random numbers, 25 patients were allocated to simple closure and 25, to closure in combination with PGV. The median follow-up was 56 months.

No intraoperative complications were seen. One patient died after PGV due to myocardial infarction, and 1 died after simple closure from peritoneal sepsis. Five (20%) nonfatal postoperative complications were observed after PGV and 2 (8%), following simple closure. Forty-five patients were reexamined. Three died of unrelated causes, 1 developed Zollinger-Ellison syndrome, and 1 was unavailable for follow-up. Four (16%) patients developed recurrent ulcers after PGV and closure; after simple closure 13 (52%) developed recurrence. Nine (69%) patients with recurrence after simple closure were reoperated on, 8 underwent elective PGV due to unsuccessful H_2-blocker treatment, and 1 underwent PGV and closure for a reperforation 6 months following initial surgery. Recurrent ulcer was diagnosed endoscopically in all patients operated electively for recurrence and in 5 patients who received medical treatment. According to Visick's classification, 77% of patients obtained excellent or good results after PGV compared with 26% after simple closure. No long-term sequelae were observed.

These results indicate that PGV and closure for perforated duodenal ulcer can be done as safely as simple closure. It could be argued that routine PGV and closure may cause 43% of the patients to have an unnecessary PGV. This will be acceptable only if PGV and closure can be performed as safely as simple closure. This was the case in this series of patients.

► These results seem absolutely clear. The problem with applying the lesson from this study in major teaching hospitals in America, however, is that there are insufficient numbers of elective operations for duodenal ulcer to allow training of residents, and in those hospitals, residents do most of the emergency operations for perforated ulcer. An emergency operation is no place at which to learn selective proximal vagotomy (called proximal gastric vagotomy in this paper). We teach our residents to do a truncal vagotomy and drainage for all good-risk patients with perforated ulcer who have any previous ulcer history. Our process of selection would exclude patients with most of the risk factors noted in the preceding paper from Hong Kong. The only qualification is that we might do an acid-reducing procedure in some patients with a major concurrent medical illness if we thought acid reduction would give the patient a better chance to handle their ulcer disease in the future, and if it appeared likely that the patient could tolerate the procedure.

The 52% recurrence rate after simple closure noted in this paper is unusually high. A 16% recurrence rate after PGV is about standard for 5-year follow-up, but most of these patients' recurrences were less than 5 years after PGV. The low incidence of complications after PGV, even in patients with ulcers sufficiently severe so as to cause perforation, is confirmed in this study.—J.C. Thompson, M.D.

Perforated Gastric Ulcers
Gregory S. McGee and John L. Sawyers (Vanderbilt Univ.)
Arch. Surg. 122:555–561, May 1987   21–8

Findings on 100 patients with perforated gastric ulcers who were treated between 1955 and 1985 were reviewed. The patients' ages ranged from 9 to 86 years with a mean age of 57 years. Ninety-one patients underwent operative therapy, and 10 were treated nonoperatively. Of the 91 patients who underwent surgery, 51 had simple patch closure (PC), with a mortality rate of 29%. Twenty-seven patients underwent primary gastric resection, with a mortality rate of 15%. Three patients underwent parietal cell vagotomy and survived the hospital stay. The remaining 10 patients were subjected to a variety of operations, including PC, vagotomy, and pyroplasty; PC and pyloroplasty; tube gastrostomy; and PC and gastroenterostomy, with a mortality rate of 40%.

Postoperative complications such as upper gastrointestinal tract bleeding, gastric outlet obstruction, and reperforation occurred within 1 month of operation in 70% of patients and within 6 months in 90% of patients. Overall operative mortality was 24%, with no reduction during the last 10 years of the study. Mortality in the nonoperative patients was 100%. Patients suffering from perforated acute ulcers had a greater mortality rate than patients with chronic ulcers (29% vs. 16%). Mortality and complications were reduced when primary gastric resection rather than patch closure was performed. Primary gastric resection is the procedure of choice for repair of perforated gastric ulcers in patients without evidence of hemodynamic instability.

▶ This article is included because of the large number of patients that it reports to have this relatively infrequent problem, and because it illustrates, in my opinion, the difficulties with retrospective chart review. The 51 patients with a simple patch closure had a mortality twice that of the 27 patients who underwent gastric resection. Although the authors attempt to equate the two groups by analyzing their risk factors, it is impossible to avoid wondering whether or not the sickest patients were not treated by closure, reserving resection for those in better shape. A recent review of operative mortality in patients with perforated duodenal ulcer (Boey et al.: *Ann. Surg.* 205:22–26, 1987, included in this section) reported a 7.8% mortality rate in 2,559 patients treated with simple closure and a 2.1% mortality rate in 1,276 patients treated by definitive operation. No one, I believe, would suggest that simple closure of a duodenal ulcer is more risky than is definitive operation. The problem clearly is that definitive operation was performed only in good-risk patients. The 90% incidence of postoperative complication reported in this series within 6 months is surprising. Were these patients given H_2-receptor blockade? If not, should they have received it? Were the complications due to progression of some other disease, to technical problems with the surgical procedure, or to persistence of the primary gastric pathology, whatever that was? The authors' conclusion that gastric resection is a procedure of choice in the treatment of perforated gastric ulcer may be correct, but since we are not sure that the patients with simple closure were not relegated to that treatment because they were sicker, how can we be sure? Retrospective chart reviews are a problem, and every time we undertake them, we must be aware of the possibility of reaching a wrong conclusion.—J.C. Thompson, M.D.

Economic and Health Aspects of Peptic Ulcer Disease and H$_2$-Receptor Antagonists

Dennis M. Jensen (Univ. of California, Los Angeles)
Am. J. Med. 81(suppl. 4B):42–48, Oct. 24, 1986   21–9

The costs of peptic ulcer disease are very high. Direct costs include those of hospitalization or clinic visits, physician's fees, and medication. Indirect costs are those involved with loss of productivity from missing work and loss of income from the death of an employee. The economic and health aspects of peptic ulcer disease and H$_2$-receptor antagonists in the United States were reviewed.

Daily costs of different medications, such as the H$_2$-receptor antagonists for intravenous treatment, acute healing, and maintenance can be easily compared. As newer antiulcer drugs have been introduced, the number of prescriptions and medication costs have increased instead of decreased. This may be due partly to the high frequency with which H$_2$ antagonists are prescribed for patients with nonulcer dyspepsia. Long-term care or drug maintenance, hospitalization, or surgery may be required for patients with chronic peptic ulcer disease. Randomized, controlled trials to compare the efficacy, safety, and costs of different therapies for patients with chronic ulcer disease or complications have not been reported. However, on the basis of good efficacy and safety for acute healing and long-term drug maintenance for painful duodenal ulcer, long-term maintenance with H$_2$-receptor antagonists is currently prescribed for many patients. No controlled trials exist documenting that long-term maintenance with H$_2$-receptor antagonists actually decreases peptic ulcer complications. By current cost estimates, long-term H$_2$-receptor antagonist treatment is less costly than ulcer surgery for uncomplicated ulcer disease for up to 8 years. However, maintenance drug therapy beyond 8 years may be more expensive than elective ulcer surgery for good surgical candidates with chronic peptic ulcer disease. Patients with complications from peptic ulcer disease represent a subset distinct from patients with symptomatic ulcer disease.

Further studies on these patient subgroups are needed to determine the most effective, safest, and least expensive treatment. Famotidine is likely to capture a significant part of the H$_2$-receptor antagonist market in the United States in the future. However, it seems unlikely that the introduction of any new antiulcer drug will reduce the direct or indirect costs of peptic ulcer disease. Nevertheless, studies to assess the impact of such drugs on the costs of this disease are recommended.

▶ This thoughtful analysis of the economic aspect of treatment of peptic ulcer disease is worth careful study. Many ulcer surgeons have regarded it as ironic that the long-awaited physiologic operation for ulcer disease (selective proximal vagotomy) arrived only after there appeared to be spontaneous diminution in the severity of ulcer disease on the one hand, and on the other, after a highly effective medical therapy became available. Jensen calls attention once again to the high rate of ulcer recurrence after cessation of H$_2$-receptor blockade (up to 70% in some series). The only reliable way to cure ulcer disease is by operation. There is, of course, a continuous rate of ulcer recurrence even after surgery, but no one has found an incidence of postoperative recurrence that is even a third of that seen after cessation of H_2-antagonist therapy. Surgeons and gastroenterologists approach the prospect of surgical treatment for peptic ulcer from such different points of view that we may never have a dispassionate evaluation of the best treatment. The vast majority of patients seen by gastroenterologists report disappearance of their symptoms after medical treatment. Of those patients that gastroenterologists do send to surgeons, usually only those who fail to do well return to the gastroenterologist. Surgeons have excellent experience with patients after selective proximal vagotomy. We cannot understand why everyone with an ulcer does not have the operation. In this light, Jensen's suggestion that maintenance drug therapy after 8 years may be more expensive than elective surgery must be carefully considered by physicians taking care of ulcer patients year in and year out.—J.C. Thompson, M.D.

Is An Aggressive Surgical Approach to the Patient With Gastric Lymphoma Warranted?
Charles B. Rosen, Jon A. van Heerden, J. Kirk Martin, Jr., Lester E. Wold, and Duane M. Ilstrup (Mayo Clinic and Mayo Found., Rochester, Minn.)
Ann. Surg. 205:634–640, June 1987   21–10

Of 84 patients seen at the Mayo Clinic from 1970 to 1979 who had abdominal exploration for primary gastric lymphoma, 44 had curative resection and 40 had either biopsy alone or a palliative procedure. They were all observed for a minimum of 5 years or until their deaths.

The survival probability for 5 years after potentially curative resection was 75% compared with 32% after biopsy with or without palliation. The operative mortality rate was 5% overall and 2% after potentially curative resection. There was a significantly higher survival rate for the patients who had tumors confined to the stomach than for those whose tumors had extended to adjacent organs or to distant abdominal sites. When lymph nodes were not involved with the tumor, the probability of 5-year survival was 68%, compared with 43% when they were involved with the tumor at the time of operation. Increased tumor size decreased the probability of survival, but the histologic classification did not.

There was no significant difference between the survival rates of patients who received radiotherapy after surgery and those who did not; nor was there any significant survival rate difference between the patients who received radiotherapy after potentially curative resection and those who had only potentially curative resection. When analyzed by the Cox proportional-hazard model, only tumor resectability affected the patient survival rate independent of other factors. Analysis of the 44 patients who had potentially curative resection demonstrated that the only independent effect on survival rate was tumor size.

An aggressive surgical attitude in treating primary gastric lymphoma is warranted, because the efficacy of radiotherapy remains to be determined.

▶ For several years, radiotherapists and medical oncologists have proposed that patients with gastric lymphoma be treated by radiation, chemotherapy, or a combination of both regimens. Although there is one series advocating primary radiotherapy (Herrmann, R., et al.: *Cancer* 46:215–222, July 1, 1980) most reports (for example, *Dig. Dis. Sci.* 27:986–992, 1982; Weingrad, D. N., et al.: *Cancer* 49:1258–1265, Mar. 15, 1982) agree with this article that survival with nonoperative treatment with chemotherapy or with radiation is not better than after operation. I am not sure of the meaning of the authors' statement that only tumor size had an independent effect on survival, when their own data show that lymph node involvement decreased the 5-year survival rate from 68% to 43%. Both size and lymph node metastasis clearly appear to affect survival. This is a good paper to have in hand when discussing proper treatment of gastric lymphoma with your colleagues in radiotherapy and medical oncology.—J.C. Thompson, M.D.

Esophagogastric Anastomosis
Willis P. Maier, Vincent W. Lauby, Francis C. Au, and Julietta D. Grosh (Temple Univ.)
Surg. Gynecol. Obstet. 164:170–172, February 1987   21–11

Lesions located in the distal esophagus and in the proximal stomach that need to be treated with esophagectomy or esophagogastrostomy are major surgical challenges. The authors describe a technique, originally used to provide a leak-proof anastomosis, that has an additional benefit of lowering or eliminating gastroesophageal reflux. Since 1978, 61 consecutive patients had esophagogastric reconstruction with this procedure.

After resection and anastomosis planning, the proximal esophagus is placed on the anterior stomach wall (Fig 21–5). Figure 21–6 shows a close-up of the details of the sutured anastomosis on the stomach's anterior wall with an interrupted end-to-side technique. Figure 21–7 illustrates the completed gastric wraparound with the end-to-side esophagogastrostomy fully enclosed by the stomach wall. To prevent compromise of the esophageal lumen, plication of the stomach is done around the esophagus. The anastomosis is completely enclosed within the stomach serosal covering.

No free anastomotic leaks were observed, as confirmed by a barium contrast roentgenogram. Before allowing solid food, an esophagogram was done. The new esophagogastric junction showed a "high pressure zone" of 12 to 16 cm of water pressure in 4 patients studied manometrically. As a result of dysphagia to solid foods, 4 other patients required dilatation within 8 weeks postoperatively. Adequate oral intake was achieved in all patients.

▶ Any time you hear of 61 consecutive patients who have undergone esophagogastric anastomosis without a leak, you should pay attention. This tech-

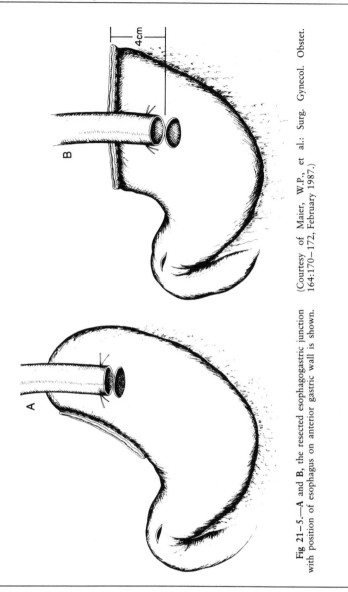

Fig 21–5.—A and **B**, the resected esophagogastric junction with position of esophagus on anterior gastric wall is shown. (Courtesy of Maier, W.P., et al.: Surg. Gynecol. Obstet. 164:170–172, February 1987.)

nique looks like a good idea, although I am surprised that it is possible to secure the degree of envelopment of the distal esophagus (shown in Figure 21–7), since the gastric wall must be edematous and thickened by this stage of the operation. The possibility of encroaching on the esophageal lumen with this gastric plication seems great, and therefore I think that it would be a good addition to position a large Maloney dilator at the same time as the gastric wrap so as to maintain the lumen in a manner exactly analogous to protection of the lumen during a Nissen fundoplication. The authors say that the technique has been successful even when 70% of the proximal stomach has been resected. I do not imagine you would end up with a very long wrap, but

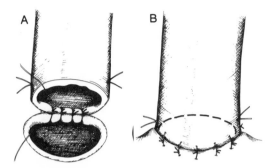

Fig 21–6.—**A**, details of the interrupted suture anastomosis, and **B**, the completed esophagogastric anastomosis, are shown. (Courtesy of Maier, W.P., et al.: Surg. Gynecol. Obstet. 164:170–172, February 1987.)

it still looks like a good idea and additionally appears to protect against reflux.—J.C. Thompson, M.D.

Percutaneous Endoscopic Gastrostomy: Procedure of Choice
Robert E. Miller, Bart A. Kummer, Donald P. Kotler, and Howard I. Tiszenkel (St. Luke's–Roosevelt Hosp. Ctr., New York)
Ann. Surg. 204:543–545, November 1986   21–12

Although operative gastrostomy (OG) is a time-proved procedure, it is often associated with significant morbidity and occasionally with mortality. The authors noted a 7% major complication rate in their own results with OG. A recent alternative is percutaneous endoscopic gastrostomy (PEG), developed by Gauderer and associates in 1980. In 1984 a simpler method, a stepwise technique thoroughly described (Figs 21–8 and 21–9), was introduced by Russell and associates. Using the Russell method, from November 1, 1984, through January 31, 1986, 98 patients were treated: 2 required a second PEG following tube displacement. The patients' average age was 75 (range, 18 to 93 years). The operation, including the endoscopy, averaged 16.5 minutes (range, 10–45 minutes); the operative component averaged 5 minutes. No patient died as a result of the procedure.

A fully inflated stomach; clear endoscopic visualization of finger indentation of the gastric wall, not referred motion; perpendicular placement of the needle, wire guide, dilator, and sheath; and fairly snug traction on the Foley catheter to appose the stomach to the abdominal wall are the keys to a successful PEG. Close cooperation and meticulous attention to detail between the endoscopist and surgeon are essential; the procedure is facilitated by a video monitor attached to the endoscope.

The Russell procedure was preferred because it requires a single endoscopy, avoids the need to pull the gastrostomy tube through the mouth and esophagus, and requires use of a Foley catheter, which is inexpensive and easy to replace. In the Gauderer-Ponsky method a mushroom cathe-

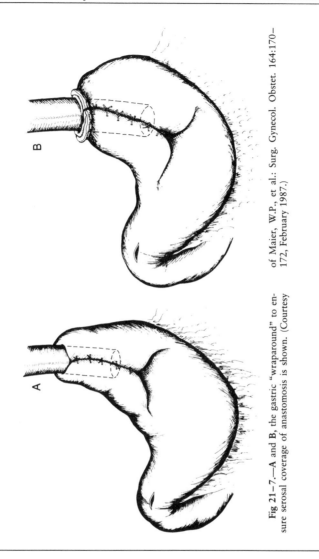

Fig 21–7.—A and B, the gastric "wraparound" to ensure serosal coverage of anastomosis is shown. (Courtesy of Maier, W.P., et al.: Surg. Gynecol. Obstet. 164:170–172, February 1987.)

ter contaminated by passage through the mouth and esophagus is used, while in the Russell method a sterile Foley catheter is inserted percutaneously.

In addition to reduced morbidity and mortality, advantages of PEG are that it is simple to perform; can be used earlier in the patient's course, avoiding nasogastric feedings or parenteral alimentation; can easily be performed at the patient's bedside or in an endoscopy unit; does not require general anesthesia; and costs less than an OG. The PEG is contraindicated in complete pharyngeal or esophageal obstruction, uncorrectable coagulopathy, or inability to perform endoscopy. The PEG technique is

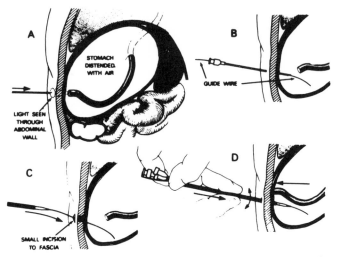

Fig 21–8.—Endoscopically controlled gastrostomy. **A,** gastric distention with needle directed at light source. **B,** guide wire passed through the needle into the stomach followed by needle removal. **C,** small incision is made along the guide wire to the peritoneum. **D,** dilator and sheath over the guide wire are advanced as a unit into stomach (gastric distention, rotary motion, and counter pressure aid this maneuver). (From Miller, R.E., et al.: Ann. Surg. 204:543–545, November 1986. Courtesy of American Journal of Surgery.)

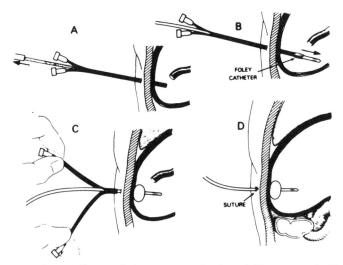

Fig 21–9.—Endoscopically controlled gastrostromy. **A,** wire and dilator removed with sheath observed remaining in stomach. **B,** lubricated Foley catheter advanced through the sheath. **C,** Foley balloon inflated (leakproof) and sheath peeled away. **D,** catheter is sutured to the skin under slight tension to oppose the stomach and anterior abdominal wall. (From Miller, R.E., et al.: Ann. Surg. 204:543–545, November 1986. Courtesy of American Journal of Surgery.)

safer, faster, and much less expensive than OG: when possible, it should be the procedure of choice if gastrostomy is indicated.

▶ Many surgeons are disturbed whenever a nonoperative method replaces an operation. We all must learn to be selective. Some operations are a great chore, and gastrostomy is certainly one of them. The incidence of complications is high, and occasionally the complications are catastrophic. The report of 100 serial percutaneous gastrostomies with no complications (except for tube displacement) and no deaths, merits close attention. The authors provide a careful recipe of how to perform the gastrostomy and avoid trouble. This method seems to provide a simple and brisk solution to a nagging problem.—J.C. Thompson, M.D.

22 The Small Intestine

Effect of Transection and Pacing on Human Jejunal Pacesetter Potentials
Harry M. Richter III and Keith A. Kelly (Mayo Clinic and Mayo Med. School, Rochester, Minn.)
Gastroenterology 91:1380–1385, December 1986   22–1

Intestinal pacing appears promising as a way of controlling gut motility and luminal transit of chyme. The effect of transection and pacing on human small intestinal electrical activity has not been fully investigated. This study was undertaken to learn whether human jejunal transection slows the pacesetter potential (PP) frequency distal to the cut, whether electrical stimuli can be entrained by human jejunal PPs, and whether human jejunal pacing is facilitated by proximal transection.

Direct recordings from surgically implanted electrodes of jejunal myoelectric activity were obtained from 11 patients. In 8 patients whose jejunum appeared healthy and who underwent Roux gastrectomy, three temporary stainless steel wire bipolar electrodes were sewn into the jejunal tunica muscularis at sites 5 cm proximal to and 10 cm and 20 cm distal to the jejunal transection. Three patients who did not undergo Roux transection served as controls and had electrodes applied at similar areas.

Jejunal PPs were observed in all control recordings, with configuration, amplitude, and frequency varying slightly from minute to minute and study to study. Recordings from the Roux limb in the 8 patients did not differ qualitatively from those obtained in the same patients from the jejunum proximal to the transection or from the jejunum of controls. In the controls, the grand mean ($\pm$SEM) PP frequencies for the proximal, mid, and distal jejunal sites were similar at 12.0 ± 0.3 cycles per minute (cpm) for two and 11.9 ± 0.3 cpm for the other. In Roux patients, the figure for proximal frequency was 11.3 ± 0.2 cpm. From the Roux limb distal to the transection, the more orad recoding site gave tracings satisfactory for PP frequency determination in 6 patients; in 7 patients, the more distal site yielded suitable records. The grand mean ($\pm$ SEM) PP frequency distal to the transection was 0.3 cpm less than the proximal frequency. The authors succeeded in entraining the PPs in only 1 of 9 patients in whom pacing was attempted. In this patient, a control, the PP frequency was increased from 12.2 to 13.0 cpm during pacing.

These results indicated that conventional distal gastrectomy produced a small decrease in proximal PP frequency. Pacing did not readily entrain the PPs in either intact or transected jejunums.

▶ Does this mean that pacing is an impractical method for controlling gut motility or does it mean that we have not yet learned how to do it? Dr. Kelly and his colleagues have been highly productive in identifying and characterizing pacemakers in the stomach and proximal duodenum. One of the aims of this study was to determine whether it might be possible to slow rapid intestinal transit in patients with the short bowel syndrome by retrograde pacing. Failure to regularly entrain the bowel in either normal or postoperative patients suggests that some other approach will be needed. Since the PP recordings from the Roux limb were similar to those of control patients, operative denervation does not seem to be the problem, so we will have to await the development of new techniques.—J.C. Thompson, M.D.

Recurrence of Crohn's Disease After Resection: Are There Any Risk Factors?

V. Speranza, M. Simi, S. Leardi, and M. Del Papa (Univ. of Rome and Univ. of L'Aquilo, Italy)
J. Clin. Gastroenterol. 8:640–646, December 1986   22–2

There is a very high risk of recurrence after the surgical treatment of Crohn's disease. Two studies of the risk of recurrence are reported.

A retrospective study involved 90 patients who had undergone surgery for Crohn's disease 1–22 years previously. The recurrence rate among these patients was calculated to be 62.2% after 10 years and 86.4% after 15 years. The site of recurrence was the same as the original site in a significant number of cases. Length of bowel involvement, extent of resection, operative indications, fistulas, abscesses, and granulomas were not related to recurrence.

A prospective study involved 22 patients operated on for Crohn's disease to examine the influence of microscopic lesions at the margins on recurrence. There was no correlation between the histologic grade of the margin and the rate of recurrence. There appears to be little chance of minimizing or influencing recurrence of Crohn's disease. Therefore, conservative surgical management, that is, resection limited to grossly diseased areas, is advocated.

▶ This study is included in order to emphasize the fact there is no medical or surgical cure for Crohn's disease; all treatment is palliative. The idea is well accepted, yet now and again surgeons will do a wide resection "to get beyond the disease." It may seem surprising that as late as 1986 there was still some question about the matter. The idea is still not universally accepted, and it is worthwhile to look at retrospective and prospective studies like this that confirm it. There is no reason to get a frozen section biopsy of the resected margin. The only thing that does seem to be related to recurrence is operation. Recurrence is higher after operation than before. This probably means only that the worst cases get operated upon.—J.C. Thompson, M.D.

Intussusception: Current Management in Infants and Children

Karen W. West, Bryon Stephens, Dennis W. Vane, and Jay L. Grosfeld (Indiana Univ. and James Whitcomb Riley Hosp. for Children, Indianapolis)
Surgery 102:704–710, October 1987   22–3

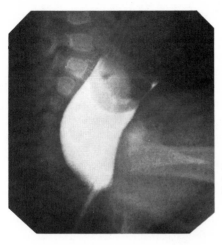

Fig 22–1.—Although the intussusception is identified by the coiled-spring sign in the sigmoid colon, complete hydrostatic reduction was possible. (Courtesy of West, K.W., et al.: Surgery 102:704–710, October 1987.)

Intussusception remains a leading cause of bowel obstruction in early infancy and childhood. The patient characteristics and diagnostic and treatment modalities of 83 patients with intussusception seen at a tertiary referral center from 1970 to 1985 are presented.

There were 51 boys and 32 girls, aged 2 months to 22 years. Ten patients had 14 separate recurrences, 9 of which occurred during the initial hospitalization. Most common symptoms on presentation were vomiting, abdominal pain, a palpable abdominal mass, rectal bleeding, and lethargy or sepsis. Fluid resuscitation and nasogastric decompression were performed on all children. Fifteen children, with symptoms for more than 5 days, presented with high grade, small bowel obstruction on plain abdominal radiographs; all underwent laparotomy without contrast studies. In the remaining 68 patients, diagnosis was confirmed by barium enema (Fig 22–1), and hydrostatic reduction was achieved in only 34 patients (42% success rate). Symptoms were present for more than 48 hours in 55% of the reduction failures. Sixty-three patients underwent laparotomy: the intussusception spontaneously reduced in 5, manual reduction was achieved in 32, and resection was required in 26, including 18 who required temporary stomas. Pathologic lead points were found in 11 patients. There were no recurrences after operation, but 10 (12%) patients developed recurrences after barium reduction. There were no deaths, but a significant morbidity rate was noted with a delay in diagnosis. Patients with successful barium enema reduction had the shortest hospital stay; 1.5 days, as compared to 9.6 days after manual reduction and 13.8 days after resection.

A high index of suspicion, early recognition, and diagnostic barium enema often allow a prompt diagnosis and nonoperative reduction of intussusception in children. Adequate preoperative preparation and prompt surgical intervention are recommended for patients with symptoms lasting more than 72 hours and severe obstructive pattern on plain abdominal radiographs.

▶ Although hydrostatic reduction by barium enema is said to be the mainstay of treatment of intussusception in this and in other studies, it is often successful in fewer than half of the patients (42% in this series). Bowel infarction is common (41% of these patients required bowel resection). Several items are worthy of attention. Even though we think of childhood intussusception as being idiopathic, a pathologic lead point was found in 11 patients. Twelve percent of patients developed recurrences after barium reduction and none after operation. Three patients who had not undergone barium enema had perforation of the colon with peritoneal soilage at the time of operation. Two patients underwent perforation during attempted barium enema reduction. Success of hydrostatic reduction was related to duration, and failure was common after 48 hours. A recent report from China (*J. Pediatr. Surg.* 12:1201–1203, 1986) reports air-pressure enema reduction in 6,396 cases in 13 years with only 2 deaths. Even though the procedure can be monitored fluoroscopically, it would seem preferable to use a radiopaque medium such as barium in order to visualize reduction with greater exactitude.—J.C. Thompson, M.D.

Gastrointestinal Lesions in Hereditary Hemorrhagic Telangiectasia
Poul Vase and Otto Grove (Odense Univ. Hosp., Odense, Denmark)
Gastroenterology 91:1079–1083, November 1986   22–4

Next to epistaxis, the gastrointestinal tract is the most frequent site of hemorrhage in patients with hereditary hemorrhagic telangiectasia (HHT). The authors evaluated differential diagnostic problems and clinical and endoscopic findings in addition to determining the age of onset of gastrointestinal bleeding. The blood group pattern of patients with HHT with gastrointestinal telangiectases was compared with the pattern of patients without signs of gastrointestinal bleeding. The blood group pattern of the total HHT group was compared with that of the background population.

Gastrointestinal telangiectases were seen in 27 of 34 endoscopically examined patients with HHT. Twenty-eight patients with HHT and gastrointestinal telangiectases came from 21 families. For 5 patients (18%) no familial history was present. Epistaxis was the first symptom in 19 patients; in 7, it was gastrointestinal bleeding; and in 2, it was cutaneous telangiectases. In these 28 patients, the median age at onset of the gastrointestinal bleeding was 55.5 years. Eighteen patients were able to provide a well-defined age at onset of epistaxis (median, 11 years). The predominant localization of gastrointestinal telangiectases was the stomach and duodenum, with positive findings in 89% and 61% of patients, respectively. The typical endoscopic finding was multiple nodular angiomas, which did not differ regarding form and size. In 15 patients, an anemic halo surrounded some of the telangiectases. Regarding heredity and clinical manifestations, there was no intrafamilial or interfamilial variation. The blood group distribution of patients with HHT with gastrointestinal telangiectases did not differ from that of HHT patients with no gastrointestinal bleeding. Blood group O did occur significantly more often in HHT patients than in the comparative background population.

It is concluded that diagnosis of gastrointestinal telangiectases in patients with HHT depends on the endoscopic technique, knowledge of hereditary factors, and clinical manifestations. To insure proper diagnosis and treatment, hereditary possibilities and external telangiectases should be considered.

▶ This condition, also known as Osler-Weber-Rendu disease, usually comes to the attention of a surgeon who has been racking his brain trying to decide the source of occult gastrointestinal hemorrhage in a patient who appears to be bleeding to death. The most important thing is to remember the possibility of telangiectatic lesions, and the next thing is to ask the patient whether they have had nose bleeds or whether they know about a tendency to bleed from a mucosal surface. Two of the patients that I have cared for knew they had the disease and gave the information on questioning. Upper and lower endoscopy is the salient study with 79% success in this series. Lesions may be anywhere from the esophagus to the rectum and rarely appear in only one segment. If the bleeding lesion can be identified endoscopically, the lesion may well respond to photocoagulation with a laser or to local injection of a vasoconstrictor. If bleeding persists, operation is indicated. Since identification of the specific bleeding point may be difficult at laparotomy, tattooing the mucosa with India ink (which can be identified by transillumination) may be helpful.—J.C. Thompson, M.D.

Acute Gastrointestinal Manifestations of Systemic Lupus Erythematosus
Algis Jovaisas and Gunnar Kraag (Ottawa Civic Hosp.)
Can J. Surg. 30:185–188, May 1987   22–5

Systemic lupus erythematosus (SLE) involves many organ systems and is a common disorder of young women. Gastrointestinal (GI) tract symptoms are a frequent clinical manifestation. When SLE is not considered in the diagnosis of the patient, infection is usually the presumptive diagnosis.

In this series of four patients with acute abdominal pain, all were initially treated for bacterial peritonitis with broad-spectrum antibiotics and all failed to respond to treatment until steroids were used. Abdominal pain and other GI tract symptoms are variable and nonspecific, ranging from nausea, vomiting, and mild abdominal pain to an acute abdominal crisis. Other common GI tract manifestations of SLE are fever, which is found in all cases, guarding, rebound tenderness, absent bowel sounds, diarrhea, and distention.

When a patient presents with either acute or chronic abdominal pain, drug-related causes should be considered and ruled out. When cholecystitis or other common disorders are excluded, the possibility of SLE should be considered. Routine laboratory investigations are not helpful. Leukocyte counts do not correlate with the clinical presentation, and the effect of steroids may be attributable to their fluctuation. In diagnosing lupus enteritis, radiologic investigations are useful, while the value of angiography is controversial. Perforation and infection must be ruled out. Spontaneous bacterial peritonitis ranges from 1% to 5% in patients with SLE and may be higher if the patient is receiving corticosteroids; thus, a diagnosis of SLE does not exclude the possibility of this complication.

That patients with lupus peritonitis or enteritis should respond to steroids within 12 to 24 hours is emphasized. If the patient's condition deteriorates, there should be prompt surgical intervention. The prognosis for patients with infarcted or perforated bowel is poor but improves with early surgery; in this study, all the patients survived. Steroids produced quick results, while antibiotics provided no improvement. Steroids may prevent perforation by controlling vasculitis if given early and in adequate doses but can have disastrous effects if the infection is not recognized.

In young women presenting with acute abdominal pain SLE should be considered in the diagnosis, and when this disease is suggested, surgical consultation and abdominal paracentesis for culture should be included in its management. A high dosage of steroids, with or without broad-spectrum antibiotics, should be started, and without a notable response within 24 hours or with suspicion of a perforated viscus, immediate laparotomy should be done.

▶ The message of this paper is given in the last sentence of the abstract: severe abdominal pain with signs of peritonitis in patients with lupus calls for high dose intravenous steroid therapy. Although the authors recommend operation within 24 hours if the patient shows no notable improvement, none of the four patients reported were operated upon, although their course was certainly stormy and prolonged. All patients did show rapid improvement on steroids, but they continued to be quite ill for some time, and one required plasmapheresis and immunosuppression. Antibiotics alone are insufficient but should be added to steroid therapy since infection is difficult to recognize in these patients. The clue to success is early administration of massive doses of steroids (between 60 and 500 mg per day of prednisone intravenously in divided doses).—J.C. Thompson, M.D.

Malignant Carcinoid Tumors: An Analysis of 103 Patients With Regard to Tumor Localization, Hormone Production, and Survival
Ingrid Norheim, Kjell Öberg, Elvar Theodorsson-Norheim, Per Gunnar Lindgren, Gudmar Lundqvist, Anders Magnusson, Leif Wide, and Erik Wilander (Univ. Hosp., Uppsala, Sweden, and Karolinska Hosp., Stockholm)
Ann. Surg. 206:115–125, August 1987   22–6

Carcinoid tumor is the most frequent of all endocrine gut tumors with malignant potential. Of 103 patients with histologically and clinically verified metastatic carcinoid tumor analyzed prospectively, the most common sites of the primary tumor were the ileum (73%), bronchi (7%), and jejunum (4%). In all patients local metastases were verified, and 96 also had metastases to the liver.

Diarrhea was the first symptom in 32% of patients, in 25% it was ileus/subileus, and in 23% it was flush. Overall frequency of diarrhea was 84%, and frequency of flush was 75%. In 33% of the patients, heart insufficiency resulting from cardiac valve disease was seen. Sixty-nine patients had complete carcinoid syndrome with flush, diarrhea, and elevated urinary 5-hydroxyindole acetic acid (5-HIAA) concentrations. Sixty-four of the 69 had carcinoid tumors of midgut origin. Either abdominal computed tomographic (CT) scan or ultrasound was used in 101 patients; metastases to the liver were found in 93 of them. In 91 patients, elevated levels of urinary 5-HIAA were found; 89 displayed liver metastases.

In 67 patients, the plasma concentration of the tachykinin neuropeptide K (NPK) was elevated, and 63 patients had tumors of the midgut region. Serum pancreatic polypeptide levels were elevated in 43%, and human chorionic gonadotropin α levels were elevated in 28%; the highest gonadotropin α levels were found in those patients with metastatic bronchial carcinoid tumors.

Of the 103 patients, 39 have died during the observation period; tumor progression was the cause of death in 18, and cardiac insufficiency was the main reason in 14. Of the 39 patients who died, the median time from carcinoid symptoms until death was 3.5 years; from histologic diagnosis it was 2 years. From the time of histologic diagnosis, the estimated median survival time was 14 years; from the time of carcinoid syndrome, it was 8 years.

This study demonstrates that midgut tumors—except appendiceal tumors—often become malignant. Diarrhea and flushing are the most frequent clinical symptoms when liver metastases have appeared; cardiac insufficiency is seen often, especially in patients with midgut carcinoid tumors and carcinoid syndrome. Nearly all patients exhibited at least one tumor-secreted product that could be used as a marker for both diagnosis and follow-up.

▶ This is the largest series of patients with malignant carcinoid tumors that I have seen and certainly the highest incidence (67%) of the carcinoid syndrome. These tumors secrete multiple vasoactive agents of which serotonin is the most common. The authors found that serotonin receptor antagonist therapy was effective in eradicating the diarrhea but not the flush; a somatostatin analog (SMS 201-995) blocked the flush and reduced plasma levels of the tachykinin, NPK. This study confirms again that the vast majority of metastatic disease originates in the midgut. The great majority of appendiceal carcinoids are benign. The estimated 5-year survival rate of 65% in this series of patients with malignant carcinoid tumor is the highest that I have seen and is, I believe, the highest ever reported. The authors suggest that this improvement may result from the use of interferon in 92 of the patients (see *N. Engl. J. Med.* 30:129–

133, 1983) and to the somatostatin analogue (see section on Endocrinology). This huge series from Uppsala reflects the Swedish policy of referral of specific diseases to a specific site. There are vast problems in having government involved in medicine, but this is surely one of the benefits. The vast array of detailed information presented here could only come from the accumulation of huge series of patients.—J.C. Thompson, M.D.

Protection From Radiation Enteritis by an Absorbable Polyglycolic Acid Mesh Sling

Dennis F. Devereux, Donald Thompson, Linda Sandhaus, William Sweeney, and Alexander Haas (Rutgers Med. School, New Brunswick, N.J.)
Surgery 101:123–129, February 1987   22–7

Pelvic irradiation results in radiation-associated small bowel injury (RASBI) in 5% to 50% of patients. To date, most surgical techniques aimed at preventing the problems of small bowel descent into the pelvis following abdominal or pelvic surgery have failed. The authors evaluated a new technique for physically removing the small bowel from the pelvis to allow the use of tumoricidal radiation doses without RASBI.

A low anterior resection was performed in 20 cebus monkeys. Ten monkeys served as postsurgical controls, and 10 animals were randomized to receive placement of a polyglycolic acid (PGA) mesh sling sewn circumferentially around the interior of the abdominal cavity, to form a supporting apron for keeping the small bowel out of the pelvic region. Ten days after surgery, all 20 animals were irradiated with 2,000 rads to the site of anastomosis. Randomly selected monkeys were killed at 1, 3, 6, 9, and 12 months, and the small bowel and rectum were histologically evaluated. Blood and 24-hour stool fat tests were performed at 1, 6, and 12 months as physiologic measures of small bowel function. Two monkeys who did not undergo surgery or irradiation were controls for normal histology and physiology.

Throughout the follow-up period, monkeys with polyglycolic acid (PGA) mesh slings had normal small bowel function and histology. Changes in the rectum substantiated that the animals had been exposed to radiation. The mesh sling was totally absorbed at 6 months, and the small bowel was floating free in the abdominal cavity. There were no infections or obstructions in these animals. In comparison, histologic evidence of acute radiation damage and laboratory results suggesting malabsorption were seen in the nonmesh-treated monkey killed at 1 month. At 2 months, all monkeys in this group had weight losses 15% to 30% of their radiation therapy weight and had died. Autopsy revealed necrosis and mucosal sloughing in the small bowel.

These results demonstrate the safety and efficacy of absorbable PGA mesh sling for protecting the small bowel from radiation-associated injury. This technique may have important therapeutic application in patients who require radiation therapy following surgery for malignant pelvic tumors.

▶ As can be confirmed by review of the last three volumes of this journal, radiation enteritis is the most important factor in limiting radiation therapy of pelvic neoplasms. Radiation therapists are often faced with the dilemma of whether to deliver a calculated tumoricidal dose to the uterus, ovary, or rectum and cause permanent, perhaps lethal, damage to the small bowel or to use a subtumoricidal dose. If the results of this study can be duplicated in humans, we may have a solution to one of the major problems in cancer treatment. I see no contraindication to the method. If the sling is sewn circumferentially around the abdominal wall at the level of the pelvic inlet, the small bowel should be kept well away from harm and the course of irradiation can be easily completed before the sling dissolves. This method seems to offer as much promise as anything I can remember.—J.C. Thompson, M.D.

23 The Colon and the Rectum

Colovesical Fistula
S.G. Pollard, R. MacFarlane, R. Greatorex, W.G. Everett, and W.G. Hartfall (Addenbrooke's Hosp. and Ipswich Hosp., Cambridge, England)
Ann. R. Coll. Surg. Engl. 69:164–165, July 1987   23–1

The authors review data on 66 patients with colovesical fistula. The most common cause of the fistula was diverticular disease; other causes were due to malignancy, Crohn's disease, radiotherapy, appendicitis, and trauma. Although many tests were performed, the most sensitive diagnostic test was barium enema, which revealed abnormality in 98% of patients. Thirty-two patients underwent a single-stage resection. There was no perioperative mortality and little morbidity. Fourteen patients underwent a two-stage procedure. Two patients died of cardiorespiratory complications. Seven patients underwent a three-stage procedure. No patient who had a successful repair had a recurrence.

Invasion of the bladder by colorectal carcinoma does not have a poor prognosis if resection of the colon and bladder is performed. Single-stage resection can give very good results, as seen in this series of patients. Single-stage resection is recommended to treat uncomplicated colovesical fistula due to diverticular disease or invasion from colonic carcinoma.

▶ One day a man will walk into your office and, with a surprised look on his face, will tell you that in the midst of urination he has noticed air passing (bubbling) from his urethra. That man has a colovesical fistula, the most common cause of which is diverticulitis (although fistula formation is actually an uncommon complication [2%] of diverticulitis [*Surg. Gynecol. Obstet.* 130:1082–1090, 1970]). Pneumaturia was present in 85% of patients in this series. The first diagnostic study after the physical examination should be sigmoidoscopy, but it is unusual to find the fistulous opening (7% of cases in this series). As noted, barium enema is the study of choice, and in rare cases of failure, the next step is cystography and cystoscopy. One-stage resection is usually routine in these patients, but colostomy may be necessary in the face of severe inflammation. The outlook is good in most patients, and recurrent colovesical fistula is uncommon.—J.C. Thompson, M.D.

Inhibition of Intestinal Carcinogenesis by Dietary Supplementation With Calcium

G.V.N. Appleton, P.W. Davies, J.B. Bristol, and R.C.N. Williamson (Bristol Royal Infirmary, Bristol, England)
Br. J. Surg. 74:523–525, June 1987   23–2

Increased dietary calcium lowers the rate of cell proliferation in colonic crypts. The authors examined the effect of dietary calcium supplementation on the development of azoxymethane-induced intestinal tumors in Sprague-Dawley rats.

Sixty male Sprague-Dawley rats received six injections of azoxymethane, 15 mg/kg of body weight per week. Half the animals had 80% midjejunoileal resections, and half had jejunal transections. Half the animals in each group received calcium lactate, 24 gm/L, in their drinking water. All rats were killed within 27 weeks of operation. Midbowel transection doubled the yield of duodenal tumors. Calcium supplementation reduced the tumor incidence by half and eliminated the effect of the transection. Small bowel resection doubled the occurrence of colorectal cancer. Calcium supplements halved the cancer rate and eliminated the effect of the resection.

These results demonstrate that calcium inhibits chemical carcinogenesis in the colon and duodenum. The anticancer activity of calcium may be due to its ability to bind fatty acids and bile acids. It is possible that a small oral dose of calcium could lower the incidence of colorectal cancer in human beings.

▶ In 1985, Lipkin and Newmark were able to decrease the rate of epithelial cell proliferation in the colonic crypts in individuals at high risk for familial colonic cancer by adding extra calcium to the diet (*N. Engl. J. Med.* 313:1381-1384, 1985). This study is a follow-up of that observation and clearly shows that calcium blocks the added carcinogenicity induced by massive small bowel resection. What is the mechanism? My colleague, Courtney M. Townsend, Jr., suggests that it may be due to binding of bile acids by calcium, thereby preventing bile enteritis. He is studying the phenomenon by decreasing dietary calcium to determine whether this will increase the incidence of cancer. Should we all be taking daily calcium supplements? You could probably mount a better justification for that than is available for massive vitamin C intake.—J.C. Thompson, M.D.

Flow Cytometric DNA Patterns From Colorectal Cancers: How Reproducible Are They?

Nigel A. Scott, Joseph P. Grande, Louis H. Weiland, John H. Pemberton, Robert W. Beart, Jr., and Michael M. Lieber (Mayo Graduate School of Med., Rochester, Minn. and Cancer Research Campaign, London)
Mayo Clin. Proc. 62:331–337, May 1987   23–3

Cancers with a DNA diploid pattern can be distinguished from tumors with a DNA nondiploid pattern by flow cytometric DNA analysis of cells or isolated nuclei from colorectal cancers. Studies have shown a better probability of survival for patients with DNA diploid carcinomas than for patients with DNA nondiploid carcinomas. Whether or not the DNA ploidy analysis would yield reproducible results if a full-thickness specimen was obtained from any one of several possible sites within a cancer was uncertain.

The heterogeneity of DNA ploidy patterns was investigated by analysis of 261 different samples from 30 fresh colorectal cancers. The same DNA was found in all specimens of 19 (63%) tumors studied. Moderate to marked heterogeneity for DNA ploidy pattern was found in 4 (13%) tumors, and minimal heterogeneity was found in 7 (23%) carcinomas. When full-thickness specimens were obtained from any one of five possible sites, the DNA pattern was the same from 79% of the carcinomas studied. Flow cytometric DNA analysis of superficial cup biopsy specimens could have determined the DNA ploidy pattern of most of the carcinomas.

These results indicate that individual colorectal cancer can be determined to be DNA diploid or nondiploid by using a variety of sampling techniques. The application of DNA ploidy determination to clinical research studies of the treatment of colorectal cancer patients can be done with some degree of confidence.

▶ Wolley and colleagues in 1982 (*J. Natl. Cancer Inst.* 69:15–22, 1982) showed that flow cytometric analysis of human colorectal cancer cells (nuclei) allowed differentiation between a DNA diploid pattern and a DNA aneuploid pattern. Subsequent studies have shown a better survival rate in patients whose DNA pattern was diploid than in those with a DNA aneuploid pattern (*Br. J. Surg.* 72:828–830, 1985; *JAMA* 255:3123–3127, 1986). Since many of the studies are performed by resurrecting tissue from embedded paraffin blocks, the authors studied multiple samples from the same tissue block and found that the pattern of DNA ploidy was sufficiently homogenous that clinical decisions may be made with some confidence. The obverse of this, of course, is that some heterogeneity was present, so that one determination of a diploid pattern does not necessarily confer good prognosis.—J.C. Thompson, M.D.

Influence of Tumor Cell DNA Ploidy on the Natural History of Rectal Cancer

King-Jen Chang, Warren E. Enker, and Myron Melamed (Mem. Sloan-Kettering Cancer Ctr., New York, and Natl. Taiwan Univ. Hosp., Taipei, Taiwan)
Am. J. Surg. 153:184–188, February 1987   23–4

The authors examined the prognostic significance of ploidy in locally excised rectal cancer in 11 men and 19 women, aged 42–84 years (mean, 66 years). Flow cytometry assays of tumor cell DNA were performed on specimens of archived, paraffin-embedded tissue.

Two patients had cancer that invaded the muscularis mucosae: aneuploid in 1 and diploid in 1. In 15, invasion was into the submucosa: aneuploid in 7 and diploid in 8. In 13 patients, the muscularis propria was invaded: aneuploid in 8 and diploid in 5. Sixteen patients had aneuploid cancer, and 14 patients had diploid cancer. Twelve patients had recurrent disease: 10 cancers were aneuploid and 2 were diploid. Of the 18 patients who remained free of disease, 12 had diploid cancer and 6 had aneuploid cancer. Seven of the 12 patients with recurrent disease died. There was no difference in DNA ploidy between survivors and those who died. While ploidy predicted tumor recurrence after local treatment, it did not predict survival after repeat excision or salvage abdominoperineal resection for recurrent disease. After at least a 5-year follow-up, 17 patients were alive and free of disease (10 with diploid disease), 5 had died of other causes (3 with diploid disease), 6 had died of disease (5 with aneuploid disease), 1 was alive with disease (aneuploid disease), and 1 had died from other causes with recurrent cancer (aneuploid disease). Of 22 patients alive or dead without disease 13 had diploid disease; 7 of 8 patients who died or were dying of cancer had aneuploid disease.

The aggressive clinical behavior of tumors having aneuploid DNA was not otherwise predictable by standard histologic features. Aggressive tumor behavior seems to correlate closely with aneuploidy in locally treated rectal cancers, compared with no correlation in the patients here who were treated with major resection. The fact that these cancers were treated by local excision may permit the prognostic impact of DNA content to reflect the natural history of cancer.

▶ As the authors point out, the likelihood of recurrence after local excision of these mobile cancers is small in the absence of histologically positive margins of resection, mural penetration, or aggressive histologic characteristics. Unfortunately, most surgeons treat these local tumors by ablation (electrocoagulation, laser vaporization, fulguration, or radiation implant) so that postoperative information on the histology of the tumor is often not available. This retrospective study suggests that determination of DNA ploidy by flow cytometry of preoperative or operative biopsies might provide reliable prognostic information. This paper and the preceding one suggests that flow cytometry determination of DNA ploidy may be an important and valuable tool in assessing the prognosis of colorectal cancer.—J.C. Thompson, M.D.

Stimulation of Growth of a Colon Cancer Cell Line by Gastrin
Christine J. Kusyk, Nancy O. McNiel, and Leonard R. Johnson (Univ. of Texas, Houston)
Am. J. Physiol. 251:G597–G601, November 1986   23–5

Gastrointestinal peptides have been reported to affect the in vivo growth of the mucosa of the digestive tract. Among these, gastrin has been reported to stimulate the growth of gastrointestinal tract tumors. The authors investigated the effect of gastrin on the growth of a human colonic adenocarcinoma cell line, LoVo cells.

Gastrin significantly stimulated thymidine incorporation into LoVo cells. This incorporation peaked at 5–8 hours after release from synchronization and exposure to gastrin. During this S phase, gastrin-treated cells incorporated 80% more [3H]thymidine than controls.

Physiologic quantities of gastrin can stimulate the growth of a human colon cancer cell line, the LoVo cell line. This model will be useful in the study of gastrin cell interactions and cell growth.

▶ Years of argument have failed to fully answer the question of what is a "physiologic" level of an active agent. We ordinarily take the concentration of the agent that is achieved after a normal physiologic stimulus (for example, eating) to be the physiologic level. The difficulty with that definition is that it assumes that the agent is active all by itself, when in fact it may require cooperation of other agents to achieve its physiologic effect. When administered exogenously alone in a concentration designed to achieve the "physiologic" level, the agent, lacking its coactive factor of factors, may not be active. There is good evidence to suggest that some secretory (and probably endocrine and muscle) cells may not function with full efficiency until multiple membrane receptors are occupied. Occupation of a single receptor after exogenous administration of an agent may not bring about a measurable effect until a much higher concentration of the single agent is achieved. This is one of the reasons that in vitro studies frequently require a much higher concentration of an agent than is required for in vivo studies in order to achieve an effect. The effector cell in vitro is removed from all sorts of stimulatory and inhibitory mechanisms (for example, contact with the autonomic nervous system) and may be extraordinarily lethargic in cell culture. The wonder of this study is that an effect of gastrin was achieved in vitro at a concentration of 10^{-9} M (that is, nanomolar concentration) that is only 100 to 1,000 times greater than the concentration found in postprandial serum (usually picomolar or 10^{-12} M). Most investigators do consider an in vitro activity at 10^{-9} M to be physiologic, and this demonstration is an important one. As shown in studies by Courtney M. Townsend, Jr., and his colleagues (*Surg. Forum* 33:384–385, 1982) and by others (*Biomedicine* 33:259–261, 1980) the growth of human colon cancer clearly is stimulated by gastrin. This study shows that the effect can be achieved in vitro with "physiologic" concentrations of gastrin.—J.C. Thompson, M.D.

Prevention of Colorectal Cancer: Role of Association Between Gallstones and Colorectal Cancer
Matteo Gafà, Leopoldo Sarli, Giuliano Sansebastiano, Ernesto Longinotti, Fabio Carreras, Nicola Pietra, and Anacleto Peracchia (Institute of Clinica Chirurgica II e Terapia Chirurgica and the Inst. of Igiene of Parma Univ., Parma, Italy)
Dis. Colon Rectum 30:692–696, September 1987   23–6

Some authors have reported an association between gallstones and an increased risk of colorectal cancer. Since the confirmation of such an association can improve measures of primary or secondary prevention of colon cancer, a case-control study was undertaken of 168 patients who underwent laparotomy for colorectal adenocarcinoma and 168 patients operated on for benign disease.

Overall prevalence of concomitant gallstones was significantly higher in patients with colorectal cancer than controls. This association was particularly significant in the right colon (odds ratio = 4), female patients (odds ratio = 3.14), and patients older than age 65 years (odds ratio = 3).

This study confirms the association between gallstones and colorectal cancer, which can be advantageous in terms of primary or secondary prevention of colorectal cancer. For example, an excessive intake of animal fats, cholesterol, and calories is associated with gallstone formation. Since a high fat and low fiber diet is associated with high levels of fecal bile acids (substances that are known colon tumor promoters in animal studies) in the large bowel, a diet low in meat, fats, cholesterol, and calories can be a primary prevention of colorectal cancer. Another preventive measure is the inclusion of gallstone patients, particularly those older than age 65 years and female, in the mass screening for patients at high risk for colorectal cancer.

▶ One of the most difficult problems to investigate is the putative relationship between one disease and another. The question always is: what is the proper control? For example there is an increased incidence of peptic ulcer disease in cirrhotic patients if you compare them with normal controls, but if you compare them with a group of chronically ill patients with a long-standing metabolic disease, the relationship evaporates. For the last several years there have been suggestions of a relationship between colorectal cancer and cholecystectomy (*Cancer* 45:392–395, 1980) and colorectal cancer and cholelithiasis (*Cancer* 50:1015–1019, 1982). The present paper is a retrospective comparison between the incidence of cholelithiasis in 168 patients operated upon for colorectal cancer as compared with 168 patients who underwent laparotomy for benign disease. Cholelithiasis was almost two and one half times as prevalent in colon cancer patients as in patients with benign disease. What does this mean? Who knows? The multiple suggestions advanced in the paper to explain the relationship in the paper are highly speculative. I would remain skeptical until the relationship is demonstrated in a prospective study.—J.C. Thompson, M.D.

Patient Management After Endoscopic Removal of the Cancerous Colon Adenoma
William O. Richards, William A. Webb, Steven J. Morris, R. Carter Davis, Linda McDaniel, Leroy Jones, and Susan Littauer (Univ. of Maryland, Baltimore; East Alabama Med. Ctr., Opelika, Ala., and Crawford W. Long Mem. Hosp., Atlanta)
Ann. Surg. 205:665–667, June 1987   23–7

The management of patients after endoscopic removal of cancerous adenomas is controversial. To provide recommendations for management of these patients, a retrospective review was conducted of 121 patients with 126 malignant adenomas removed by colonoscopic polypectomy between 1971 and 1985.

Carcinoma in situ was found in 41 patients, and invasive carcinoma was found in 80. A synchronous colon cancer was found in 5 patients. At a minimum follow-up of 1 year after polypectomy, none of the patients with carcinoma in situ had evidence of residual tumor or metastatic disease as evidenced by colon resection in 3 and endoscopic surveillance in 38 patients. Forty-four patients with invasive carcinoma underwent colon resection: 34 showed no evidence of tumor in the resected bowel or mesenteric lymph nodes, and 10 had either residual cancer or regional lymph node metastasis. Each of these patients exhibited risk factors based on the criteria of Christie, such as incomplete excision, poorly differentiated tumor, invasion of the line of resection, invasion of the polyp stalk, and invasion of venous or lymphatic channels.

Colon resection with regional lymphadenectomy is recommended for patients with one or more of the above risk factors following endoscopic removal of an invasive malignant adenoma. Endoscopy should be repeated as early as 3 months after curative polypectomy in patients without any of these risk factors to evaluate the polypectomy site. Total colonoscopic evaluation is recommended at 1 year after polypectomy to identify synchronous lesions missed at the initial procedure and ensure that the patient's surveillance program begins with a cancer-free colon.

▶ The question posed is whether it is safe ever to locally excise an invasive carcinoma of the colon, and the authors provide a cautious positive answer. The answer is qualified, and they provide the five criteria which, if present, require segmental resection of the colon (or, if in the rectum, at least a wider local excision with histologic monitoring of the excised tissue). The authors' recommendations appear sound, and the keystone of surveillance is colonoscopy. With the recent experience of the President, colonoscopy has become a household word and nearly everyone understands its importance.—J.C. Thompson, M.D.

Intraoperative Ultrasonography in Screening for Liver Metastases From Colorectal Cancer: Comparative Accuracy With Traditional Procedures

Junji Machi, Hiroharu Isomoto, Yuichi Yamashita, Toshihiko Kurohiji, Kazuo Shirouzu, and Teruo Kakegawa (Kurume Univ., Kurume, Japan)
Surgery 101:678–683, June 1987   23–8

Assessment of liver metastases is an integral part of colorectal cancer management. The authors describe a comparison of high-resolution real-time intraoperative ultrasonography, preoperative ultrasound, computed tomography (CT), and surgical exploration in the diagnosis of liver metastases in 84 patients with colorectal cancer.

No metastatic tumors were detected in the liver in 72.6% of the patients. In the other 23 patients, 46 metastatic tumors were identified. Ultrasound and CT detected 50% of these tumors. The addition of surgical

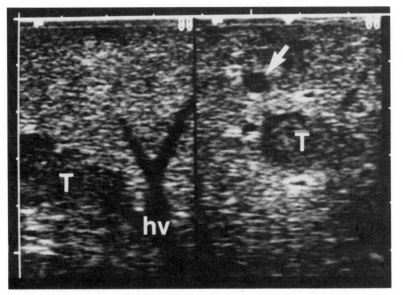

Fig 23–1.—Operative sonogram of multiple metastatic tumors. Two large tumors *(T)* were diagnosed preoperatively, while a smaller one *(arrow)* was identified for the first time by operative ultrasonography. This tumor could not be palpated and ultrasonically showed hypoechogenicity. The size was 0.4 × 0.5 cm, and the depth from the surface was 1.3 cm. Distance between each marker on top and left is 1.0 cm. *(hv,* middle hepatic vein). (Courtesy of Machi, J., et al.: Surgery 101:678–683, June 1987.)

exploration and palpation brought the total number of identified tumors to 32. Intraoperative sonography alone identified 31 of these tumors and also detected 14 additional tumors. These tumors were 0.4 × 0.4 to 1.0 × 1.6 cm in size and were 1.0–5.0 cm deep. These tumors revealed either hypoechogenicity or a bull's-eye appearance (Fig 23–1).

Intraoperative ultrasonography was significantly more sensitive than preoperative ultrasound, CT, or surgical exploration. The overall accuracy of intraoperative ultrasonography was significantly higher than the other screening procedures. High-resolution intraoperative ultrasonography is a safe, simple, and accurate procedure for the screening of liver metastases during surgery for colorectal cancer.

▶ Intraoperative ultrasonography appears clearly to be the method of choice in detecting liver metastases, and every surgeon who operates on patients with intra-abdominal malignancy should learn the technique. The only negative points are the cost of the machine and the time required to learn the method. There is no shortcut: the only way to learn is to practice on a series of patients in order to learn the feel of the probe and to learn how to interpret those gray squiggly lines. The sensitivity of 98% reported here shows that intraoperative ultrasonography is a hands-down favorite over preoperative ultrasound or CT (really no contest with either) and, in the hands of these authors, gives 40% better results than surgical exploration. Many surgeons are reluctant to adopt high tech methods. This appears unavoidable.—J.C. Thompson, M.D.

Initially Unresectable Rectal Adenocarcinoma Treated With Preoperative Irradiation and Surgery

William M. Mendenhall, Kirby I. Bland, William W. Pfaff, Rodney R. Million, and Edward M. Copeland III (Univ. of Florida, Gainesville)

Ann. Surg. 205:41–44, January 1987   23–9

The authors present their experience with locally advanced rectal adenocarcinoma. Between March 1970 and April 1981, 23 patients with lesions believed unresectable at initial evaluation were treated with preoperative irradiation and surgery. Five (22%) patients underwent exploratory laparotomy and diverting colostomy before radiation therapy. Irradiation was administered to the pelvis at 180 rads per fraction per day, with a continuous-course technique to total doses of 3,500–6,000 rads (mean, 4,800 rads; median, 5,000 rads). All patients underwent surgery 2 to 11 weeks later (mean, 4.9 weeks).

Preoperative irradiation was well tolerated, with no or minimal side effects in 12 patients, mild diarrhea or dysuria requiring medication in 5, and moderate diarrhea or dysuria or desquamation of the inguinal areas, perineum, or both, in 2. Postoperatively, 11 patients had an apparently complete resection of their cancer, while 12 did not. Reasons for complete resection included positive margins in 7 patients, discovery of diffuse peritoneal seeding in 2, and liver metastases with positive margins in 2. One patient had a late complication of a small bowel obstruction. No apparent relationship was observed between preoperative irradiation dose and the likelihood of local recurrence or persistence over the range of doses used. The 5-year absolute survival rate for patients with complete resection was 18% (2 of 11 patients). The 5-year absolute and determinate survival rates for the whole study were 9% (2 of 23 patients) and 9% (2 of 22 patients), respectively. In the incomplete resection group, 1 patient died postoperatively, secondary to sepsis and diffuse intravascular coagulation.

The prognosis when preoperative irradiation and surgery are used for clinically unresectable rectal cancer is poor. Yet, the chance of local control and long-term survival is minimal only with surgery. Thus, the authors recommend preoperative irradiation and surgery for patients with locally advanced unresectable rectal adenocarcinoma.

▶ Reports of results of studies with these unresectable lesions have given vastly divergent results, and many of the survival statistics are confusing. As the authors suggest, the 5-year survival rate after operation is probably the best and certainly the most stringent of criteria that have been used. In the series they review, this rate varies from 9% (their own series) to 28% (*Cancer* 52:814–818, 1983). All sorts of warnings are necessary to anyone who seeks to evaluate these series. As the authors state, the first thing to standardize is whether or not the tumor is truly unresectable to begin with. Some of the series report tumors that are "tethered," that is, those that have diminished mobility but are not absolutely fixed. Then others talk about tumors that are "borderline resectable." The present authors emphasize that the tumors in this series were truly fixed and were clinically nonresectable. In creating a plan for patients with absolutely fixed tumors, one might first create a permanent colostomy, sequester the unresectable tumor in a short Hartmann's pouch, and elevate the small bowel out of the pelvis with a Dexon sling (see Abstract 22–7) so as to keep the small bowel out of harm's way during the irradiation of the rectal tumor. The tumor could then be excised at a later operation. This technique might allow for safe application of a truly tumoricidal dose of radiation to the rectum.—J.C. Thompson, M.D.

Local Recurrence of Rectal Adenocarcinoma Due to Inadequate Surgical Resection: Histopathological Study of Lateral Tumour Spread and Surgical Excision

P. Quirke, P. Durdey, M.F. Dixon, and N.S. Williams (Univ. of Leeds, England)
Lancet 2:996–999, Nov. 1, 1986   23–10

The incidence of local recurrence after resection of rectal adenocarcinoma varies from 4% to 50%, as shown from previous studies. But the main cause remains unproved, especially in patients who have undergone curative resection, defined as that in which the surgeon was confident all macroscopic tumor had been removed and in which there was no evidence of metastatic spread at operation, on preoperative ultrasound, or on computed tomography (CT) of the liver. The degree of lateral spread of 52 patients with biopsy-proved rectal adenocarcinoma whose operations took place between 1983 and 1985 were investigated prospectively. Abdominoperineal resection was done in 25 patients; a sphincter-saving operation was done in 26, and a Hartmann's operation was done in 1. Median follow-up was 23 months (range, 9 to 29).

Six of 52 specimens showed lateral resection margin involvement, designated LRM-positive, on the single primary slice, while 14 or 52 were noted to be affected when all the tumor was embedded and examined. In 7 the spread was visible only microscopically, and in the other 7 it was visible macroscopically. There was local recurrence in 11 of 13 who were lateral resection margin patients (LRM)-positive and in 1 of 38 who were LRM-negative overall. The sensitivity, specificity, and positive predictive values of the total embedding methods were 92%, 95%, and 85%, respectively, in predicting local recurrence. Increasing Duke's stage, decreasing tumor differentiation, and the pattern of the invasive border were associated with clinical local recurrence. There was a recurrence rate of 26% for abdominoperineal excisions and 18% for sphincter-saving operations. The local recurrence rate after the different operations did not differ in the curative and palliative subgroups (Fig 23–2).

In the retrospective series of 52 patients, 24 had local recurrences, and 17 had liver metastases. There were also significant associations with clinical recurrence, similar to those of the prospective group, Duke's stage, and the histologic grade. The rate of local recurrence was no higher in sphincter-saving resections than in the abdominoperineal resec-

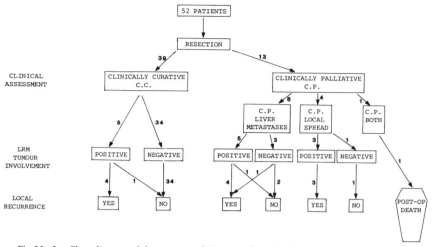

Fig 23–2.—Flow diagram of the outcome of 52 cases of rectal adenocarcinoma related to involvement of the lateral resection margin. (Courtesy of Quirke, P., et al.: Lancet 2:996–999, Nov. 1, 1986.)

tions. There was involvement of other pelvic organs in 4, compared with 6 in the prospective series.

The finding of involvement of the LRM by carcinoma in 25% of the unselected cases of rectal adenocarcinoma and its subsequent local recurrence in 85% of these cases shows that local recurrence arises beyond doubt mainly as a result of incomplete surgical resection. Distance of clearance around the tumor seems much less important than frank involvement of the margin to determine recurrence at any stage, for the recurrence rate in the prospective group closely matches that already found in the retrospective group after long follow-up. Single slice examination underestimated lateral spread by 50%, but the incidence of LRM involvement doubled after histologic examination.

▶ Local recurrence is one of the two leading causes of death in patients with rectal cancer. Surgeons are not expert in assessing lateral spread. In this series of patients from Leeds, careful retrospective study of whole-mount specimens allowed gross and histologic evaluation of lateral spread. The lateral margins of resection were involved in one of every four cases, and of those patients, 85% developed a local recurrence. Of interest is the finding that the rate of local recurrence after abdominoperineal resection was greater (although not significantly so) than it was for sphincter-saving operations (26% vs. 18%). Clearly local recurrence, as we have always known, follows incomplete resection. Plastic surgeons, using the Mohs' technique for chemosurgical resection of squamous cell carcinoma of the face, have for years used multiple frozen-section biopsies to guide their extirpative efforts and to protect against leaving cancer in place. Similar efforts might greatly improve excision of these rectal tumors. We might even be able to lure the pathologists into the operating room, witness the excision, and take the specimen to look for involvement of the margins.—J.C. Thompson, M.D.

Improved Survival in Epidermoid Carcinoma of the Anus in Association With Preoperative Multidisciplinary Therapy

Warren E. Enker, Martin Heilwell, Abbe J. Janov, Stuart H. Quan, Gordon Magill, Maus W. Stearns, Jr., Brenda Shank, Robert Leaming, and Stephen S. Sternberg (Mem. Sloan-Kettering Cancer Ctr., New York)
Arch. Surg. 121:1386–1390, December 1986   23–11

The authors report the outcome of treatment of epidermoid carcinoma in two groups of patients who were treated with or without multidisciplinary preoperative protocol. From 1973 to 1983, 78 patients with primary anal cancers were treated. Forty-four patients were administered fluorouracil intravenously (750 mg/sq m for 5 days), mitomycin (10–15 mg/sq m on day 1), followed sequentially by 3000 rads of external beam irradiation to the pelvis over 3 weeks. After examination 3 to 5 weeks later, if gross residual tumor was present, abdominoperineal resection was performed. Thirty-four patients were treated without preoperative multidisciplinary therapy, usually surgically.

Within the protocol group, 20 (4.5%) were initially treated by local excisions. In 24 (54.5%) patients, abdominal resection was performed. In nonprotocol patients, 2 underwent fulguration, 8 (33%) underwent local excisions, and 14 (58%) underwent abdominoperineal resection. Five patients did not have surgery for various reasons. At a median follow-up of 42 months in the protocol group, 5 patients were dead, 17 were censored (whose last observation was short of the median), and 22 (81.5%) of 27 were alive or past the median. In the nonprotocol group, 14 patients were dead, 6 were censored, and 14 (50%) of 28 patients were alive at the median. At 60 months or longer, 8 (80%; 1 with disease) of 10 protocol patients were alive and 4 (50%; 1 with disease) of 8 nonprotocol patients were alive. Of protocol-treated patients, 18 (41%) had residual tumor on the resected or excised specimen compared with 24 (70.6%) in the nonprotocol group. Tumor recurrence was seen in 10 (23%) protocol patients and 17 (50%) nonprotocol patients.

Clinically estimated tumor size significantly influenced the outcome. Survival differences according to size also were attributable to protocol treatment. Documentation of pathologically positive inguinal lymph nodes included 2 (4.5%) protocol patients and 4 (12%) nonprotocol patients. Poor survival was associated with age; patients aged younger than 60 years showed a survival advantage. Survival seemed to slightly favor women. Eleven (69%) of 16 protocol patients had deep infiltration on pathologic examination compared with 19 (91%) of 21 nonprotocol patients.

As dramatic clinical and pathologic tumor regression was seen in most patients, with no residual tumors in 60% treated by protocol, the authors attribute differences between the groups to treatment used. Sex, age, size, nodal status, level of invasion, and clinical stage should be considered in the randomization and stratification scheme of future studies.

▶ Last year in this section, the highly promising improvement in the primary treatment of anal carcinoma (achieved by means of combined chemotherapy and irradiation followed by local excision [*Cancer* 51:1826–1829, 1983]) was described with the conclusion that if these early results were substantiated by later experience, the cure rate would be greatly improved. This report from the Memorial Sloan-Kettering Cancer Center in New York is difficult to interpret for several reasons: the two series (protocol and nonprotocol) of patients are not comparable, patients are not randomly assigned, patients are not necessarily similar in severity (69% of protocol patients showed deep infiltration on histologic exam, and 91% of nonprotocol patients had deep infiltration), and patients underwent different operations. At the time of operation 75% of the protocol group was free of disease, compared to 32% of the nonprotocol group. These results provide continuing support for the early enthusiasm for this combined regimen; we will probably have to wait another 5–8 years before we can be certain. Nonetheless, anyone treating patients with squamous cell carcinoma of the anus should avail their patients of this treatment.—J.C. Thompson, M.D.

Technical Modifications Making On-Table Washout Easier
A.H.R.W. Simpson and W.H.F. Thomson (Gloucestershire Royal Hosp., Gloucester, England)
Br. J. Surg. 74:464, June 1987   23–12

On-table colonic lavage is a routine procedure. This brief report describes two modifications to facilitate this technique. Instead of amputating the appendix and intubating the stump, the appendix is slit transversely and intubated (Fig 23–3). The second modification involves evacuating the contents of the large bowel rectally through a large, cuffed endotracheal tube into a bucket placed between the patient's legs (Fig 23–4). Before transection, the bowel is cross-clamped and then irrigated with antiseptics.

This procedure can be used even when the bowel is partially obstructed. This method clears any fecal material that remains after preoperative purgation.

▶ Intraoperative colonic lavage has been widely used in the United Kingdom for several years (*Br. J. Surg.* 67:80–81, 1980). The method is often used so as

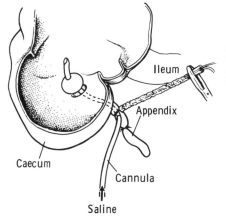

Fig 23–3.—The appendix is (dilated if necessary and then) intubated in a similar manner to the cystic duct for cholangiography. (Courtesy of Simpson, A.H.R.W., and Thomson, W.H.F.: Br. J. Surg. 74:464, June 1987.)

Ileum

Appendix

Caecum

Cannula

Saline

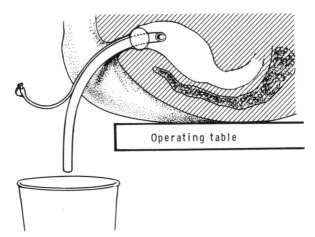

Fig 23–4.—The anal canal is intubated with a large endotracheal tube. (Courtesy of Simpson, A.H.R.W., and Thomson, W.H.F.: Br. J. Surg. 74:464, June 1987.)

to allow primary anastomosis of an obstructed colon. American surgeons have been slow to adopt the technique: one of the main reasons has been dissatisfaction with the usual mess involved in conducting the lavage. This brief snippet provides a simple method for irrigating the entire colon and draining the irrigant through the rectum, avoiding the threat of spill at the operating table. The entire colon is thereby lavaged, from cecum to rectum.—J.C. Thompson, M.D.

Colectomy With Ileorectal Anastomosis for Familial Adenomatous Polyposis: The Risk of Rectal Cancer
Richard G. Sarre, David G. Jagelman, Gerald J. Beck, Ellen McGannon, Victor W. Fazio, Frank L. Weakley, and Ian C. Lavery (Cleveland Clinic Found., Cleveland)
Surgery 101:20–26, January 1987   23–13

The management of familial adenomatous polyposis is controversial. The authors advocate treating this condition by abdominal colectomy with ileorectal anastomosis, leaving 12 to 15 cm of rectum in situ. The case records of 133 patients who underwent resection with ileorectal or ileosigmoid anastomosis were evaluated. Postoperative follow-up was usually done every 6 months with proctoscopy and fulguration of excision of any polyps seen. Once clear of polyps, proctoscopy was performed annually. The risk of developing cancer in the rectal stump was studied using actuarial determination of net survivorship in patients who were free of cancer and was analyzed with respect to various factors.

At the time of diagnosis, all patients had at least one rectal polyp. The net survivorship rate for those free of cancer was 96% at 10 years. At 20 years, 68% of women and 93% of men were free of cancer, for a total of 88%. Median length of follow-up was 65 months (range, 0–441 months). For patients with fewer than 20 polyps at initial surgery, 97% were free of rectal cancer at 20 years. The figures were 77% and 78% for those with more than 20 polyps and those with innumerable polyps, respectively. In 26 of 117 patients, total regression of rectal polyps was noted during the first postoperative year. One or more cancers in the resected colon at initial colectomy were seen in 22 patients. At 20 years' follow-up, there was little, if any, increase in the risk of developing rectal cancer specifically related to the presence of a previous colon cancer. At 20 years' follow-up, 84% of patients aged older than 40 years at the time of colectomy and 93% of patients aged younger than 40 years were free of rectal cancer. In 111 patients whose rectal stump was measured, there was no significant difference between those with anastomosis less than 15 cm from the anus compared with those with an anastomosis 15 cm or greater. Rectal cancer developed in 10 patients after colectomy and ileorectal anastomosis, with a mean interval of 10 years.

Advantages of colectomy and ileorectal anastomosis include safety and good functional result regarding bowel habit. The authors believe that the incidence of rectal cancer development is low enough to justify this procedure as long as a strict follow-up is enforced. The establishment of a registry for families with polyposis seems to have encouraged improved compliance with follow-up.

▶ This is a huge collection of patients with this rare condition (also known as Gardner's syndrome). The question today would be whether these patients should be treated by total abdominal colectomy, mucosal proctectomy, and ileoanal anastomosis, or whether it is sufficiently safe to do a total abdominal colectomy with anastomosis of the ileum to the rectum. The authors make a strong case for the latter procedure, reporting 96% of their patients to be free of rectal cancer at 10 years and 88% to be free of cancer at 20 years. Patients with a rectal stump of less than 15 cm did significantly better than those whose remaining rectal segment was longer. As with patients with hereditary multiple polyposis of the colon, anything less than complete removal of all the mucosa at risk means that the surgeon must assume responsibility for lifelong maintenance of close observation with repeated 6-month to annual proctoscopic examination of the remaining rectal mucosa. The operation of total abdominal colectomy, mucosal proctectomy, and ileoanal anastomosis obviates that risk, but the procedure is associated with many more complications and only a relatively small number of surgeons have great experience with the operation. This means that except for certain centers, most all patients with malignant polyp syndromes will undergo abdominal colectomy and ileorectal anastomosis. The patient, the patient's family, and the surgeon must all undertake the responsibility of lifelong monitoring.—J.C. Thompson, M.D.

S-Pouches vs. J-Pouches: A Comparison of Functional Outcomes
S.M. McHugh, N.E. Diamant, R. McLeod, and Z. Cohen (Toronto Western Hosp. and Toronto Gen. Hosp.)
Dis. Colon Rectum 30:671–677, September 1987   23–14

Seventy patients who underwent restorative proctocolectomy with loop ileostomy closure were evaluated with respect to the functional outcomes of three pouch constructions used: the J-pouch long rectal cuff of 8 to 10 cm, the J-pouch short rectal cuff of 2 to 3 cm, and the S-pouch short rectal cuff of 2 to 3 cm. Both objective and subjective, i.e., self-monitoring diary, measures were used.

The S-pouch patients appeared to have better early functional results than the J-pouch subjects; however, no significant differences were found between the functional results of both groups at least 1 year after ileostomy closure. Virtually all subjects preferred their pouch surgery to conventional ileostomy and would recommend the same procedure to others contemplating surgery. However, a number of subjects had significant social, recreational, and work disability that correlated with increased total bowel movement frequency, nocturnal bowel movement frequency, and more episodes of fecal soiling. Bowel habit worries were reported by one third of patients and were associated with behavioral changes to accommodate a bowel habit that was not entirely predictable. Greater than normal frequency of bowel activity was associated with stools that were usually watery and with decreased abilities to discriminate flatus from stool. Fecal soiling was present in 84% of patients but was a significant problem in only 20%.

The actual significance of these symptoms is difficult to determine at present. It appears that further efforts should be directed toward features separate from pouch size to improve the functional outcome. The quality of life of individuals with restorative proctocolectomy should be compared to those having surgery.

▶ Which pouch is best? What criteria are pertinent in evaluating bowel function after mucosal proctectomy and ileoanal anastomosis? These problems have been discussed in these pages for the last 3 years, and if any solution is available, it is not yet apparent. One cannot help but wonder just how different the results would be if a straight anastomosis was made between the ileum and the anus, avoiding pouches. Surely with all the troubles found in long-term studies of patients with various reservoirs it should be worth trying the simplest procedure. Each different ileoanal maven has his own set of rules, rules regarding indications for operation, staging or nonstaging of procedures, loop or diverting ileostomy, the proper length of the rectal segment, and the correct criteria needed in order to decide which patient is a success and which patient is not. We will need some time to get it straight. Nearly everyone agrees that patients who have had an abdominal ileostomy that is converted to ileoanal anastomosis much prefers the latter if it works at all well. Perhaps a convention of patients, operated upon by different surgeons, might be convened in order to compare experiences and provide a guiding light.—J.C. Thompson, M.D.

The Colostomy Plug: A New Disposable Device for a Continent Colostomy
Flemming Burcharth, Akeel Ballan, Frederik Kylberg, and Sten Nørby

Rasmussen (Univ. of Copenhagen; Coloplast Ltd., Espergaerde, Denmark; Karl-stad Hosp., Sweden; and Aalborg Hosp. North, Denmark)
Lancet 2:1062-1063, Nov. 8, 1986   23–15

In 1984 the authors invented a disposable device for colostomy control, a colostomy plug that could be used by many patients. This colostomy continence device is a disposable two-piece system consisting of an adhesive base plate and disposable colostomy plug. A hole in the plate's center allows the seal to be cut to the stoma's size. A coupling flange is around this hole, permitting it to be effectively linked to the plug or a colostomy bag. The plug is composed of open-cell polyurethane foam, enabling bowel gas to pass and be released but preventing feces and fluid passage. This plug is fixed to a water-impermeable cover with a carbon filter and then compressed in a water-soluble film. A few seconds after insertion, the film disintegrates and the plug expands to its natural size. A colostomy bag may be applied to the plate upon plug removal, or bowel irrigation may be done. A new plug is applied following evacuation.

This plug was tested in 53 consecutive patients. All were able to use it, and 50 reported insertion to be simple. Thirty-seven (70%) found the plug easy to apply to the base plate. Complete fecal continence was obtained with 445 (86%) of the plugs. Intestinal gas passed freely in 466 (90%). In 130 cases (25%) the plug was replaced when obstructed partially by feces or mucus. With 90% of the plugs, gas passed noiselessly, and with 477 (92%) gas passed with no odor. Some abdominal discomfort was felt by meteorism or intestinal colic with 15% of plugs. Forty (75%) patients had a plug in position for more than 5 hours; 79% of plugs were used for more than 5 hours. A significant difference was observed between groups using irrigation and natural evacuation in the numbers of plugs used for more than 5 hours. No complications were observed.

This system appeared effective in storing fecal matter inside the intestine. Only a few patients found it ineffective.

▶ This sounds like a splendid idea. Where do you buy it? I guess from Coloplast Limited in Espergaerde, Denmark. These are the people who invented the disposable colostomy bag that is used all over the world, and I imagine this apparatus would also work well.—J.C. Thompson, M.D.

Simple In-Office Sphincterotomy With Partial Fissurectomy for Chronic Anal Fissure
Bruce S. Gingold (St. Vincent's Hosp. and Beth Israel Med. Ctr., New York)
Surg. Gynecol. Obstet. 165:46–48, July 1987   23–16

Anal fissure is a common painful condition of the anorectum. The author describes a simple in-office treatment for this condition that has been used successfully in 86 patients.

The patient is placed on the proctoscopy table and prepared with io-

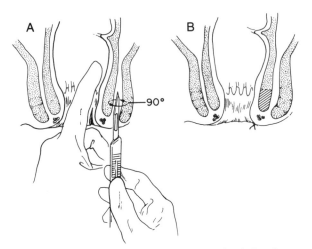

Fig 23–5.—Partial lateral internal sphincterotomy. **A**, insertion of scalpel, and **B**, appearance at conclusion of sphincterotomy. (Courtesy of Gingold, B.S.: Surg. Gynecol. Obstet. 165:46–48, July 1987.)

dine antiseptic. The patient is anesthetized with 0.25% bupivacaine. Wheals are raised in the subcutaneous perianal and submucosal areas with a 30 gauge needle. Additional anesthetic is applied to the raphe between the internal and external sphincter muscle and to the area of the fissure. A no. 11 scalpel blade is inserted in the intersphincteric groove (Fig 23–5,A) and advanced higher than the fissure. The blade is rotated so that the sharp edge faces the canal and the blade is withdrawn, transecting the internal sphincter muscle. If bleeding persists, it is controlled with a single 3-0 Vicryl suture (Fig 23–5,B). A Hill-Fergueson retractor is used to expose the fissure (Fig 23–6,A). Scar tissue or a sentinal tag is excised with a cautery wire loop tip (Fig 23–6,B). Granulation tissue is removed by scraping with a small curette. The base of the fissure does not have to be excised (Fig 23–6,C), minimizing the risk of a keyhole deformity. A pressure dressing is applied, and the pa-

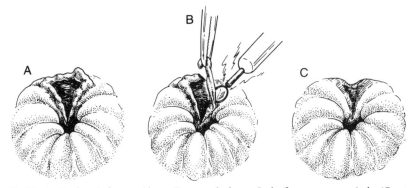

Fig 23–6.—**A**, chronic fissure with tag. **B**, removal of scar. **C**, the fissure postoperatively. (Courtesy of Gingold, B.S.: Surg. Gynecol. Obstet. 165:46–48, July 1987.)

tient is allowed to recover for 15–30 minutes. The entire procedure takes 10 minutes. Patients must lie flat for that day but can resume normal activities the next day. They must avoid heavy lifting and high dietary residue items for 1–2 weeks until healing can occur.

The median time of patient follow-up was 2 years. There have been no recurrences in 96.4% of these cases. There were no significant complications. Partial lateral sphincterotomy should be the treatment of choice for routine anal fissures that do not respond to medical management.

▶ This looks like a good solution to a difficult problem. I have trouble getting anywhere close to the fissure in some patients, and I am surprised at the apparent efficacy of local anesthesia, which means of course that the anesthetic agent is applied slowly and profusely. How easy is it to find the intersphincteric groove in a patient in whom you have injected local anesthetic? It is all probably easy as pie once you have seen it done.—J.C. Thompson, M.D.

24 The Liver and the Spleen

Intraoperative Ultrasound of the Liver: An Important Adjunctive Tool for Decision Making in the Operating Room
Matthew D. Rifkin, Francis E. Rosato, H. Mitchell Branch, Jonathan Foster, Shuin-Lin Yang, Donna J. Barbot, and Gerald J. Marks (Thomas Jefferson Univ., Philadelphia)
Ann. Surg. 205:466–472, May 1987   24–1

Intraoperative ultrasound has recently become a complementary procedure for many routine and complicated surgical procedures. Delineation of hepatic, biliary, and pancreatic tissue can be clearly demonstrated, and the efficacy of this technique is becoming more widespread. A study was done using prospective diagnosis and retrospective analysis of data to evaluate the benefits of intraoperative ultrasound of the liver in 49 patients with possible hepatic pathology.

The patients were examined during surgery with a 7.5-MHz linear array transducer attached to a specially produced intraoperative ultrasound machine, an Aloka 330. Disposable, sterile sheaths were used to cover the transducer. The entire liver was imaged in longitudinal and transaxial orientations. When unsuspected nonpalpable lesions were found, ultrasound-guided biopsies were done. This technique required an average of 10 to 15 minutes of additional operating time. In 55% of subjects, no new information was obtained by this technique. In 19%, new information was obtained that changed the surgical approach. In another 14%, new information was obtained, but no change in therapeutic approach was needed. In 12% of the patients, no new information was gathered, but a change in surgical approach and management of the patient was made possible by the use of intraoperative ultrasound. The effectiveness of the various imaging techniques was compared, and, overall, operative ultrasonography was found to be the most sensitive.

This study demonstrated that the routine use of ultrasound during operative procedures, particularly those involving hepatic structures, is clinically useful. In a significant proportion of the patients, it can change the course of management.

▶ There is increasing evidence that intraoperative ultrasonography is an important adjunctive procedure. It provides definition of common duct stones and facilitates hepatic resection at surgery. Cosgrove and associates (*JCU* 15:231, 1987) showed that the portal, venous, and arterial supply, plus the hepatic veins, can be defined ultrasonographically, thus expediting the selection of lines of resection. In the cirrhotic patients, the use of intraoperative ultrasound has permitted definition of small hepatocellular carcinomas and allowed a resection that minimized tissue loss. An article in *World J. Surg.* 11(5), 1987, is devoted to a symposium addressing advances in intraoperative ultrasound. Bismuth et al. (*World J. Surg.* 10:614, 1987) evaluated operative ultrasound in 77 patients submitted for surgery for primary liver tumors. His technique provided more detailed information about the liver tumors than can be obtained by any preoperative investigation. Makuuchi (*World J. Surg.* 11:615, 1987) evaluated 386 patients receiving intraoperative ultrasonography. This procedure led to the development of new, liver-sparing hepatectomy procedures. It was regarded as indispensable in liver surgery, not only for diagnosis of tumor spread in the liver, but also as a direct guide for hepatectomy. Boldrini et al. (*World J. Surg.* 11:622, 1987) reported that previous undetected neoplastic nodules were visualized as a result of the systematic use of operative ultrasonography for liver scanning during colorectal surgery.—S.I. Schwartz, M.D.

The Use of Operative Ultrasound as an Aid to Liver Resection in Patients With Hepatocellular Carcinoma

Masatoshi Makuuchi, Hiroshi Hasegawa, Susumu Yamazaki, Kenichi Takayasu, and Noriyuki Moriyama (Natl. Cancer Ctr. Hosp., Tokyo)
World J. Surg. 11:615–621, October 1987   24–2

Real-time operative ultrasonography has been used since 1979 for detecting small tumor nodules. Of 391 patients having laparotomy for hepatectomy in 1979–1985, 386 underwent intraoperative sonography and 347 had hepatic resection. Hepatocellular carcinoma was present in 245 patients, 152 of whom had tumors less than 5 cm in diameter.

A total of 203 small hepatocellular carcinomas were identified, and 191 of them were resected from 145 patients. Operative ultrasonography was significantly more sensitive than preoperative ultrasonography, an-

DIAGNOSIS OF DAUGHTER NODULES OR INTRAHEPATIC METASTASIS IN 152 PATIENTS WITH SMALL HEPATOCELLULAR CARCINOMA

	Intraoperative ultrasonography	Preoperative ultrasonography	Angiography	Computed tomography
Sensitivity (%)	41.7	12.5	14.0	22.4
Specificity (%)	82.2	92.2	92.0	89.2
Predictive value of positive test (%)	48.8	40.0	41.2	50.0
Predictive value of negative test (%)	76.9	69.6	69.2	70.5
Overall accuracy (%)	69.1	66.7	66.0	67.5

(Courtesy of Makuuchi, M., et al.: World J. Surg. 11:615–621, October 1987.)

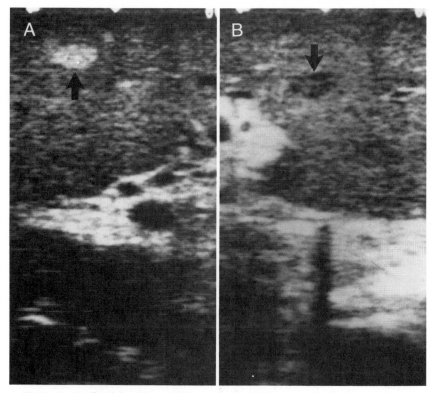

Fig 24–1.—Small nodules of hepatocellular carcinoma which were not found on preoperative examination. Patient is a 62-year-old man with hepatocellular carcinoma in the anterosuperior area and chronic hepatitis. **A,** other than the main tumor of the liver, echogenic tumor *(arrow)* is seen in the left medial segment. This tumor is a hepatocellular carcinoma of Edmondson's grade 1. **B,** the third tumor *(arrow)* is seen in left lateral segment. It is hypoechoic, and the histologic diagnosis is a hepatocellular carcinoma of Edmondson's grade 2. (Courtesy of Makuuchi, M., et al.: World J. Surg. 11:615–621, October 1987.)

giography, and computed tomography (Fig 24–1). In patients with small tumors, the intraoperative study was two to three times more sensitive than the preoperative studies (table). More than 40% of hepatocellular carcinomas were not visible or palpable from the liver surface. The ability to distinguish tumor, vessels, and lines of liver transection promoted the use of systematic subsegmentectomy (Fig 24–2) and of hepatectomy preserving the inferior right hepatic vein. Intraoperative ultrasonography demonstrates the inferior right hepatic vein more clearly than preoperative examination.

Intraoperative ultrasonography is indispensable in liver surgery, both for diagnosing tumor spread in the liver and for guiding transection and vessel puncture. More precise resective surgical procedures are possible using this method.

▶ This is an appropriate consideration of the state of the art. Bismuth et al. (*World J. Surg.* 11:610, 1987) evaluated operative ultrasonograms in 77 pa-

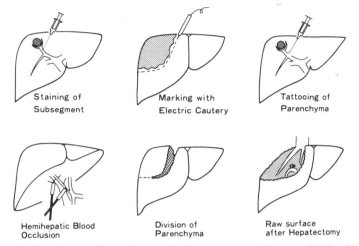

Fig 24–2.—Operative procedure of systematic subsegmentectomy. (Courtesy of Makuuchi, M., et al.: World J. Surg. 11:615–621, October 1987.)

tients submitted to operation for primary liver tumor. Preoperative ultrasonography, computed tomography, and hepatic arteriography were performed in all patients. The operative ultrasonogram provided additional information in 33% of cases. Often the information modified the intended surgical procedure and facilitated a subsegmental resection. Boldrini et al. (*World J. Surg.* 11:622, 1987) advised routine use of intraoperative ultrasonography for detection of liver metastases during colorectal surgery. Previously undetected nodules, including lesions that escaped visualization, were noted.—S.I. Schwartz, M.D.

Cavernous Hemangioma of the Liver: A Single Institution Report of 16 Resections
Seymour I. Schwartz and Wendy Cowles Husser (Univ. of Rochester, N.Y.)
Ann. Surg. 205:456–465, May 1987   24–3

Cavernous hemangioma is the most frequent primary liver tumor. Sixteen patients had resection of cavernous hemangioma of the liver at one institution from 1959 to 1986. In the same period, 12 patients were not operated on. Three fourths of all patients were women. Symptoms were not characteristic of a hepatic lesion. A liver mass was palpated in half of the operated patients. One patient noted a rapidly enlarging mass in early pregnancy (Fig 24–3).

The indications for surgery were an abdominal mass, pain, or both. A wide range of resective procedures was employed (Fig 24–4). The lesions averaged 10 cm in size, compared with less than 5 cm in unoperated patients. In some cases an ultrasonic scalpel was used for parenchymal dissection or to enucleate a central lesion. Twelve patients received transfusions. Two patients developed subphrenic abscess, and 1 was reexplored for bleeding, but there were no operative deaths. In the patients who did

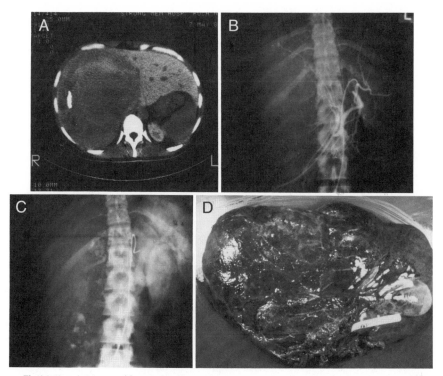

Fig 24–3.—A 31-year-old woman with rapid appearance of hemangioma during the first trimester of pregnancy. **A,** computed tomographic scan shows tumor replacement of right lobe and organized clot within the tumor. **B,** arterial phase of hepatic artery angiogram shows relatively avascular mass replacing the right lobe of the liver and displacement of the hepatic arterial system into the left upper quadrant. **C,** venous phase of hepatic artery angiogram shows typical pooling of dye in segments of the tumor, the majority of which does not opacify. The portal vein has been displaced into the left upper quadrant. **D,** specimen consisting of right lobe and medial segment of left lobe (3,700 gm). (Courtesy of Schwartz, S.I., and Husser, W.C.: Ann. Surg. 205:456–465, May 1987.)

not undergo surgery, no progression of symptoms was observed and there were no adverse sequelae of the liver lesion. All the patients who had surgery were asymptomatic when last evaluated.

The possibility of rupture is not an indication for resection of a cavernous hemangioma of the liver. All the present patients who were observed rather than being operated on have done well. When treatment is indicated, surgical excision is the only consistently effective approach. Hepatic artery ligation has not reduced the size of these lesions.

▶ In a parallel report, Bornman et al. (*Surgery* 101:445, 1987) came to the same conclusion that resection in asymptomatic cases should be carried out only in those cases that require a diagnostic laparotomy and where the lesion is easily resectable. These authors described four surgically treated giant hemangiomas and indicated that an important diagnostic triad (clinical signs of acute inflammatory process of the liver, accompanied by normal liver function tests and a white blood count) should alert the clinician to the diagnosis. None of our

NO.	AGE	SEX	INDICATION	LESION DIAMETER EXTENT OF RESECTION	BLOOD RE-PLACEMENT	COMPLICATION
1	61	F	Mass + ITP	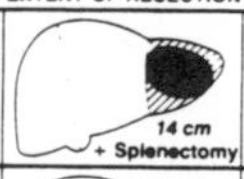 14 cm + Splenectomy	1000 (ml)	—
2	56	F	Mass	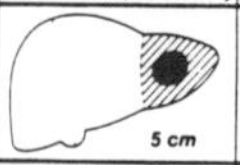 5 cm	2000 (ml)	—
3	53	F	Pain	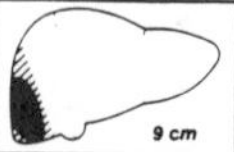 9 cm	—	—
4	51	M	Pain	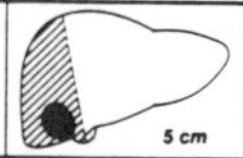 5 cm	4000 (ml)	—
5	42	F	Pain	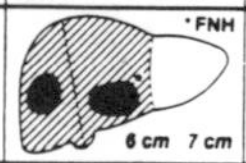 · FNH 6 cm 7 cm	1000 (ml)	Postoperative Bleed
6	48	F	Mass + Pain	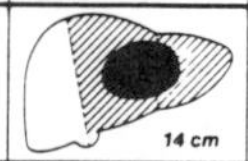 14 cm	4000 (ml)	—
7	36	F	Mass	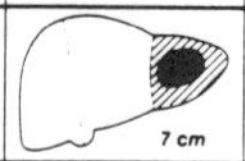 7 cm	500 (ml)	—
8	53	M	Diagnosed Hepatocellular Carcinoma	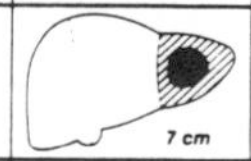 7 cm	1000 (ml)	—
9	32	F	Mass + Pain	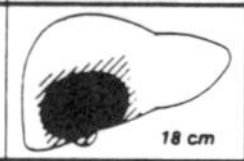 18 cm	3500 (ml)	—
10	57	F	Pain	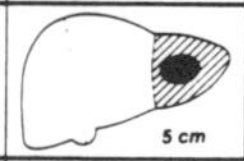 5 cm	—	—
11	80	M	Incidental	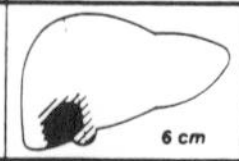 6 cm	—	—
12	31	F	Mass (Rapid Growth) Pregnancy	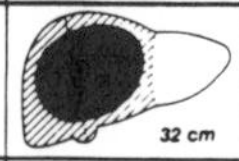 32 cm	3500 (ml)	Subphrenic Abscess
13	43	M	Pain	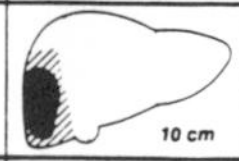 10 cm	5000 (ml)	Subphrenic Abscess
14	71	F	? Metastatic Tumor	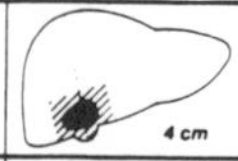 4 cm	500 (ml)	—
15	43	F	Pain + Mass	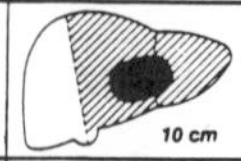 10 cm	2000 (ml)	—
16	50	F	Pain + Mass	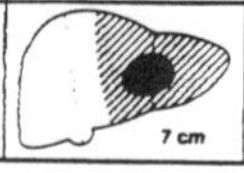 7 cm	—	—

Fig 24—4.—Cavernous hemangioma. Sixteen hepatic resections. (Courtesy of Schwartz, S.I., and Husser, W.C.: Ann. Surg. 205:456–465, May 1987.)

patients have had rigor and pyrexia, although they often had pain and hepatomegaly. We also have not encountered the situation in which the angiogram, coupled with infusion computed tomography scan, fails to delineate the lesion. We feel that magnetic resonance imaging is the preferred initial diagnostic modality.—S.I. Schwartz, M.D.

Human Liver Regeneration After Major Hepatic Resection: A Study of Normal Liver and Livers With Chronic Hepatitis and Cirrhosis
Naofumi Nagasue, Hirofumi Yukaya, Yuichiro Ogawa, Hitoshi Kohno, and Teruhisa Nakamura (Hiroshima Red Cross Hosp. and Shimane Med. Univ., Izumo, Japan)
Ann. Surg. 206:30–39, July 1987   24–4

Normal liver has remarkable regenerative capacity after major resection. Cirrhotic livers are less able to regenerate, and major resection is contraindicated in the presence of liver cirrhosis. Nevertheless, some patients with cirrhosis have been able to tolerate extensive hepatic resection, and it therefore is wiser to select candidates for major resection from patients with cirrhosis by quantitative evaluation of hepatic reserve in each case. The regenerative process was assessed in 28 adults undergoing major hepatic resection. Liver size, function, and histology were considered.

Twenty-one patients had hepatocellular carcinoma, 4 had secondary liver cancer from colorectum, 1 had carcinoma of the gallbladder, 1 had Klatskin tumor, and 1 had Caroli's disease. Twenty-two were men and 6 were women, aged 17 to 74 years. All patients with hepatocellular carcinoma had underlying liver disease: 14 with liver cirrhosis and 7 with chronic hepatitis. Extended right lobectomy was performed in 10 cases, right lobectomy in 16, and left lobectomy in 2. In 15 patients, residual liver size was serially estimated by computed tomography (CT). Six had normal liver, 5 had chronic hepatitis, and 4 had cirrhosis. In 2 patients with normal livers, a complete restoration of the residual liver size was seen in 3 and 6 months, respectively. In all patients with the parenchymal diseases, the liver was enlarged, but more slowly, compared with normal liver. In patients with normal livers, liver functions were restored to normal within 2 to 3 weeks. Nevertheless, hyperbilirubinemia persisted longer in those with chronic hepatitis and cirrhosis. A continuous rise of bilirubin signaled liver failure and subsequent death in 5 patients with cirrhosis. Serum α-fetoprotein did not rise in accordance with regeneration. Histologic evidence of active regeneration with increased mitotic activity was seen at 10 and 35 days in patients with normal livers. Mitosis was not found in a specimen taken at 7 days. Enlarged cuboidal hepatocytes and cells with basophilic cytoplasm or two nuclei were generally seen in all specimens. Livers with cirrhosis or hepatitis also had histologic evidence of regeneration in the first 2 months, but it was substantially less compared with normal liver, supported by CT volumetric studies of the liver remnants.

This study demonstrated that normal liver regenerates much faster than previously assumed. Cirrhotic livers or livers with chronic hepatitis enlarged more slowly but completed restoration in some patients with these parenchymal disorders. Patients for liver resection should be selected on the basis of quantitative—not qualitative—evaluation.

▶ This is perhaps the most detailed assessment of hepatic regeneration after major resection. The demonstration that the cirrhotic liver regenerates, albeit at a slower rate, is of interest. But it would have been helpful if the authors had defined the extent of cirrhosis, the etiology of the cirrhosis in each instance, and the extent of hepatic dysfunction at the time of resection. Our own anecdotal experience with hepatic resection in a patient with extensive cirrhosis is that a major resection is intolerable; this liver has shown little evidence of significant regeneration. Our patient with cirrhosis had alcoholic nutritional cirrhosis and hyperbilirubinemia preoperatively and mild ascites.—S.I. Schwartz, M.D.

Optimizing Surgical Management of Symptomatic Solitary Hepatic Cysts
John D. Edwards, Frederic E. Eckhauser, James A. Knol, William E. Strodel, and Henry D. Appelman (VA Med. Ctr., Ann Arbor, Mich., and Univ. of Michigan)
Am. Surg. 53:510–514, September 1987   24–5

The clinical course of ten patients with symptomatic solitary cysts of the liver are reviewed in this report. The average age of these patients was 49 years. The most common symptoms included pain, a palpable mass, and early postprandial satiety. Liver function tests were normal. Either ultrasound or computed tomography could be used for diagnosis.

Eight patients had simple cysts and two patients had multilocular complex cysts. In the patients treated by needle aspiration, incision, and internal drainage or external catheter drainage, the cyst recurred, requiring reoperation. The cysts did not recur in patients treated by unroofing the cyst or excision. One patient had a carcinoma in the cyst wall.

Extensive unroofing of solitary hepatic cysts minimizes cyst recurrence and the need for hepatic resection. Multilocular cysts should be treated by excision. All cysts with neoplasms should be treated by excision.

▶ Only a very large or symptomatic solitary cyst requires surgical intervention. Percutaneous drainage is usually associated with recurrence. In most instances, large cysts containing clear fluid can be managed simply by an extensive unroofing procedure. This obviates the need for hepatic resection. Multilocular cysts and cysts that have been associated with intracystic bleeding usually are more readily managed by hepatic resection. The reported finding of an unsuspected carcinoma in the cyst wall is quite uncommon, particularly in the case of unilocular cyst containing clear fluid.—S.I. Schwartz, M.D.

Role of Surgery in the Treatment of Primary Carcinoma of the Liver: A 31-Year Experience

T.-Y. Lin, C.-S. Lee, K.-M. Chen, and C.-C. Chen (Natl. Taiwan Univ., Taipei)
Br. J. Surg. 74:839–842, September 1987   24–6

Review was made of 225 major hepatic resections done for symptomatic primary liver cancer in 1954–1985. The series included 115 right hepatic lobectomies and 94 left hepatic lobectomies. Another 107 partial hepatic resections were carried out in 89 patients having small asymptomatic hepatocellular carcinomas.

Operative mortality was 8% in the patients having major hepatic resection and 5.6% in those having partial resection. Five operations were for cholangiocarcinoma rather than hepatocellular carcinoma. The finger fracture technique was consistently used. Hepatic clamping and the Pringle maneuver were utilized in selected cases. The 5-year survival after major hepatic resection was 18%. Twenty-eight of the 89 patients undergoing partial resection for small asymptomatic carcinomas died within 4 years after surgery from a second new growth. None of these patients died of liver failure after primary liver surgery.

Very satisfactory long-term results have been obtained by major hepatic resection in patients with primary liver cancer. The chief cause of late deaths was recurrence in the remaining lobe of the liver. Intraoperative ultrasonography will make it possible to detect deep-seated metastatic nodules in the contralateral lobe before lobectomy is undertaken.

▶ This extensive report comes from the experience of Professor Lin, whose name is associated with the promulgation of the finger fracture technique. A 5-year survival rate of 18% is in keeping with most reports. Nagasue et al. (*Br. J. Surg.* 74:836, 1987) reported 38 patients with hepatocellular carcinoma smaller than 3 cm in diameter, all superimposed on hepatic disease. A radical resection was performed in 32 cases, and the survival rate at 4 years was 59%. In the Oriental populations surveillance is carried out in patients with hepatitis. Using alpha-fetoprotein as a marker and ultrasonography as an imaging technique, early lesions are detected. This situation rarely occurs in our patient population.—S.I. Schwartz, M.D.

Hepatic Resection for Hepatocellular Carcinoma: Clinical Features and Long-Term Prognosis

Takeshi Nagao, Shinichiro Goto, Nobuhiro Kawano, Sumio Inoue, Tetsuaki Mizuta, Yasuhiko Morioka, and Yoshimichi Omori (Tokyo Univ.)
Ann. Surg. 205:33–40, January 1987   24–7

The incidence of hepatocellular carcinoma (HCC) has greatly increased during the last decade. Although long-term survival of patients cannot be expected with any treatment other than resection, the resection rate remains considerably low. From 1963 to 1985, 98 hepatic resections for HCC were done on 94 patients and the results were reviewed.

There were 19 deaths (19%) among the 94 patients. Ten died within 30 days after operation; the main causes were hepatic failure and postoperative bleeding. The survival rate of the other 75 patients at 1, 3, and 5 years was 73%, 42%, and 25%, respectively; including the hospital deaths, the rates were 58%, 33%, and 20%, respectively.

Macroscopically, 63% of the main tumors were encapsulated by fibrous tissue, which is different from other malignant tumors. The predictive value of preoperative laboratory data was investigated on long-term survival. An analysis of serum albumin level, linearity index of oral glucose tolerance test, and maximal removal rate of indocyanine green indicated no differences in survival patterns; nor was there any significant difference in survival pattern on the basis of Child's classification.

In 17% of the patients, HBs antigen was positive; in 70%, preoperative serum alpha-fetoprotein was more than 20 ng/ml, and in 75%, liver cirrhosis was present. Significant differences of survival patterns were seen when analyzed on the basis of preoperative alpha-fetoprotein level ($\leq$ 200 vs. > 200 ng/ml), tumor size ($\leq$ 5 vs. > 5 cm), and tumor capsule. Survival patterns were not influenced by microscopically proved concomitant liver diseases, such as cirrhosis, fibrosis, and chronic hepatitis. Carcinoma recurrence was the main cause of death in 56% (42 patients) who died after their hospital discharge.

The authors' recent standard operations for HCC are lobectomy for noncirrhotic liver and, whenever functional reserve of the liver permits, segmentectomy for cirrhotic liver.

▶ It must be emphasized that the Japanese literature has to be considered different from the experience of Western civilization. In this series, the tumor was smaller than 5 cm in 60% of patients, all of whom had liver disease. Also, 63% of the tumors were encapsulated. These two features are most unusual in our experience. With the use of intraoperative ultrasonography the Japanese have performed very limited resections, whereas most American series are based on major hepatic resection. The limited resections performed by the Japanese account for the fact that the Child's C patients do relatively well in the immediate postoperative period. Kinami et al. (*World J. Surg.* 10:294, 1986) reported on hepatic resection for hepatocellular carcinoma associated with cirrhosis in the Japanese population. The fact that the 5-year survival rate for large tumors was 0 enforces my bias that a major hepatic resection in a patient with cirrhosis has little to offer and represents a significant risk to the patient.—S.I. Schwartz, M.D.

Hepatic Resection for Colorectal Liver Metastases: Influence on Survival of Preoperative Factors and Surgery for Recurrences in 80 Patients
Bernard Nordlinger, Rolland Parc, Eric Delva, Marc-Antoine Quilichini, Laurent Hannoun, and Claude Huguet (Hôpital St. Antoine, Paris, and Princess Grâce Hosp., Monaco)
Ann. Surg. 205:256–263, March 1987   24–8

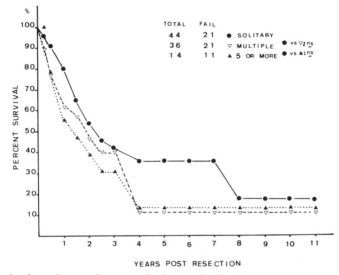

Fig 24–5.—Survival curves of patients with solitary and multiple liver metastases. (Courtesy of Nordlinger, B., et al.: Ann. Surg. 205:256–263, March 1987.)

In certain patients with liver metastases of colorectal origin, surgical resection may be the only efficient treatment. Determining the clinical factors that could predict the surgical outcome would improve patient selection. Data concerning 80 patients who underwent liver resection for metastatic colorectal carcinoma were analyzed. All primary colorectal cancers were resected.

Liver metastases were solitary in 44 patients and multiple in 36; metastases were unilobar in 76 patients and bilobar in 4. In 33 patients the tumor size was less than 5 cm; in 30 it was 5–10 cm and in 17, larger than 10 cm. There were 43 synchronous and 37 metachronous liver metastases with a delay of 2–70 months. Major liver resection was done in 55 patients and wedge resection, in 25. Usually, portal triad occlusion was used, with complete vascular exclusion of the liver performed for resection of larger tumors.

In-hospital mortality after liver resection was 5%. Including postoperative mortality, the respective 2-year, 3-year, and 5-year survival rates were 50%, 40.5%, and 25%. There was no difference in length of survival among patients with solitary liver metastases, those with multiple metastases, and those having more than four resected metastases (Fig 24–5). For patients with liver metastases smaller than 5 cm, the survival curve was not different from that for patients with larger metastases; nor was the stage of the primary tumor a determinant of survival. No difference was noted between synchronous and metachronous liver metastases with respect to survival.

During the study, 51 patients had recurrent disease, 20 during the first 6 months, and 13 had it during the next 6 months. In 21 patients the disease recurred in the liver; 17 patients had recurrence in extrahepatic sites, and 13 had recurrence in both locations. Ten patients had surgery for cancer recurrence after resection of liver metastases: 4 for extrahepatic recurrence, 2 for exploration for unresectable local retroperitoneal recurrence, 1 for a lung metastasis, and 1 for both adrenal and pulmonary metastasis.

Thus, the size and number of metastases, Duke's stage of the primary cancer, and length of delay between the diagnosis of colon cancer and the diagnosis of liver metastasis did not affect outcome after resection. The increased safety of major liver resections when performed by experienced surgeons, as well as the use of chemotherapy, may allow a more aggressive approach to the management of these patients.

► Bozzetti and associates (*Ann. Surg.* 205:264, 1987) also studied the patterns of failure following surgical resection of colorectal cancer. The stage is the most important parameter related to overall recurrence rate (47% in stage I, 62% in stage II, 81% in stage III). In stage I the extrahepatic and intrahepatic relapses were similar; in stages II and III disease intrahepatic relapses occurred more frequently. The authors concluded that resection alone is an inadequate form of therapy in the case of colorectal cancer and metastases of the liver, and they suggested including adjuvant therapy.—S.I. Schwartz, M.D.

Intrahepatic or Systemic Infusion of Fluorodeoxyuridine in Patients With Liver Metastases From Colorectal Carcinoma: A Randomized Trial
Nancy Kemeny, John Daly, Bonnie Reichman, Nancy Geller, José Botet, and Paula Oderman (Mem. Sloan-Kettering Cancer Ctr., New York)
Ann. Intern. Med. 107:459–465, October 1987   24–9

Direct infusion of a chemotherapeutic agent into the hepatic artery may be effective because hepatic metastases of colorectal cancer are supplied chiefly by this vessel. The efficacy of infusion of fluorodeoxyuridine directly was compared with systemic chemotherapy in patients having histologically verified colorectal adenocarcinoma and measurable liver metastases. Patients with evidence of extrahepatic disease were excluded. A pump was inserted with either a hepatic artery catheter or an Infuse-a-port for systemic infusion (Fig 24–6). Fluorodeoxyuridine was given for 2 weeks and saline for the same interval. The starting dose was 0.3 mg/kg daily for the intrahepatic group and 0.15 mg/kg daily for the systemic group.

Responses were significantly more frequent after hepatic arterial infusion than with systemic chemotherapy (50% vs. 20%). The only complete response was in one of the intrahepatic patients. More patients given intrahepatic therapy had a reduced level of carcinoembryonic antigen. Extrahepatic progression occurred more often in the intrahepatic group, but more systemically treated patients had disease progression in the liver. Median survivals were 17 months for the intrahepatic group and 12 months for the systemic group. Toxicity in the intrahepatic group

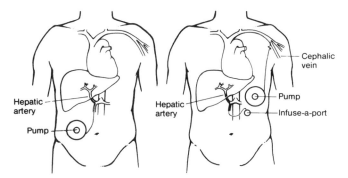

Fig 24–6.—Placement of hepatic artery catheter and pump for hepatic infusion *(left)* and placement of pump and Infuse-a-port for systemic infusion *(right)*. (Courtesy of Kemeny, N., et al.: Ann. Intern. Med. 107:459–465, October 1987.)

included four cases of biliary sclerosis, which was reversible in three instances.

Direct hepatic arterial infusion of fluorodeoxyuridine produced better results than systemic treatment in these patients with liver metastases from colorectal carcinoma. Further study of this modality is warranted.

▶ This randomized study has been conducted well and provides meaningful data. Our own experience with the use of intra-arterial chemotherapy via the implantable pump has been less encouraging. Only 15% of patients had a 50% reduction in size of tumor mass defined by imaging technique, and three quarters of the patients had significant symptoms. As a consequence of this and other poor experiences, we have kept the pump on the back burner and reserve it for patients in whom, having undergone exploration for resection, the lesion was deemed unresectable. It is to be stressed that in the present series, there is no statistically significant difference in the median survival. Daly et al. (*Arch. Surg.* 122:1273, 1987) conducted a randomized trial comparing hepatic arterial infusion with portal venous infusion and demonstrated significantly improved response after hepatic arterial infusion.—S.I. Schwartz, M.D.

Recognition and Clinical Implications of Mesenteric and Portal Vein Obstruction in Chronic Pancreatitis
Andrew L. Warshaw, Gongliang Jin, and Leslie W. Ottinger (Massachusetts Gen. Hosp. and Harvard Univ., Boston)
Arch. Surg. 122:410–415, April 1987   24–10

Occlusion of the superior mesenteric or portal veins (SMV-PV), or both, has not been appreciated in the literature, whereas splenic vein obstruction is a well-described feature of chronic pancreatitis. Only six reports of patients with mesenteric-portal venous obstruction associated with chronic pancreatitis have been found. In this article are described 14 patients with SMV-PV with proved chronic pancreatitis without cancer, of whom 11 were known alcoholics.

In 4 of the 14, portal hypertension was first suspected because of variceal bleeding; in 10 it was suspected because of unexpected varices at laparotomy. They required a total of more than 40 operations for complications of chronic pancreatitis. In only 1 case were varices detected in barium swallow examination; by endoscopy, varices were detected in 5 of 14 cases. In 1 of 13 cases, the venous phase of the superior mesenteric arteriogram showed a high-grade portal vein stenosis; and in 12 cases it showed SMV-PV occlusion or both, with surrounding retroperitoneal variceal collaterals. In 8 of 13 patients who had angiograms the splenic vein was also occluded. In all cases the liver was normal. It was estimated that in approximately 5% to 10% of the surgically treated chronic pancreatitis population SMV-PV was found: an unexpectedly high figure, given the rarity of previously reported cases.

In 6 patients splenectomy alone was performed: 4 of these patients had bled from varices. In 2 of these 4, bleeding recurred after the procedure. Transgastric ligation of varices was successfully carried out in 1 of the rebleeders. To the present time, 10 patients have not bled from varices, including 7 who have had no treatment pertinent to controlling them or reducing portal hypertension. With a follow-up ranging from 6 months to 11 years, 13 of the 14 are still alive after their diagnosis of SMV-PV obstruction.

Major problems caused by SMV-PV occlusion have become the differentiation from pancreatic cancer and the necessity of working through the fragile periportal and peripancreatic varices when operating for other complications of chronic pancreatitis. Preoperative diagnosis of SMV-PV occlusion may be difficult without routine angiography, but the authors have not yet accepted that conclusion, principally because of cost and possible morbidity.

The clinical importance of SMV-PV occlusion in chronic pancreatitis lies in its presentation by variceal bleeding, probable necessity for non-shunting means of control for bleeding varices, increased difficulty of operations on the pancreas because of portal hypertension, and possible confusion with pancreatic cancer. The authors emphasized that SMV-PV narrowing and occlusion within the pancreas does not necessarily indicate presence of cancer.

▶ This paper reports an unusual clinical situation. In our experience the recognition of varices in patients with chronic pancreatitis is a very rare event, and clinical gastrointestinal bleeding caused by these varices has not occurred. My prejudice is not to perform splenectomy as treatment for angiographically defined varices that have not bled. Nor would I think that varices that have caused gastrointestinal bleeding and have been demonstrated endoscopically would respond to splenectomy alone in the face of occlusion of superior mesenteric or portal vein, or both. It is well known that splenectomy in this situation does not alter the hemodynamics. We have reported a series of patients with extrahepatic portal vein thrombosis and occlusion of the mesenteric and splenic vein manifest by gastrointestinal bleeding. These patients were followed for a prolonged period of time of intermittent bleeding, but no surgical intervention was attempted (Grauer, S.E., and Schwartz, S.I.: *Ann. Surg.* 189:566, 1979).—S.I. Schwartz, M.D.

Shunt Surgery Versus Endoscopic Sclerotherapy for Long-Term Treatment of Variceal Bleeding: Early Results of a Randomized Trial

Layton F. Rikkers, David A. Burnett, Gary D. Volentine, Kenneth N. Buchi, and Robert A. Cormier (Univ. of Nebraska at Omaha and Univ. of Utah)
Ann. Surg. 206:261–271, September 1987   24–11

An attempt was made to determine whether shunt surgery or endoscopic sclerotherapy is best for cirrhotic patients with bleeding varices. A prospective trial enrolled 57 patients who survived initial bleeding. Twenty-three patients had a distal splenorenal shunt operation, and 4 had nonselective portal decompression. Thirty patients had chronic sclerotherapy. The two groups were initially comparable. More than 80% of all patients had alcoholic cirrhosis; one third were Child's class C patients.

Two-year survival was 65% in the shunt group and 61% in the sclerotherapy group. Eight of 12 deaths in the latter group were due to recurrent hemorrhage. Six of 10 deaths in the shunt group were secondary to liver failure. Rebleeding occurred in 57% of sclerotherapy patients and in 19% of the shunt group during a mean follow-up of 25 months. Only two sclerotherapy failures were salvaged surgically. Portal perfusion and portal pressure at 1 year were best maintained in the sclerotherapy group (table). Liver function and encephalopathy were similar in the two groups, as were total medical costs.

Endoscopic sclerotherapy is an acceptable alternative to shunt surgery for the management of cirrhotic patients with variceal bleeding. It is not, however, a superior treatment. Patients with limited liver function might do better with chronic sclerotherapy than with shunt surgery.

▶ Results reported by Warren et al. (*Ann. Surg.* 203:454, 1986) were somewhat different. In that report, 16 of 37 patients randomized to sclerotherapy either died or failed that therapy. Another difference was that the Emory group showed significant improvement in hepatocyte function in the sclerotherapy group. The improved hepatic function in the sclerotherapy group, coupled with the ability to surgically salvage sclerotherapy rebleed failures, gave a significantly improved survival rate to that group. At all points in time the survival curve of the sclerotherapy group was significantly ($P < .03$) better than that of the shunt group.—S.I. Schwartz, M.D.

Endoscopic Sclerotherapy Versus Portacaval Shunt in Patients With Severe Cirrhosis and Acute Variceal Hemorrhage: Long-Term Follow-Up

John P. Cello, James H. Grendell, Richard A. Crass, Thomas E. Weber, and Donald D. Trunkey (Univ. of California, San Francisco, and San Francisco Gen. Hosp.)
N. Engl. J. Med. 316:11–15, Jan. 1, 1987   24–12

SERIAL HEPATIC HEMODYNAMIC DATA							
	Shunt				Sclerotherapy		
	N	Preoperative	1 Year	N	Preoperative	1 Year	
EHBF (mL/min)	11	1418 ± 109	1191 ± 93	14	1294 ± 112	1155 ± 49	
PPG	7	2.0 ± 0.3*	2.6 ± 0.5*	8	1.8 ± 0.4	1.9 ± 0.4	
CSP (mmHg)	6	15.3 ± 2.6†	9.7 ± 1.3†	8	13.6 ± 1.8	16.4 ± 1.8	

*P = .03.
†P = .04.
(Courtesy of Rikkers, L.F., et al.: Ann. Surg. 206:261–271, September 1987.)

A previous article reported the preliminary results of a randomized trial comparing endoscopic sclerotherapy with portacaval shunt surgery for active variceal hemorrhage in patients with Child's class C cirrhosis. That article noted that the 28 patients assigned to sclerotherapy required less operative time and less blood during their hospitalization compared with the 24 assigned to emergency therapeutic portacaval shunt. Although there was no difference in hospital mortality or in long-term survival, those treated by sclerotherapy were noted to have significantly lower total health care costs than those treated by portacaval shunting. On the basis of those preliminary long-term results, 12 additional patients were entered. This article reports the follow-up data on all patients discharged alive for a minimum of 9 months of observation.

The study population consisted of 64 patients with Child's class C cirrhosis and variceal hemorrhage requiring six or more units of blood who were randomly assigned to receive either a portacaval shunt (32 patients) or endoscopic sclerotherapy (32 patients). The duration of the initial hospitalization and the total amount of blood transfused during hospitalization tended to be substantially less among the patients who received sclerotherapy. Fifty percent of the sclerotherapy group was discharged alive, compared with 44% of the shunt-surgery group; thus, there was no difference in short-term survival. After randomization, both groups were followed for a mean of 530 days. Rebleeding from varices, the duration of rehospitalization for hemorrhage, and transfusions received after discharge were all markedly higher in the sclerotherapy group. Of the sclerotherapy-treated patients, 40% who were discharged alive (7 of 16 patients) ultimately required surgical treatment for bleeding varices, despite a mean of 6.1 treatment sessions. The health care costs and long-term survival did not differ significantly between the groups.

It is concluded that although endoscopic sclerotherapy is as good as surgical shunting for the acute management of variceal hemorrhage in poor-risk patients with massive bleeding, sclerotherapy-treated patients in whom varices are not obliterated and in whom bleeding continues should be considered for elective shunt therapy.

▶ In the classic article, Warren et al. (*Ann. Surg.* 203:454, 1986) demonstrated that distal splenorenal shunt and endoscopic sclerotherapy had essentially equivalent results as far as long-term survival was concerned in patients with bleeding varices. It is important to define the extent of hepatocellular dysfunction, and the strength of this article is that it considers the Child's class C patients. Orloff has been the strongest proponent of an immediate shunt, and recently he and Bell (*Am. J. Surg.* 151:176, 1986) presented the largest series of patients subjected to an emergency shunt, i.e., one created within 8 hours of admission to the hospital for bleeding. Those results indicate a very acceptable survival and essentially no rebleeding.—S.I. Schwartz, M.D.

Injection Sclerotherapy in Adult Patients With Extrahepatic Portal Venous Obstruction
D. Kahn, J. Terblanche, S. Kitano, and P. Bornman (Univ. of Cape Town, South Africa)
Br. J. Surg. 74:600–602, July 1987   24–13

Extrahepatic portal venous obstruction, the most common cause of portal hypertension in children, may also be encountered for the first time in adults. The natural history of this condition is not well understood. Patients may stop bleeding or bleed less severely and less frequently as they age. This possibility has engendered a more conservative management policy for patients with extrahepatic portal venous obstruction. Experience with injection sclerotherapy in a group of adults and teenagers was reviewed.

The study group included 22 males and 17 females aged 12–69 years. Before the study began, 26 patients experienced a total of 77 variceal hemorrhages. Seventeen patients had 39 episodes of variceal bleeding in 781 patient months at risk before treatment, or 1 episode per 20 months, compared with 5 episodes in 600 months at risk during the treatment period, or 1 per 120 months. Esophageal varices were eradicated in 33 patients after a mean of 7 injections (range, 1–17) during a mean of 14.5 months (range, 1–48 months). Fewer injections were required to eradicate varices in older patients. Variceal bleeding occurred 13 times in 9 patients before eradication and 4 times in 4 of the 33 patients in whom varices were eradicated. Follow-up ranged from 3 months to 105 months, with a mean of 44 months. No patient died during the study. Complications caused by treatment, noted in 25 patients, included injection site leak in 5, stenosis in 7, and mucosal ulceration in 23. These complications were usually minor.

In this series, no deaths occurred in the 9-year study period, morbidity was acceptable, and recurrent variceal bleeding was markedly decreased. Injection sclerotherapy would appear to be the treatment of choice for patients with extrahepatic portal venous obstruction.

▶ This is an impressive series, and the good results would be anticipated. Many of these patients, who have persistent varices for years, bleed sporadically, have spontaneous cessation of the bleeding, and have a normal life expectancy with operative intervention (Grauer, S., and Schwartz, S.I.: *Ann. Surg.* 189:566, 1979). In patients with multiple episodes of bleeding a shunting procedure may well represent the most expeditious method of management. A recent study by Alagille et al. (*J. Pediatr. Gastroenterol. Nutr.* 5:861, 1986) assessed 42 children with portal obstruction without liver disease and underwent a portal systemic shunt. Psychometric tests were identical in shunted and control groups. Minimal portal-systemic encephalopathy appeared to be undetectable by either electroencephalogram or venous ammonia levels.—S.I. Schwartz, M.D.

Emergency Portacaval Shunt for Variceal Hemorrhage: A Prospective Study
Jean-Pierre Villeneuve, Gilles Pomier-Layrargues, Lester Duguay, Réal Lapointe, Serge Tanguay, Denis Marleau, Bernard Willems, P.-Michel Huet, Claire Infante-Rivard, and Pierre Lavoie (Saint-Luc Hosp., Montreal, and Univ. of Montreal)
Ann. Surg. 206:48–52, July 1987   24–14

In patients with cirrhosis, variceal hemorrhage is a life-threatening complication of portal hypertension. Because of the high operative mortality, emergency portacaval shunt has not been recommended. The authors describe the use of emergency portacaval shunt to treat variceal bleeding after hemodynamic stabilization in patients with mild to moderate liver disease. In this procedure, bleeding is controlled with balloon tamponade if necessary.

Of 79 patients admitted for variceal hemorrhage, 62 rebled after treatment with propranolol failed. Nine patients died of massive hemorrhage; of the 53 survivors, 11 had severe liver disease and were not considered for shunt surgery. Emergency shunt surgery was performed on 36 patients. In most patients, surgery was performed within 24 hours of endoscopic diagnosis.

The operative mortality rate was 19%; 1- and 2-year survival rates were 78% and 71%, respectively. Postoperative hepatic encephalopathy occurred in 36% of patients. All patients responded well to protein restriction and lactulose. When other treatments for the prevention of rebleeding have failed, emergency portacaval shunt produces an acceptable long-term survival rate in patients with mild or moderate liver disease.

▶ For a period of time it was suggested that portacaval shunts should be deleted from the armamentarium directed at the management of bleeding varices. The present article emphasizes that the procedure performs a distinct role and can have an acceptable survival rate in appropriately selected patients. Cello et al. (*Surgery* 91(3):333, 1982) presented evidence that portal decompression may be the best treatment for improving the survival of class C alcoholic cirrhotics who have substantial variceal bleeding that cannot be controlled on a medical regimen.—S.I. Schwartz, M.D.

Prospective Evaluation and Long-Term Results of Mesocaval Interposition Shunts

K.-J. Paquet, J.-F. Kalk, and P. Koussouris (Heinz-Kalk Hosp., Bad Kissingen, West Germany)
Acta Chir. Scand. 153:423–429, July–August 1987   24–15

A prospective series of mesocaval interposition shunt operations was undertaken in 86 patients with portal hypertension resulting mainly from hepatic cirrhosis. Patients with residual perfusion of 15% to 30% and no active liver disease were included in the series. Residual portal perfusion was demonstrated intraoperatively in all cases. Visceral angiography excluded hepatic arterial stenosis and "portal pseudoperfusion" preoperatively. A 14- or 16-mm Dacron prosthesis was utilized.

Operative mortality was 8%, with five of seven deaths resulting from liver failure. Encephalopathy developed in 10% of surviving patients but was severe in only one instance. Shunt thrombosis was detected in 8 patients within 2 years of surgery; the long-term patency rate was 90%. Liver function was normal generally within 1–2 weeks of operation. Injection sclerotherapy was effective in 4 patients with thrombosed shunts who had recurrent variceal bleeding shortly after operation. Life expectancy at 5 years was nearly 70%, and the 10-year survival exceeded 50%

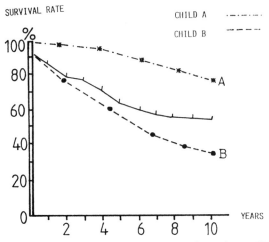

Fig 24–7.—Cumulative survival rates in total patient series and according to Child classification (A, B). (Courtesy of Paquet, K.-J., et al.: Acta Chir. Scand. 153:423–429, July–August 1987.)

(Fig 24–7). Mortality was low in Child class A cases. Most low risk patients are presently leading normal lives.

The mesocaval interposition shunt has a role in the elective or semiurgent management of patients with portal hypertension. The operation is technically the simplest portal-systemic shunt and carries the lowest operative mortality. The mesocaval shunt will be especially useful if the incidence of encephalopathy does not exceed 10% and if long-term shunt patency is assured by subcutaneous heparin administration.

▶ The authors used a Dacron prosthesis that is smaller than that generally used in this country. It is interesting that they showed residual portal perfusion in 75% of cases after the shunt was inserted and 60% at 6 months. The total encephalopathy rate is also low. Another important finding of this study is that the reduction of residual portal perfusion was not associated with a rising encephalopathy rate. Rypins (*Ann. Surg.* 207:706, 1984) used 8- to 14-mm portacaval H-grafts and was able to effect adequate reduction in portal pressure with maintenance of prograde portal flow and low incidence of encephalopathy.—S.I. Schwartz, M.D.

Effects of Altered Portal Hemodynamics After Distal Splenorenal Shunts
Layton F. Rikkers, Robert A. Cormier, and Nghia M. Vo (Univ. of Nebraska at Omaha and Univ. of Utah)
Am. J. Surg. 153:80–85, January 1987   24–16

In this study, 58 cirrhotic patients who had undergone distal splenorenal shunts as treatment for bleeding esophageal varices were grouped based on preoperative and postoperative changes in their hepatic portal perfusion and portal pressure.

Patients were classified into four groups, based on their postoperative hemodynamic studies: group 1, 23 patients (40%), had portal perfusion present, grades 1 through 3, and corrected sinusoidal pressure maintained with 3 mm Hg of preoperative value; group 2, 10 patients (17%), had portal perfusion present and corrected sinusoidal pressure increase of more than 3 mm Hg above the preoperative value; group 3, 18 patients (31%), had portal perfusion present and corrected sinusoidal pressure decrease of more than 3 mm Hg below the preoperative value; and group 4, 7 patients (12%), had hepatic portal perfusion absent, grade 4. The preoperative values were similar with no significant differences among the groups, nor were preoperative values for prothrombin time and serum albumin, total bilirubin, glutamic oxaloacetic transaminase, glutamic pyruvate transaminase, and alkaline phosphate levels significantly different among the groups.

For groups 2 and 4, early postoperative morbidity as quantified by duration of postoperative hospitalization was significantly greater (19 ± 4 days, $P < .001$; and 27 ± 6 days, $P < .001$, respectively) than for group 1 (11 ± 1 days) and group 3 (12 ± 1 days). For group 2 (30%, $P < .05$), group 3 (33%, $P < .05$), and group 4 (71%, $P < .001$), severe early postoperative ascites were significantly more frequent than in group 1 (0%). In group 1 (13%), group 2 (33%), group 3 (6%), and group 4 (25%), encephalopathy complicated the late postoperative course, but these frequencies were not significantly different. For group 4, the 1-year survival rate was significantly less than for the other groups ($P < .05$).

In 40% of the patients, both hepatic portal perfusion and a postoperative corrected sinusoidal pressure were maintained within 3 mm Hg of the preoperative value. When these hemodynamic conditions pertained, none died in the early postoperative interval, severe postoperative ascites did not occur, late postoperative encephalopathy developed in only 13%, and their long-term survival was better than in any other of the groups. Loss of hepatic portal perfusion secondary to complete portal vein thrombosis was the acute hemodynamic change with the most adverse consequences (group 4).

When both hepatic portal perfusion and sinusoidal pressure were maintained near preoperative levels (group 1), morbidity was least. Survival was significantly better than for group 4, who lost portal flow to the liver during the early postoperative interval. The worst survival and greatest morbidity were among patients with absent hepatic portal perfusion. Intermediate results were achieved in the two groups who had postoperative preservation of portal perfusion but significant preoperative to postoperative alterations in sinusoidal pressure. Although survival curves for these two groups were not significantly different, morbidity was greater, especially for patients with an increase in sinusoidal pressure (group 2) than for those in group 1.

▶ This study provides interesting data but in part adds to the confusion of the already confused arena, i.e., the effects of altered portal hemodynamics on survival following decompressive procedures. There were no major differences in the long-term results in the first three groups. There was no explanation why an increase in postoperative postsinusoidal pressure should be associated with a turbulent course. The authors state that survival for patients who maintained portal perfusion was significantly better than for patients who lost portal flow to the liver during the early postoperative interval. This is in contrast to other studies that showed identical survival for end-to-side portacaval shunts and selective shunts. I know of no study that shows improved survival related to the maintenance of hepatic portal perfusion. Most studies concentrate on a decreased incidence of encephalopathy (Langer, B., et al.: *Gastroenterology* 88:424, 1985).—S.I. Schwartz, M.D.

Simultaneous Retrohepatic Inferior Vena Cavoplasty and Side-to-Side Portacaval Shunt for Recurrent Thrombosed Mesoatrial Shunt in the Budd-Chiari Syndrome
Sam S. Ahn, Leonard I. Goldstein, and Ronald W. Busuttil (Univ. of California at Los Angeles)
Surgery 101:165–171, February 1987   24–17

Budd-Chiari syndrome comprises less than 5% of surgically correctable causes of portal hypertension and can be one of the most difficult to treat; recurrence, which is associated with a thrombosed mesoatrial shunt, can be even more difficult to manage because of the patient's debilitated condition, hypercoagulable state, and altered anatomy from the previous thoracic and abdominal operations. A patient was seen with a recurrent thrombosed mesoatrial shunt, tightly stenotic retrohepatic inferior vena cava, and occluded hepatic veins with severe portal hypertension.

Man, 29, had thrombosis of the hepatic veins and retrohepatic inferior vena cava. A month later he underwent decompressive mesoatrial shunt. After an uneventful recovery, the patient was discharged, and sodium warfarin, Coumadin, aspirin, and dipyridamole were prescribed. Liver function returned to normal. Four months later, ascites and abnormal liver function redeveloped. The mesoatrial shunt, which had thrombosed, was then revised with a modified silicone rubber cuff-reinforced Dacron graft. The patient was readmitted for evaluation of recurrent ascites 12 months after this second operation. In August 1984, the patient underwent one-stage Gore-Tex patch angioplasty of the retrohepatic inferior vena cava and a side-to-side portacaval shunt with a short interposition Dacron graft. An incontinuity median sternotomy-bilateral subcostal incision was made to achieve adequate exposure of the entire retrohepatic vena cava, and the diaphragm was split to the suprahepatic vena cava. The thrombosed mesoatrial shunt was removed, and the liver was lifted out of its bed and retraced to the left. The retrohepatic vena cava was widened with a large Gore-Tex patch (Fig 24–8). After caval reconstruction, a 12-mm woven Dacron interposition graft was placed between the portal vein and the infrahepatic vena cava. An enlarged caudate lobe and a scarred immobile portal vein prevented a direct portal vein to caval anastomosis. The patient continued to have excellent results at 26 months' follow-up.

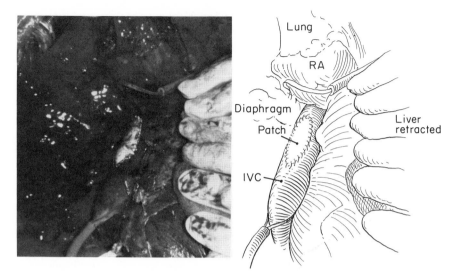

Fig 24–8.—Photograph obtained intraoperatively shows the retrohepatic inferior vena cava after completion of the Gore-Tex patch cavoplasty. The liver is retracted anteriorly and to the left. The redundant loose tape tourniquet is around the intrapericardial vena cava, and the nonredundant tourniquet surrounds the suprarenal inferior vena cava. The diaphragm was split and the mesoatrial shunt removed to allow exposure of the entire retrohepatic vena cava. *RA,* right atrium; *IVC,* inferior vena cava. (Courtesy of Ahn, S.S., et al.: Surgery 101:165–171, February 1987.)

The choice of prosthetic material may be criticized. However, the convenience and expediency of the prosthetic material probably outweigh the theoretical, and perhaps even clinical, advantages of autologous tissue in these difficult cases. With either material, autologous or prosthetic, direct caval repair and use of a short portacaval interposition graft should result in a low incidence of early graft thrombosis.

▶ There are almost as many articles on innovative operations for this procedure as there are patients. A variety of portosystemic shunts and peritoneovenous shunts has been used. Orloff and Johansen (*Ann. Surg.* 188:494, 1978) reported that side-to-side anastomosis was the treatment of choice, superior to the peritoneal venous shunt because it treats the liver disease. Warren et al. (*Surg. Gynecol. Obstet.* 159:101, 1984) initially used a mesoatrial shunt and then performed a side-to-side portacaval shunt as a two-stage procedure. Cameron et al. (*Ann. Surg.* 198:335, 1983) reviewed an experience with 12 patients treated with a mesenteric-systemic shunt. In five of these a mesocaval shunt was performed, and in seven a mesoatrial shunt. Shunt thrombosis occurred in many of these patients. The current approach is most analogous to the radical operation described by Nakao et al. (*J. Cardiovasc. Surg.* 25:216, 1984), in which the inferior vena cava is opened to allow direct examination of the length of the obstruction, and a Fogarty catheter is used to remove thrombi from the hepatic vein. A patch of pericardium reinforced with Teflon prostheses is secured over the side of the inferior vena cava after removal of the thrombus and the scar.—S.I. Schwartz, M.D.

The Place of Sugiura Operation for Portal Hypertension and Bleeding Esophageal Varices

George M. Abouna, Hussam Baissony, Basil M. Al-Nakib, Amir T. Menkarios, and O.S.G. Silva (Kuwait Univ. and Al-Sabah Hosp., Kuwait City)
Surgery 101:91–98, January 1987   24–18

Surgical therapy of portal hypertension and bleeding esophageal varices is needed to prevent exsanguination; nevertheless, the high mortality and common complication of encephalopathy make shunting procedures disadvantageous. The Sugiura operation first described in 1973 is a two-stage procedure consisting of extensive devascularization of the abdominal and thoracic esophagus, esophageal transection, splenectomy, vagotomy, and pyloroplasty. The Sugiura procedure has been modified from a two-stage to a single-stage, transabdominal operation, and its use in patients with portal hypertension and bleeding esophageal varices is reported (Fig 24–9).

Fifty patients aged 10 months to 72 years with variceal hemorrhage were treated using a modified Sugiura operation (26 cases), with an emergency mesocaval shunt if bleeding could not be stopped (10 cases) or with a distal splenorenal shunt if bleeding could be stopped. Follow-up lasted 1.5 to 6 years: it consisted of monthly checkups, upper gastrointestinal tract series, and occasionally an endoscopy at 3 months and annually following operation.

In the patients undergoing Sugiura operations (group 3), hospital mortality, recurrent hemorrhage, encephalopathy, and late death were markedly lower than for the patients undergoing shunt procedures (table). By 3 months after the Sugiura operation, varices were present in only 5% of the patients, and hypersplenism was not present in any patient. Major

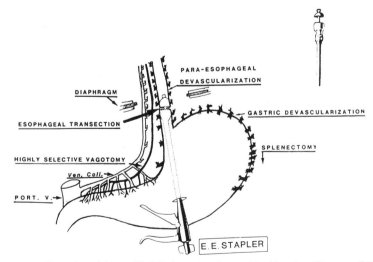

Fig 24–9.—Illustration of the modified Sugiura operation used in this series. (Courtesy of Abouna, G.M., et al.: Surgery 101:91–98, January 1987.)

COMPARISON OF THE RESULTS OF SURGICAL TREATMENT IN THE THREE TREATMENT GROUPS

Group	No. of pts.	Hospital deaths No. (%)	Recurrent hemorrhage No. (%)	Encephalopathy No. (%)	Late death No. (%)	Alive No. (%)	Duration (yr)
1	10	2 (20)	3 (30)	3 (30)	2 (20)	6 (60)	2-6
2	14	2 (14.3)	2 (14.3)	2 (14.3)	1 (7.2)	1 (85)	2-6
3	26	2 (7.7)	1 (3.4)	0 (0)	0 (0)	24 (92)	1-5

(Courtesy of Abouna, G.M., et al.: Surgery 101:91–98, January 1987.)

complications were gastric and esophageal leaks in 2 patients, 1 of whom died, and temporary dysphagia in 6 patients.

The authors conclude that the modified Sugiura nonshunt operation is the best treatment for variceal hemorrhage in the nonalcoholic patient. This operation focuses on arresting variceal bleeding, the true danger, rather than portal hypertension.

▶ Inokuchi (*World J. Surg.* 9:171, 1985) reviewed 3,136 cases of direct interruption of esophageal varices; 70% survived. The incidence of recurrent variceal bleeding was 7%, and that of Eck's syndrome was 5%. Spence and Johnston (*Surg. Gynecol. Obstet.* 160(4):323–329, 1985) reviewed 100 consecutive cases with stapled esophageal transection for varices. More than 80% remained free from variceal bleeding at 5 years after treatment. There is little question that patients with schistosomiasis tolerate poorly a complete portacaval decompression and that the two operations applicable are the Sugiura and the Warren shunt.—S.I. Schwartz, M.D.

Experience With the Esophagogastric Devascularization Procedure
Donna J. Barbot and Ernest F. Rosato (Univ. of Pennsylvania, Philadelphia)
Surgery 101:685–690, June 1987   24–19

Many modalities have been used to treat portal hypertension with subsequent variceal bleeding. Devascularization procedures and esophageal transection procedures have been periodically revived for treating patients with bleeding esophageal varices. Limited long-term success or technical difficulties have hindered their wide adoption. At one institution, 28 consecutive unselected patients were treated for esophageal varices by a modified Sugiura procedure between 1978 and 1985.

Using Child's classification, 59% of the patients were class A, 11% were class B, and 30% were class C. The etiology of cirrhosis was alcohol abuse in 42% of patients, hepatitis in 33%, granulomatous disease in 7%, and cryptogenic disease in 18%. One patient had extrahepatic portal hypertension from unknown causes. In all cases, surgical treatment involved esophageal and gastric devascularization. The operation was done through a left eighth intercostal thoracic incision with access to the abdominal cavity through a circumferential diaphragmatic incision. Esophagogastric devascularization was completed initially by transection of the vessels on the lesser curvature of the stomach. Devascularization along the lesser curvature was modified: the vessels were ligated at the omental level instead of at the gastric wall. Ligation of the right gastric artery in the lesser omentum above the pylorus was added to the procedure. Truncal vagotomy and ligation of the collateral azygous veins were also included. The esophageal transection was done in the first half of the group, using an end-to-end anastomosis autosuture stapling device. Transection and anastomosis were subsequently accomplished with a continuous suture technique used on the transected mucosal tube, with interrupted closure of the muscular layer. Four patients died of sepsis related to gastric or esophageal leakage from the transection site itself or from the gastrotomy site used for end-to-end anastomosis autosuture placement. Average operative time was 4.5 hours; average blood replacement during surgery was eight units. Operative mortality was 32%: 2 patients of 16 in class A; 1 of 3 in class B; and 6 of 9 in class C. Morbidity was 33%. Six of the 18 patients who survived surgery died later: only 1 death was presumed to be from recurrent variceal hemorrhage. Significant bleeding occurred in 2 patients from recurrent varices and in 2 from peptic ulcer disease. Encephalopathy, present in 2 patients preoperatively, was still manifest after surgery but well controlled. The 12 surviving patients currently have stable liver function.

Sugiura's esophagogastric devascularization procedure has been associated with a higher operative mortality in non-Japanese patients. Nevertheless, this study documented the effective long-term control of bleeding and suggested modifications that made the operation technically easier to perform.

▶ The reports from Japan regarding the use of the Sugiura procedure are extremely impressive and have a high index of success. As the authors point out, the procedure has not met with equivalent success in Western countries, which is due in part to the difference in the patient population. The omission of esophageal transection in the face of sclerotherapy performed is interesting but is open to question because transection and esophageal devascularization more thoroughly interrupts variceal flow. Another modification of the procedure that seems quite logical is substituting a highly selective vagotomy for a truncal vagotomy and avoiding performance of a pyloroplasty. The addendum by Ginsberg et al. (*Ann. Thorac. Surg.* 34:258, 1982) is most appropriate: a fundoplication following esophageal devascularization to prevent leakage. The caveat for application of this procedure on a broad scale as pointed out by the authors does not address the issue of gastric varices.—S.I. Schwartz, M.D.

Selective Management of Blunt Splenic Trauma
Peter Mucha, Jr., Richard C. Daly, and Michael B. Farnell (Mayo Clinic and Mayo Found., Rochester, Minn.)
J. Trauma 26:970–979, November 1986   24–20

Classic teaching continues to embrace splenectomy as the only assured means for preventing the immediate or delayed life-threatening conse-

235 Patients

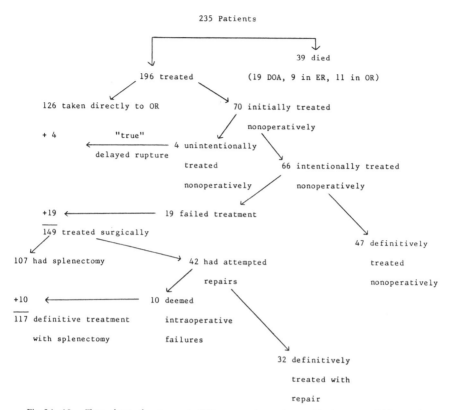

Fig 24—10.—Flow chart of outcome in 235 consecutive patients with documented blunt splenic trauma. *DOA,* dead on arrival; *ER,* emergency room; *OR,* operating room. (Courtesy of Mucha, P., Jr., et al.: J. Trauma 26:970–979, November 1986.)

quences of splenic injury, but the role of splenectomy must now be balanced against a fuller appreciation of the physiologic importance of the spleen. Of 196 patients treated in accordance with an evolving selective management program, 117 (60%) had splenectomy, 32 (16%) underwent splenorrhaphy repair, and 47 (24%) had nonoperative treatment (Fig 24–10).

The median Injury Severity Score was 10 points higher among patients requiring operation (splenectomy or repair) than that for patients successfully treated nonoperatively (P <.001). Also, the percentage of patients with hemodynamic instability or documented systolic blood pressure of less than 100 mm Hg after injury was also significantly higher (P <.001) in those who underwent splenectomy or repair. Correlating with hemodynamic status, there was a significant difference (P <.001) in the number of blood transfusions needed by the three treatment groups: 42.5% of nonoperatively treated patients, 87.5% of those having repair, and 92% of those having splenectomy.

Of 47 patients who had definitive nonoperative treatment, radionuclide spleen scans (done usually before 1981) diagnosed the splenic injury in 22; in 23 patients the diagnosis was made by abdominal computed tomography. Mortality (2%) was significantly lower in this group than among patients who underwent splenectomy (10%) or repair (9%). There was only one death in the nonoperatively managed patients, this resulting from CNS trauma. Also, morbidity was significantly higher among those who were operated on. No hemostatic failures occurred in patients undergoing definitive repair postoperatively.

There seems to exist a spectrum of blunt splenic trauma, as manifested by the degree of associated injuries, the hemodynamic status, and blood transfusion requirements, that enables application of a rational selective management program. Comparative analysis among the three treatments showed differences that were more a reflection of the overall magnitude of total bodily injury than the specific manner in which an injured spleen is managed. Recommendations for selection criteria for nonoperative management include absolute hemodynamic stability, no or only minimal peritoneal signs, and a maximum requirement of 2 units of blood. Splenorrhaphy or repair is preferred, but this should be abandoned if hemostasis is inadequate, less than a third of the functioning splenic tissue can be preserved, or associated life-threatening injuries take precedence. Splenectomy remains the most appropriate course of action in many patients who sustain blunt splenic trauma.

▶ It is critical to distinguish between pediatric and adult cases because the results of nonoperative management differ in the two groups. Selective nonoperative management in children is associated with a much higher incidence of success than is that with adults. In an experience reported by Tibi et al. (*Contemp. Surg.* 26:73, 1985) a subset of 43 patients was selected for review; splenic trauma was the only serious injury in these patients. Twenty-three patients underwent splenectomy, 8 patients underwent splenorrhaphy, and in 12 a nonoperative course of management was initially undertaken. In all instances, the splenic injury resulted from blunt trauma. There were no deaths in any group. The 12 patients not operated on had a mean blood replacement of two units and a 12-day stay. Nonoperative therapy was successful for 10 of the 12 patients. Splenectomy was necessary in 2 patients after evidence of persistent bleeding was diagnosed by the failure of patients to stabilize after presumed adequate blood replacement. In retrospect, both patients displayed evidence of continued bleeding from the time of presentation.—S.I. Schwartz, M.D.

Pyogenic Splenic Abscess in Intravenous Drug Addiction
Manohar N. Nallathambi, Rao R. Ivatury, Daniel H. Lankin, Irene L. Wapnir, and William M. Stahl (Lincoln Med. and Mental Health Ctr. and New York Med. College, New York)
Am. Surg. 53:342–346, June 1987   24–21

Infectious complications from intravenous (IV) drug abuse range from simple local infections to life-threatening systemic sepsis. Splenic abscess is considered a rare complication. Experience with five such patients, all treated within 1 year, is reported.

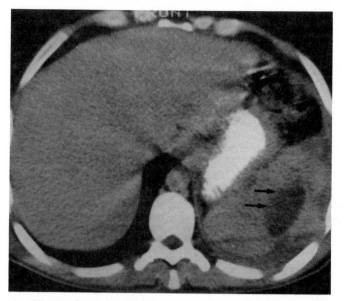

Fig 24–11.—CT scan of upper left quadrant showing a low density area *(arrows)* consistent with splenic abscess. (Courtesy of Nallathambi, M.N., et al.: Am. Surg. 53:342–346, June 1987.)

The patients, all men aged 26 to 41 years, had IV drug addictions. All but one had varying degrees of abdominal pain. All had fever. Splenomegaly was noted in one patient; left upper quadrant tense abdominal mass was felt in another. Leukocytosis was present in two patients. Only two patients had abnormal chest radiographs. Three patients had concomitant bacterial endocarditis. Sonography and computed tomography were used in diagnosis (Fig 24–11): there were no false-positive or false-negative results. At surgery, four patients, including the three with endocarditis, were noted to have multiple abscesses. In three, the abscesses had ruptured into the subdiaphragmatic space without generalized peritonitis or pus in the peritoneal cavity. Splenectomy was done in all patients. Active suction drainage of the splenic bed was done routinely. Three patients had uneventful postoperative courses and were discharged. Two patients died; one, treated for concomitant bacterial endocarditis, continued to be septic after splenectomy; and the second patient, who underwent clipping of the middle cerebral artery aneurysm, developed recurrent intracerebral hemorrhage 28 days after surgery. *Stapyhlococcus aureus* septicemia was present in four patients at the time of splenectomy (table).

Clinicians should be alert to the possibility of pyrogenic splenic abscess in patients with IV drug addictions, especially when patients present with vague abdominal signs and persistent sepsis. Noninvasive imaging methods—computed tomography scan and ultrasound—were found to facilitate early diagnosis in these patients.

▶ Splenic abscess is a lesion appearing with increasing frequency related to its presence in immunosuppressed patients and its occurrence as a consequence of intravenous drug addiction. More common complications related to drug

SUMMARY OF FIVE PATIENTS WITH SPLENIC ABSCESS

Case	Age/Sex	Presentation	Imaging Methods	Organism	Clinical Course*	Outcome
1†	34 M	H/O old trauma, fever, tender LUQ mass *no endocarditis*	Ultrasound	Staph aureus	Preoperative rupture of abscess contained	Recovered
2	36 M	H/O old trauma, fever, abdominal pain and tenderness, no mass *no endocarditis*	Ultrasound (Fig. 1) CT scan (Fig. 2)	Klebsiella	Preoperative rupture of abscess contained	Recovered
3	33 M	Disorientation, fever splenomegaly *endocarditis*	Ultrasound (Fig. 3) CT scan (Fig. 4)	Staph aureus (methicillin resistant)	None	Recovered
4	41 M	Fever, tenderness left abdomen *endocarditis*	Ultrasound CT scan	Staph aureus (methicillin resistant)	Continued sepsis Candidemia	Expired
5‡	26 M	Altered mental status, fever, abdominal tenderness *endocarditis*	Ultrasound CT scan	Staph aureus	Preoperative rupture of abscess contained. Craniotomy for bleeding from a mycotic aneurysm. Recurrent intracranial bleeding	Expired

*All patients underwent splenectomy.
†In addition, distal pancreatectomy.
‡In addition, segmental resection left lobe liver.
(Courtesy of Nallathambi, M.N., et al.: Am. Surg. 53:342–346, June 1987.)

abuse are vascular injury and infection. Vasculitis, mycotic visceral aneurysms, and fungal endocarditis all have been reported. Distal gangrene may be a consequence of intra-arterial drug injection (Yeager, R.A., et al.: *J. Trauma* 27:305, 1987).—S.I. Schwartz, M.D.

Late Septic Complications in Adults Following Splenectomy for Trauma: A Prospective Analysis in 144 Patients
J.B. Green, S.R. Shackford, M.J. Sise, and P. Fridlund (Univ. of California, San Diego, and Naval Hosp., San Diego)
J. Trauma 26:999–1004, November 1986   24–22

Although much of the data concerning overwhelming postsplenectomy infection (OPSI) comes from case reports and retrospective series of patients who had splenectomy for hematologic disease, the true incidence among healthy adult patients of OPSI following splenectomy is unknown. Through an asplenic registry, 144 patients were followed prospectively for development of late septic complications after splenectomy for trauma. The mean follow-up was 61 months (range, 12–144 months).

Blunt trauma was the indication of the splenectomy in 111 patients, penetrating trauma in 6, and intraoperative injury in 27. There were 16 major septic complications in 14 patients, with 2 deaths occurring in the follow-up period—1 from a drug overdose and 1 from fatal OPSI (a 27-year-old man 3 years after his splenectomy). Pneumonia was the most common major infectious complication (5 patients), followed by septicemia (4 patients), abscesses (3 patients), and infection of a prosthetic heart valve, meningitis, and fever of unknown origin (1 each). All but 2 infections were due to encapsulated organisms. The septicemia, pneumonia, or meningitis incidence in this asplenic group was 8.3%, or 166 times the rate expected in the general population (expected incidence, 0.05%).

Following incidental splenectomy, major late septic complications occurred more frequently than for those following splenectomy for blunt or penetrating trauma (18.5% and 5.9%, respectively; $P < .05$). In this series, mortality from major septic complications is lower (7%) than in others previously reported (30%–80%).

The data indicate that the risk of major infection is significantly higher for adult patients undergoing splenectomy for trauma than that of the general population. Because of this risk, surgical management of the injured spleen indicates a conservative approach, especially when injury is incidental to an elective operative procedure. The difference in the low mortality rate in this series may be due to the close follow-up patients received by nature of being in the asplenic registry. All the patients were informed about potential risks of the asplenic state and were encouraged to seek medical attention at the earliest sign of minor infection.

▶ This report points out a different increased incidence of infectious complications following splenectomy for nonhematologic causes. The percentage of infections and fatal sepsis are both higher than in most reports. Schwartz and associates (*JAMA* 248:2279, 1982) studied 193 individuals who underwent splenectomy during a 25-year review period. Forty-eight splenectomies were performed for trauma, 36 were done incidental to abdominal operations, and the remainder were for hematologic disease. Only two cases of fulminant sepsis were documented for a rate of 0.1 case per 100 person years of follow-up. Infections were significantly more frequent in patients who had malignancy or were treated with immunosuppression. Malangoni et al. (*Surgery* 96:775, 1984) reviewed the data on 245 adults who underwent splenectomy for trauma: no deaths resulted from late postsplenectomy infection. Sixty-eight patients had early postoperative infections, and death was more frequent in patients with multiple injuries. The authors added the report of four other groups totaling 3,315 patient years of observation, indicating that the rate of serious infection was 1 per 331 patient years of observation; there were no sepsis-related deaths and only one fulminant infection. They concluded that splenectomy remained an appropriate treatment for trauma in adults.—S.I. Schwartz, M.D.

Splenectomy for Idiopathic Thrombocytopenic Purpura
William W. Coon (Univ. of Michigan)
Surg. Gynecol. Obstet. 164:225–229, March 1987   24–23

Splenectomy has been the treatment of choice for the majority of adults with idiopathic thrombocytopenic purpura (ITP), but the response in the individual patient is unpredictable. In this study, patients were classified as having satisfactory responses to the procedure only if they achieved immediate platelet responses of 150,000/cu mm or higher and maintained platelet counts of 150,000/cu mm or more at last follow-up examination, after intraoperative and postoperative steroid therapy had been discontinued. Failures were defined as (1) inadequate initial platelet response but development of sustained remission (platelet count of more than 150,000) while off all treatment occurring in less than 1 year, or (2) other patterns of failure.

Of 216 patients, 156 (72%) achieved a satisfactory response to the splenectomy, and an additional 7.4% had a sustained platelet count of 150,000 develop while receiving no drug therapy within the first postoperative year; 60 were considered failures, and 16 of these were in the first above-mentioned category. Of 44 patients in the second category, 18 had satisfactory and sustained platelet response develop while off all drug therapy after 1 year or more of follow-up. In the authors' experience, duration of known thrombocytopenia has had no predictive value for response to splenectomy nor did response to steroid therapy have any prognostic value. Of 202 patients receiving a steroid in pharmacologic doses and having frequent platelet counts for monitoring, only 24% of failures but 72% of successes had peak platelet responses of greater than 50,000, while 9% of failures and 47% of successes had peak platelet responses develop that were more than 100,000. There was an excellent postoperative platelet increase in 42 of 73 patients whose platelet counts did not increase to 50,000 or more on adequate steroid therapy.

Of the remaining 39 patients classed as failures in the second category, 8 had sustained remissions develop after intervals of 20 months to 13 years. At last visit, platelet counts were more than 100,000 for 16, between 50,000 and 90,000 in 13, and less than 50,000 in 10. Of the 4 deaths occurring from splenectomy in this series, only 1 patient died from subsequent thrombocytopenic bleeding.

No reliable predictive factors could be found for satisfactory remission of thrombocytopenia after operation. Although older patients and those with suboptimal responses to high-dose steroid therapy are somewhat less likely to achieve a normal platelet count, the majority of these patients had successful outcomes also. Only 8 of 39 surviving patients who failed to have normal platelet counts develop after splenectomy required prolonged treatment with prednisone or other immunosuppressive agents.

▶ The results of this large series of patients are similar to those we reported (*Surgery* 88:208, 1980). In our experience, over 80% of patients sustained platelet counts greater than 100,000/cu mm while off drug therapy within the first year. Among the responders 90% had elevation of platelet counts within 1 week of the splenectomy. In our experience, the response to steroid therapy did not have a prognostic value. In a group of patients whose platelet counts remained below 50,000/cu mm subsequent to splenectomy, recurrences of petechiae or ecchymosis, or both, have been rare, and no patient died of thrombocytopenic bleeding.—S.I. Schwartz, M.D.

Splenectomy for Primary and Recurrent Immune Thrombocytopenic Purpura (ITP): Current Criteria for Patient Selection and Results
Onye E. Akwari, Kamal M.F. Itani, R. Edward Coleman, and Wendell F. Rosse (Duke Univ.)
Ann. Surg. 206:529–541, October 1987   24–24

Splenectomy was performed in 100 of 565 patients admitted with thrombocytopenia in 1975–1985. Ninety-eight of these patients, with primary immune thrombocytopenic purpura (ITP), had failed to respond to chronic immunosuppressive therapy. Three patients with acute intracranial bleeding or with no platelets in a peripheral blood smear had splenectomy on an urgent basis. Patients were prepared with pneumococcal vaccine and with steroids.

Seventy-one patients had a good response to splenectomy, achieving a platelet count above 150,000/μl without medication. Nonresponders were older than the patients who responded. Nine patients had accessory splenectomy for recurrent or, in four cases, persistent ITP (table). Neither platelet antibody titer nor platelet survival or turnover predicted the platelet response to splenectomy (Fig 24–12).

Splenectomy continues to induce remission of ITP in most patients

ACCESSORY SPLENECTOMY: SUMMARY OF CASES, DUKE UNIVERSITY 1975–1985

		Primary Splenectomy		Accessory Spleen	
		Duration of	Time from Initial		
Patient		Response	Splenectomy	Spleen Size	
#	Age/Sex	(Months)	(Months)	(cm)	Response*
1	48/F	3	9	1.8	Excellent
2	9/F	72	506	0.6	No response
3	60/F	0	40	2.5	Good
4	34/F	24	72	2.0 (×2)	Relapsed
		0	96	2.0	Excellent
5	27/F	0	1	1.5 (×2)	Excellent
6	20/F	2	156	3.0	Fair
7	25/M	72	108	1.4 (×2)	Excellent
8	47/F	0	180	1.5 (×2)	Fair
9	7/F	360	444	7.0	Good

*Excellent = platelet count > 100,000/μl; no steroids. Good = platelet count > 100,000/μl; steroids for limited period. Fair = platelet count > 100,000/μl; receiving steroids.
(Courtesy of Akwari, O.E., et al.: Ann. Surg. 206:529–541, October 1987.)

who resist immunosuppressive therapy or who have complications of steroid therapy. Patients with persistent ITP after primary splenectomy and those who have relapses should be scanned for accessory spleens. Coon points out that many patients who do not respond to splenectomy function quite well without treatment.

▶ I would agree with Dr. Coon's discussion in the presentation. We seldom administer platelet transfusions perioperatively unless the platelet count is well below 20,000/cu mm. We have also observed that, in our nonresponding patients with persistent thrombocytopenia, prednisone maintenance is frequently

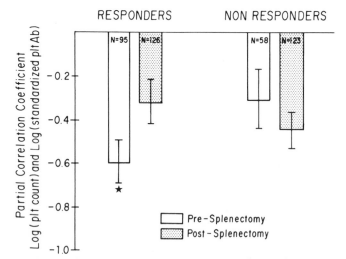

Fig 24–12.—The partial correlation coefficient between log (platelet count) and log (platelet antibody titer) in the responders before splenectomy was significantly higher (*$P < .05$) than in all other categories. The partial correlation coefficient between these two variables was not different in the nonresponders before and after splenectomy ($P > .05$). (Courtesy of Akwari, O.E., et al.: Ann. Surg. 206:529–541, October 1987.)

unnecessary, and ecchymosis and purpura rarely occur. The issue of accessory spleens has been addressed by Rudowski (*World J. Surg.* 9:422, 1985), who emphasized that accessory spleens are frequent in patients with ITP, and that removal of an accessory spleen or spleens can lead to omission and enhance the medical control of this disorder. Schneider et al. (*Arch. Surg.* 122:1175, 1987) focused on immunodeficiency-associated thrombocytopenia as a feature of the acquired immunodeficiency syndrome. Splenectomy should be performed in these patients, with acceptable morbidity and likelihood of response.—S.I. Schwartz, M.D.

25 The Biliary Tract

Aggressive Management of Cholecystitis During Pregnancy
Neal P. Dixon, David M. Faddis, and Howard Silberman (Univ. of Southern California)
Am. J. Surg. 154:292–294, September 1987   25–1

The role of primary operative therapy in symptomatic cholelithiasis during pregnancy was evaluated by reviewing the records of 44 pregnant patients with this diagnosis. Conservative treatment was used in 26 cases, and 18 patients underwent cholecystectomy.

Among the patients treated nonoperatively, 58% had recurrent episodes of biliary colic. Two patients required total parenteral nutrition for 27 and 30 days, respectively, during the third trimester. Three patients had spontaneous abortions, and three had induced abortions. The average hospital stay was 14 days. Three patients underwent cholecystectomy in the first trimester without knowing they were pregnant. All three had abortions. During their second trimesters, 14 patients were operated on. Cholangiograms were performed with fetal shielding. Twelve of these patients delivered healthy infants. The mean hospital stay in the operative group was 12 days.

Prepregnancy cholecystectomy is advised for the patient with a history of cholelithiasis. Cholecystitis occurring during the first trimester should be treated medically, with cholecystectomy scheduled for the second trimester. Biliary symptoms occurring during the second trimester should be treated operatively to avoid recurrent symptoms, multiple hospitalizations, and fetal loss. Symptoms that occur during the third trimester should be treated medically.

▶ The consensus is that a nonoperative approach is preferred for patients with biliary colic occurring during pregnancy. Hiatt et al. (*Am. J. Surg.* 150:263, 1986) reported that fetal loss occurred in five of nine patients who underwent operation during pregnancy. Four of these five patients were operated on during the first trimester, and one patient had an ectopic pregnancy. Although many reports indicate low fetal loss when operation is carried out during the second trimester, the authors of these reports generally recommend nonoperative treatment of biliary disease if possible because symptoms promptly subside in most cases treated conservatively. Hamlin et al. (*N. Engl. J. Med.* 244:128, 1951) reported that most patients go on to term.—S.I. Schwartz, M.D.

Towards a Selective Policy of Operative Cholangiography: A Prospective Clinical Study

C.J. Simpson, A. Smith, D.C. Smith, and G. Gillespie (Victoria Infirmary, Glasgow, Scotland)

J. R. Coll. Surg. Edinb. 32:15–17, February 1987   25–2

A selective approach to operative cholangiography is not uncommon, although biliary surgical opinion is that operative cholangiogram is indispensable in elective cholecystectomy to avoid overlooking silent common duct stones and unnecessary choledochotomies. A prospective study was done with 108 patients undergoing elective cholecystectomy to assess the effect of a selective policy, based on surgical judgement, on the rate and results of operative cholangiography (table).

Of 25 patients who were thought to require a cholangiogram, 13 (52%) were reported as normal. Of these, 11 (44%) had abnormal cholangiograms, including 1 false-positive and 1 false-negative examination, and all underwent duct exploration, 10 proving positive and 1, negative. Where the operative cholangiogram was thought unnecessary, 77 of 83 patients were found to be normal. Of the 5 patients found abnormal, 2 had abnormal cholangiograms and underwent choledochotomy and 2 had very small calculi, which were removed from the lower end of a normal caliber duct. The last, whose cholangiogram had indicated on three separate films a filling defect at the lower end of the common duct with failure of drainage of contrast into the duodenum, had both supraduodenal duct exploration and transduodenal sphincterotomy and duct exploration, without detection of a calculus.

In this series three (2.7%) cholangiograms were known to have been

"IS PERIOPERATIVE CHOLANGIOGRAM NECESSARY IN THIS PATIENT?"		
108 patients		
Cholangiogram not indicated	83	77%
Cholangiogram indicated	25	23%
Indication for cholangiogram:		
Common bile duct dilated	8	
Wide cystic duct, small calculi	11	
Pancreatitis	1	
Palpable stone	2	
Jaundice	10	
Abnormal liver function tests	11	
Anatomical confirmation	1	

(Courtesy of Simpson, C.J., et al.: J.R. Coll. Surg. Edinb. 32:15–18, February 1987.)

inaccurate, two being false-positive and one false-negative. The number of examinations performed using a selective policy would have been reduced by 77% and would have resulted in one negative duct exploration. In 1 patient two small calculi would have been overlooked, giving an incidence of silent, unsuspected stones of 0.9%. The only death in this series, which followed surgical sphincterotomy performed during an unsuccessful search for a stone suggested on the cholangiogram, would have been avoided.

This study is the first to define clearly the accuracy of surgical judgement, and it is not unreasonable that a significant number of normal examinations should be found in the group where a perioperative cholangiogram was thought necessary. Of fundamental importance is the 2.7% of misleading examinations in this series, exceeding the rate of 0.9% of unsuspected common duct stones. Routine cholangiography will detect unsuspected stones as evident from this series, but it also leads to an increase in the number of negative duct explorations. While other series have regarded this as safe, it was not the case in the present study. The authors suggest that a selective policy should become the accepted practice and challenge the status of mandatory operative cholangiography in elective cholecystectomy.

▶ A similar conclusion has recently been reached by Bogokowsky et al. (*Surg. Gynecol. Obstet.* 164:124, 1987). Their study included 505 patients who underwent surgical treatment of the gallbladder. Three hundred forty-three were operated on without operative cholangiography, with an incidence of retained stones of 0.03%. One hundred ten underwent operative cholangiography for similar reasons (outlined in the paper). If cholangiography were performed for each of the 100,000 cholecystectomies carried out in the U.S. during one year, the cost would be approximately $90 million. There is little question that a selective approach provides a significant saving.—S.I. Schwartz, M.D.

Influence of Intraperitoneal Drains on Subhepatic Collections Following Cholecystectomy: A Prospective Clinical Trial
J.R.T. Monson, J. MacFie, H. Irving, F.B.V. Keane, T.G. Brennan, and W.A. Tanner (St. James's Univ., Leeds, England, and Adelaide Hosp., Dublin, Ireland)
Br. J. Surg. 73:993–994, December 1986   25–3

The influence, if any, of intraperitoneal drains on the true incidence and clinical significance of subhepatic collections remains unclear. This prospective randomized study of 112 patients who had acute or elective cholecystectomy was done to assess the influence of an intraperitoneal drain on the incidence and clinical significance of subhepatic collections. Fifty-four received drains, and 58 did not. There was no significant difference with respect to age, sex, the number of cases who underwent cholecystectomy for acute cholecystitis, or the number of patients in whom the gallbladder bed was formally closed between the two groups.

In 11 (10%) of the 112 patients, subhepatic fluid collections were detected by ultrasound examination. Ten (18%) of the 54 patients who received drains had collections, while only 1 (1.8%) of the 58 in the nondrained group had developed a collection, a statistically significant difference ($P <.01$ χ^2 test). In this study, all collections were of a size in excess of that of the gallbladder fossa. None of the collections was clinically significant in that no patient developed intra-abdominal sepsis that necessitated either surgical drainage or continued antibiotic treatment, and there was no morbidity directly attributable to the presence of the retained fluid.

In 13 of the 112 patients, acute gallbladder disease was the surgical indication: 6 of these were in the drainage group, and in 1 a subhepatic collection developed. No collections were observed in the 7 undrained patients. With these cases excluded from analysis, the incidence of collections remains statistically higher in the drained group (10 vs. 1; $P <.05$). In 47 of 112 cases where the gallbladder bed was formally closed, 26 were in the drainage group and each of 4 (14.8%) had a collection. Of the 21 undrained patients, 1 (4.7%) had a collection.

Suction drains may predispose to the development of a significantly higher incidence of subhepatic collections as detected by ultrasound after cholecystectomy rather than preventing fluid collections. The wisdom of routine drainage following cholecystectomy should be questioned.

▶ This is a meaningful study, particularly since the drainage was performed by closed-system high-pressure suction drain. Raves et al. (*Am. J. Surg.* 148:618, 1984) conducted an experimental study comparing closed-suction and simple conduit drainage. They demonstrated that retrograde migration of bacteria along the drain tract occurs relatively often with a simple conduit drainage and significantly less often with closed-suction drainage. My own approach to the situation has changed over the years; in the past I routinely drained the gallbladder bed with a Penrose drain inserted into a Hollister bag. Recently I have limited drainage to those patients in whom the dissection of the gallbladder was difficult or to the circumstance in which there was significant edema. Presently I rarely drain following cholecystectomy.—S.I. Schwartz, M.D.

Management of Acute Cholangitis and the Impact of Endoscopic Sphincterotomy
T. Leese, J.P. Neoptolemos, A.R. Baker, and D.L. Carr-Locke (Leicester Royal Infirmary, Leicester, England)
Br. J. Surg. 73:988–992, December 1986   25–4

The presence of preprocedure fever or cholangitis is rarely mentioned in reports of patients undergoing endoscopic sphincterotomy, suggesting that most of these procedures have been performed on patients who are not septic and are therefore in a relatively low risk category. Of 94 patients aged 25–88 years (mean, 70 years) hospitalized with acute cholangitis since 1977, 87% were more than 60 years of age and 23% were

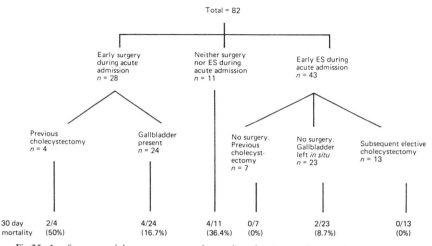

Fig 25−1.—Summary of the management and mortality of patients with acute cholangitis caused by common bile duct calculi. *ES,* endoscopic sphincterotomy. (Courtesy of Leese, T., et al.: Br. J. Surg. 73:988–992, December 1986.)

more than 80 years. Further, 82 had common bile duct calculi and 12 had other pathologies. In patients with stones, the 30-day mortality was 15%; in the remainder it was 25%; the overall 30-day mortality was 16%.

The patients who died had significantly more medical risk factors (*P* <.05), significantly lower serum albumin levels (*P* <.005), and significantly higher serum urea levels (*P* <.005), compared with survivors. The initial treatment was with antibiotics intravenously in all patients. Of the 82 patients with common bile duct calculi, 71 underwent early decompression, 28 (39%) having surgical decompression and 43 (61%) endoscopic decompression. The other 11 patients had neither procedure during their initial hospitalization because, in 7, the cholangitis resolved with antibiotic therapy alone; the other 4 died before biliary decompression could be attempted (Fig 25−1). A significantly higher 30-day mortality was associated with early surgery than with endoscopic sphincterotomy (*P* <.002) despite the fact that the patients having early sphincterotomy were significantly older (*P* <.002) and had significantly more medical risk factors (*P* <.005) but no significant differences in clinical or laboratory criteria of cholangitis severity.

Of the 60 patients with gallbladders present at the time of common bile duct decompression, 24 underwent early surgery: 23 had cholecystectomy and 1 had a large abscess drained by cholecystostomy. In 20 patients the common bile duct was explored supraduodenally, and in 12, transduodenally; 13 had T-tube drainage and 12 had internal drainage; of the latter group, 7 had choledochoduodenostomy, 4 had transduodenal sphincteroplasty, and 1 had transduodenal sphincterotomy. Thirteen of the 60 underwent early endoscopic sphincterotomy and improved; 6 elected cholecystectomy during the same admission, and 7, at a subsequent admission. Twenty-three others underwent early endoscopic sphincterotomy with the gallbladder left in situ because of their advanced age (mean, 79 years) and frailty. Follow-up for the latter group was between 1 and 7 years: 2 patients died within 30 days of the procedure, and 6 have died since from unrelated causes; 13 remain alive, 1 of whom has mild biliary colic controlled with a low-fat diet. Two others required cholecystectomy, one at 19 days after sphincterotomy because of empyema of the gallbladder and the other, at 5 months for recurrence of cholangitis.

The results suggest that acute cholangitis should be treated by urgent endoscopic biliary decompression after resuscitative measures, with emergency surgery reserved for those in whom endoscopic decompression fails or who do not improve after endoscopic sphincterotomy. Under this policy, it should be possible to keep mortality caused by acute suppurative cholangitis resulting from common bile duct calculi to less than 5%.

▶ This represents a relatively new approach to the problem. Kadir et al. (*AJR* 138:25, 1982) reported that percutaneous transhepatic drainage was performed on 18 patients with biliary sepsis. Fifteen had favorable responses. Some data suggest that when endoscopic sphincterotomy is performed for cholangitis, morbidity and mortality are significantly higher than usually quoted and are not necessarily better than the results obtained with operation.—S.I. Schwartz, M.D.

Unilateral Hepatic Duct Obstruction
Stephen G. ReMine, John W. Braasch, and Ricardo L. Rossi (Lahey Clinic Med. Ctr., Burlington, Mass.)
Am. J. Surg. 153:86–90, January 1987   25–5

In clinical practice, unilateral hepatic duct obstruction is often unrecognized because its symptoms are mild or vague, and there is a noticeable absence of literature on the subject. Of 500 patients with biliary reconstruction treated between 1965 and 1984, there were 33 with unilateral hepatic duct obstruction requiring repair—22 in women, 11 in men (median age, 56 years). Operative injury was the most common cause of stricture in 24 patients (73%), followed by unilobar intrahepatic stones in 6 (18%), sclerosing cholangitis in 4 (12%), and cholangiocarcinoma in 1 (3%). There had been 98 previous operations for biliary tract disease or complications in these patients.

Evidence of sepsis and a consistent intermittent fever and pain was the presenting symptom in 24 patients (73%): 13 (39%) of the patients had histories of intermittent jaundice with a mean bilirubin level of 4.8 mg/dl. In 6 of 9 patients, percutaneous transhepatic cholangiography and endoscopic retrograde cholangiopancreatography showed the site of the obstruction. By a ratio of 2:1, obstruction of the right duct predominated over left ductal obstruction. Complex procedures used for repair of the unilateral strictures were hepaticojejunostomy (14 patients), dilation and drainage (13), hepatic resection (3), or combined hepaticojejunostomy or dilation and segmental hepatic resection (3).

Although there were no operative or postoperative deaths, 51.5% of the patients had postoperative difficulties. Over a mean period of 5.4 years (range, 1–16 years), follow-up information was available for 28 patients. Of 7 (64%) of 11 patients in the dilation group, reoperation for recurrent stricture was necessary, and 2 patients (18%) died from septic complications related to a biliary tract procedure. Of 14 patients who had hepaticojejunostomy, 5 (36%) needed reoperation for stricture, and 1 (7%) died from sepsis postoperatively.

Operative injury was the most common cause of unilateral hepatic duct obstruction (73% of the patients). These patients underwent 131 operations, including operations for unilateral obstruction, related to biliary tract problems. Follow-up demonstrated that patients who had hepaticojejunostomy needed less frequent reoperation than those who had dilation, and they had a lower postoperative mortality rate related to biliary tract problems.

Unilateral hepatic duct obstruction occurs most commonly because of operative injury. It is best treated by hepaticojejunostomy or by resecting chronically obstructed lobes when possible.

▶ This subject is rarely presented in the literature. In considering unilateral duct obstruction, one could include the congenital stenosis of the left hepatic duct, causing the development of a cisterna in which gallstones can develop. Unilateral obstruction of a hepatic duct may be a consequence of recurrent pyogenic cholangitis, which occurs more frequently in Oriental countries. In these patients, the extent of intrahepatic unilobar disease is so great that hepatic resection may be indicated.—S.I. Schwartz, M.D.

Randomised Trial of Endoscopic Versus Percutaneous Stent Insertion in Malignant Obstructive Jaundice
Antony G. Speer, Peter B. Cotton, R. Christopher G. Russell, Richard R. Mason, Adrian R.W. Hatfield, Joseph W.C. Leung, Kenneth D. MacRae, Joan Houghton, and Christina A. Lennon (Middlesex and London Hosps. and King's College Hosp., London)
Lancet 2:57–62, July 11, 1987   25–6

A prospective trial compared the percutaneous and endoscopic approaches to treating biliary obstruction secondary to malignancy in patients who are unsuitable for open operation. Patients with obstructive jaundice due to primary carcinoma of the pancreas, gallbladder, or bile ducts were included. Thirty-nine of the first 75 patients were randomized to treatment with an endoscopic prosthesis/stent (EP), and the remaining 36 were treated with percutaneous transhepatic endoprostheses (PTE). More patients in the EP group had leukocytosis and hilar strictures, both factors adversely affecting survival.

Jaundice was relieved in 81% of the EP group and 61% of the PTE group, a significant difference. The respective 30-day mortalities were 15% and 33%. The higher mortality after percutaneous stenting resulted from complications of liver puncture, such as hemorrhage and bile leakage. Jaundice was not relieved in 3 patients having apparently successful endoscopic stenting.

Endoscopic stent insertion is more likely to succeed in relieving obstructive jaundice than is percutaneous stent placement in patients with malignant disease who are not operative candidates. The present findings are consistent with those reported by other groups. Surgical palliation may be advantageous in patients having a better prognosis than those in the present study.

▶ Results in large part are dependent upon the expertise of the endoscopist. Joseph et al. (*JAMA* 255:2763, 1986) reported a mortality of almost 90% related directly to percutaneous transhepatic biliary drainage. Emergency operations were required in 5% of patients, and in 12%, blood transfusions were needed. The overall sepsis rate was 35%. This was decreased to 16% when antibiotics were given prior to catheter insertion.—S.I. Schwartz, M.D.

Surgical Experience With Adenocarcinoma of the Ampulla of Vater
A. Chiappetta, C. Sperti, B. Bonadimani, C. Pasquali, C. Militello, P. Petrin, and S. Pedrazzoli (Univ. of Padua, Italy)
Am. Surg. 52:603–606, November 1986   25–7

Correct diagnosis is of primary importance in ampulloma since it differs from tumors of the pancreas, choledochus, and duodenum in that it has a more benign biologic activity. At earlier stages the choice between ampullectomy and pancreaticoduodenectomy (PD) has been discussed for a long time, and there is also debate at which borderline stage it is still useful to perform PD. Thirteen PDs, 1 total pancreatectomy, 2 ampullectomies, and 1 choledochoduodenostomy for neoplasia of the ampulla of Vater were evaluated, along with 1,894 PDs and 61 ampullectomies from a review of the literature.

SERIES OF AMPULLECTOMIES PUBLISHED FROM 1969 TO 1984
AND PRESENT SERIES

Author	Years of Treatment	Ampullectomies	Mortality %	% 5-year Survival
Nakase	1949–74	17	0	11
Akwari	1950–72	4	0	50
Schlippert	1940–76	7	14	14
Collected series		23	0	17
Wise	1956–68	8	12	37
Present series	1968–82	2	0	100
TOTAL		61	3	23

(Courtesy of Chiappetta, A., et al.: Am. Surg. 52:603–606, November 1986.)

In the 17 resected patients, operative mortality was zero, and the actuarial 5-year survival was 52.6%. The patient with total pancreatectomy and the 3 with regional node metastases who underwent PD died because of cancer recurrence. Seven who had PDs are still alive, and the last 3 who were without metastases also died of cancer recurrence. Only one of the 17 patients, 5.5%, was unresectable.

Of the 61 ampullectomies reviewed (table), operative death was lower (3%) than for the 1,894 PDs (14%), but the 5-year survival after ampullectomy was 23%, while for the 187 patients without node metastases who underwent PDs it was 39%. For cancer of the ampulla of Vater, PD is considered the operation of choice. Control of neoplastic growth was certainly better after PD considering that the 187 node-negative patients who had PD were probably at a more advanced stage than the 61 who underwent ampullectomy. The 52.6% survival rate in the authors' cases is similar to that of other authors' observations.

▶ Carcinoma of the ampulla of Vater certainly has a better prognosis than that associated with carcinoma of the head of the pancreas. This paper provides an excellent review of the subject. Ampullectomy is probably best reserved for localized fungating lesions in patients regarded as poor risks for pancreaticoduodenectomy.—S.I. Schwartz, M.D.

26 The Pancreas

Pancreas Transplant Result According to the Technique of Duct Management: Bladder Versus Enteric Drainage
Mikel Prieto, David E.R. Sutherland, Frederick C. Goetz, Mark E. Rosenberg, and John S. Najarian (Univ. of Minnesota, Minneapolis)
Surgery 102:680–691, October 1987   26–1

The optimal method of duct management for pancreas transplantation remains controversial, although an analysis of the Pancreas Transplant Registry shows no difference in results for the three major duct management techniques: polymer injection, enteric drainage (ED), and bladder drainage (BD). At one institution, both ED and BD techniques were used in a 28-month period. The outcome and complications associated with each are summarized.

From July 1978 to February 1987, 177 pancreas transplants were done. The technique for ED of segmental grafts involved intussuscepting the cut surface of the pancreatic neck into the end of a Roux-en-Y limb of recipient jejunum. Whole pancreas transplants involved anastomosing the graft duodenum to the side of a Roux-en-Y limb of recipient jejunum through a patch in 6 patients and the intact duodenum in 4. In 5 patients, the technique for BD of whole pancreas grafts involved anastomosing a patch of duodenum to the posterior wall of the bladder. In 28 pancreaticoduodenal grafts, a duodenocystostomy was done by anastomosing the lateral duodenum to the bladder (Fig 26–1). Up to October 1984, the 1-year patient and graft survival rates for the first 100 transplants were 88% and 27%, respectively. Beginning in November 1984, duct drainage was used for 74 of 77 transplants; BD, in 36; and ED, in 38. The 1-year patient survival rates were 89% and 92%, respectively, and graft survival rates were 58% and 42%, respectively. In both groups, the technical failure rate was 31%. Most recipients were nonuremic without kidney transplants; 1-year graft survival rates were 69% for 21 BDs and 42% for 29 EDs. Of technically successful grafts, the number of rejection episodes reversed per number diagnosed was 23 in 26 BDs and 6 in 15 EDs. Because the BD method allows monitoring of urine amylase activity, 1-year cadaveric graft survival rates were 90% for 23 BDs and 47% for 15 EDs. In patients receiving segmental transplants with ED from living related donors, 1-year graft survival rates were 57% of the total number of 18 and 88% in the 12 technically successful cases.

The technique appears to be the most successful for pancreas transplants from cadaver donors. The ability to monitor exocrine and endocrine function continuously leads to early diagnosis and treatment of re-

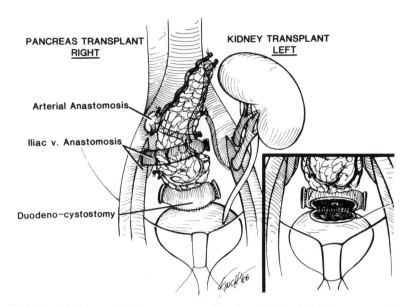

Fig 26–1.—Technique of whole pancreas transplantation with BD. A duodenocystostomy is performed by placing interrupted nonabsorbable sutures in the seromuscular layers followed by a running absorbable suture to approximate the mucosa *(inset)*. On completion of the duodenocystostomy *(full figure)*, a kidney transplant may or may not be performed, depending on the severity of diabetic nephropathy in the recipient. (Courtesy of Prieto, M., et al.: Surgery 102:680–691, October 1987.)

jection episodes. One disadvantage is metabolic acidosis induced by chronic bicarbonate loss in the urine from the pancreas graft.

▶ The number of pancreatic transplants performed in America has increased tremendously in the last 2 years, with rates of survival of the transplant at 1 year that are similar to those achieved with other organs. This study and others (for example, *Surg. Gynecol. Obstet.* 162:547–555, 1986) provide evidence that the procedure is no longer experimental but reliably therapeutic. The exocrine tissue is the burden that the pancreatic endocrine transplant carries along, and getting rid of the exocrine secretion is the big problem. Blocking the duct by ligating it or by injecting it with polymer proved unsatisfactory. Exocrine drainage is provided now by anastomosis of either whole segments of duodenum or a duodenal button to the small bowel or to the bladder. Each method has a disadvantage. Enteric anastomoses are bathed with enteric organisms and are prone to infection; drainage of pancreatic bicarbonate into the bladder results in a metabolic acidosis. The salient need in all cadaveric organ transplantation is a means of early detection of graft rejection. Monitoring the total hourly urinary amylase secretion (said by these authors to be more accurate than measuring urinary amylase concentration), coupled with glucose measurements, do usually provide this early warning, which allows adjustment of the immunosuppressive therapy so as to successfully combat the rejection. In technically successful grafts, the 1-year survival rate for cadaveric grafts drained into the bladder was twice as high (90%) as that achieved with enteric drainage. The great therapeutic promise of pancreas transplantation is that it will halt progression of diabetic pathology in all organs. The recent report (*N. Engl. J. Med.* 318:208–214, 1988) from the University of Minnesota of failure of successfully functioning pancreatic allografts to halt progression of diabetic retinopathy is a natural cause for concern. There are all sorts of anecdotal data demonstrating lack of progression of renal and neuropathic lesions. We must still await firm demonstration of the efficacy of pancreatic allografts in man.—J.C. Thompson, M.D.

Pancreas Divisum: Is It a Normal Anatomic Variant?
Choichi Sugawa, Alexander J. Walt, Domingo C. Nunez, and Hironori Masuyama (Wayne State Univ., Detroit)
Am. J. Surg. 153:62–67, January 1987   26–2

Pancreas divisum results from the failure of the dorsal and ventral pancreatic anlage to fuse during the 8th week of gestation, but surgical and endoscopic observations remain contradictory in many ways. An overall incidence rate varying from 0.8% to 5.7% has been reported in the literature, but one study reported an incidence as high as 25.6% in a subgroup of patients with idiopathic acute pancreatitis. The latter observation implicated pancreas divisum as a likely etiologic factor with a presumed pathophysiologic cause postulated to be a relative flow obstruction at the minor papilla. Thus, surgical attempts at correcting pancreas divisum have increased in order to correct upper abdominal pain of obscure cause, but results have been mixed and unpredictable.

In a review of 1,529 patients with successful pancreatograms, grouped according to incidental, unexplained upper abdominal pain, alcoholic, and idiopathic pancreatitis, 41 were found to have pancreas divisum (2.7%), with similar rates in each group. In contrast to some other reports, no increased incidence was apparent among the pancreatitis patients, whether from the alcoholic or idiopathic group. The majority of these patients (80%) who had pancreas divisum had it as an incidental finding or in association with alcoholic pancreatitis. Fourteen patients had an incomplete divisum, of which 5 were in the incidental group, 3 were in the alcoholic pancreatitis group, and 6 were in the abdominal pain group, and none were in the idiopathic pancreatitis group.

The finding of an increased incidence of ductal variation in patients with idiopathic pancreatitis is the major argument for implicating pancreas divisum as a cause of pancreatitis. Nevertheless, no increased incidence was found in any of the subgroups in this study, findings similar to those of Delhaye and associates. These findings also argue against any substantial relationship between pancreas divisum and pancreatitis. The authors believe consideration of accessory duct sphincterotomy should be limited at the present to patients with biochemically proved acute recurrent pancreatitis who have a relatively normal duct pattern on pancreatography, and they conclude that pancreas divisum is a normal anatomical variant that very seldom causes pancreatic pain.

▶ Was the great temporary interest in pancreas divisum as a cause of pancreatitis merely one of those fleeting medical fads? This paper certainly provides a strong argument against the association, and I am persuaded that the conclusions that the authors reach are correct. Cotton (*Gut* 21:105–114, 1980) provided much of the initial enthusiasm when he reported that 26% of patients with idiopathic pancreatitis had pancreas divisum. He has continued to examine the question and in a recent editorial (*Gastroenterology* 89:1431–1435, 1985) concluded that most patients with pancreatitis in association with pancreas divisum should be managed conservatively and that duct surgery should be considered only when attacks are frequent and disabling. I would bet that the number of patients fulfilling that criterion (the anatomical basis of which, he says, is the coexistence of pancreas divisum and stenosis of the orifice of the accessory duct) would be small: probably not even a blip on an epidemiologist's oscilloscope.—J.C. Thompson, M.D.

Simultaneous Treatment of Chronic Pancreatitis and Pancreatic Pseudocyst
John S. Munn, Gerard V. Aranha, Herbert B. Greenlee, and Richard A. Prinz (Loyola Univ., Maywood, Ill., and Hines VA Hosp., Hines, Ill.)
Arch. Surg. 122:662–667, June 1987   26–3

The records of 87 consecutive patients from 1975 to 1985 who had undergone lateral pancreaticojejunostomy (LPJ) for chronic pancreatitis were reviewed to determine the incidence of pseudocyst and the safety of combined pancreatic duct and pseudocyst drainage. The patients' mean age was 47 years, and there were 79 men and 8 women. Chronic pancreatitis was attributed in 85 patients to alcohol abuse, and the cause was idiopathic in the other 2. All complained of abdominal pain.

Preoperative ultrasonography was done in 19 patients who had a pseudocyst confirmed at operation. A computed tomographic (CT) scan correctly identified pseudocysts in 11 of 12 patients. The patients were divided into two groups: 26 underwent simultaneous pseudocyst drainage and LPJ (group 1), and 61 underwent LPJ without pseudocyst drainage (group 2). Four patients in group 1 had undergone previous surgical treatment for pancreatic pseudocysts, while the other 22 had pseudocysts drained for the first time during LPJ. Eight of the 61 patients in group 2 had had pseudocyst drainage previously and had no evidence of recurrence at the time of LPJ. The overall incidence of pancreatic pseudocysts in patients undergoing pancreatic ductal drainage was 39%.

In group 1, complications occurred in 5 patients, and there were two deaths: 1 patient developed an anastomotic leak and died of overwhelming staphylococcal sepsis, and 1 patient died from severe peptic ulcer disease complications. The latter also had external drainage of an infected pseudocyst. In group 2, there were 11 complications and one death, which resulted from mesenteric infarction in a patient with chronic renal failure. Of the patients in group 1, 57% were pain free at follow-up time, ranging from 3 months to 10 years; in group 2, 48% of the patients were pain free at follow-up. The percentage of patients who benefited from pancreatic drainage was 81% in group 1 and 84% in group 2. One patient in group 1 and 4 in group 2 required additional surgical procedures for pain related to pancreatitis. From the follow-up period to date, no recurrent pseudocysts have been detected.

Pseudocyst drainage with LPJ did not appear to increase the risk of operation in this series. In both groups the morbidities and mortalities were the same, as was patient outcome. The risk of internal pseudocyst drainage does not appear to increase with simultaneous LPJ; nevertheless, when infected pseudocysts are encountered, care must be taken. In such patients a two-stage approach is probably necessary.

▶ The authors pose the question of whether it is safe to simultaneously drain a pancreatic pseudocyst when performing a Puestow type pancreaticojejunostomy in a patient with chronic pancreatitis. Their answer is yes, in that the number of complications and mortality in the series of patients with the combined operation were not significantly different from that in a series of patients who had ductal drainage alone. I would have been greatly surprised if the results had been significantly different. It is our policy, whenever we consider a Puestow procedure, to carefully assess the patient for evidence of biliary obstruction caused by the pancreatitis and for pseudocysts and any other pathology and to try to address all of these at the same time. I would agree that if a pseudocyst was filled with pus it probably should not be drained through the same Roux-en-Y limb as used in the pancreaticojejunostomy. If the infected lesion is a true abscess, it will of course need external drainage. If however it is merely a slightly infected pseudocyst (that is, cyst fluid with some pus cells in it), we might either marsupialize it or bring up another Roux-en-Y limb, if we could keep the two anastomotic lines clearly separate. Whatever would best keep pus away from the anastomosis between the pancreatic duct and the Roux-en-Y limb would probably be the best choice.—J.C. Thompson, M.D.

Glucose, Fatty Acid, and Urea Kinetics in Patients With Severe Pancreatitis: The Response to Substrate Infusion and Total Parenteral Nutrition
J.H.F. Shaw and R.R. Wolfe (Auckland Hosp., Auckland, New Zealand and Univ. of Texas, Galveston)
Ann. Surg. 204:665–672, December 1986   26–4

Two important benefits of glucose infusion are suppression of endogenous glucose production and direct use as an energy source. Glucose infusion is thought to be advantageous in patients with pancreatitis, but there is little data concerning glucose metabolism in these individuals to confirm this hypothesis. The authors conducted a series of investigations evaluating glucose oxidation, fat metabolism, and the response of glucose and protein metabolism to total parenteral nutrition (TPN) in patients with pancreatitis in the basal state, during glucose infusion (4 ml/kg/min), and during TPN.

The study population included 16 normal controls and 9 patients with pancreatitis. Following appropriate priming of the bicarbonate pool, primed constant infusions of either 6-^{3}H-glucose or 6-d$_2$-glucose and either U-^{14}C-glucose or U-^{13}C-glucose were used to assess glucose turnover and glucose oxidation, respectively. Primed constant infusion of (^{15}N$_2$)-urea or U-^{14}C-urea were used for determining urea kinetics. A constant infusion of 1,2-^{13}C-palmitate was administered to evaluate free fatty acid (FFA) kinetics.

Basal state production of glucose and plasma glucose clearance were significantly higher in the patients with pancreatitis than in the controls. Glucose infusion resulted in nearly absolute suppression of endogenous glucose production in the volunteers (94%) compared with only 44% suppression in the pancreatitis group, a statistically significant difference. The percentage of available glucose oxidized decreased significantly in the patients with pancreatitis and was less than in the controls. The patients had a significantly greater rate of urea production in the basal state. Glucose infusion produced a significant decrease in this parameter in both groups. There was no difference between groups in the rate of FFA turnover nor in the effects of glucose infusion on suppressing FFA turnover. Administration of TPN to the patients with pancreatitis had no additional significant effect on endogenous glucose production, plasma urea concentration, or the rate of urea production beyond that seen with glucose infusion alone. It did result in a significant increase in the percentage of glucose uptake oxidized and glucose oxidation.

These results indicate that patients with pancreatitis are metabolically and nutritionally similar to septic patients. Patients with pancreatitis had impaired ability to oxidize infused glucose compared with normal subjects. In response to the increased glucose available through TPN, however, the patients with pancreatitis were able to increase the percentage of glucose uptake oxidized. An increased rate of net protein catabolism was also found in the patients with pancreatitis. A significant decrease in the rate of net protein catabolism followed glucose infusion in these patients, although the effect was smaller than that occurring in normal volunteers.

▶ These authors have previously shown (*Surgery* 97:557–567, 1985) that severely septic patients show an enhanced rate of glucose clearance, a decreased suppressibility of endogenous glucose production, and a decrease in the percentage of glucose uptake that is oxidized. This present work confirms all of these findings in patients severely ill with pancreatitis. Studies with TPN confirmed the findings with acute glucose infusion and showed a marked increase in the percentage of glucose uptake that was oxidized. Furthermore, even though the pancreatitis patients did not show an increased rate of lipolysis, they were heavily dependent upon fat for energy, a finding also previously reported in trauma and sepsis (*Prog. Clin. Biol. Res.* 3:89–109, 1983). This study is another elegant demonstration of the efficacy of stable isotope techniques in the study of intermediary metabolism in severely ill patients.—J.C. Thompson, M.D.

Preoperative Localization and Intraoperative Glucose Monitoring in the Management of Patients With Pancreatic Insulinoma

L. Brian Katz, Arthur H. Aufses, Jr., Elliot Rayfield, and Harold Mitty (Mount Sinai School of Medicine, New York)
Surg. Gynecol. Obstet. 163:509–512, December 1986   26–5

More than 90% of the tumors of insulinoma are benign, and the operative cure consequently is high. But because of the tumor's multicentricity (12% to 13%) and its frequently small size, some series report 15% to 30% inadequate or failed operations. Fifteen patients diagnosed with insulinoma from 1974 to 1984 were reviewed, the age range being 8 to 68. Abdominal sonography, computerized axial tomography (CT), angiography, and transhepatic portal venous sampling were the procedures used to establish the precise anatomical location of the tumor.

The patients' blood sugar levels were monitored frequently intraoperatively while they received a 5% glucose infusion. When the tumor was located, the continuous infusion was stopped, and samples of blood were drawn every 15 minutes for glucose determination. Sustained elevation of the blood sugar level of more than 125 mg% showed adequacy of resection. To prevent possible hypoglycemia, sugar levels were monitored: if the level did not increase, further exploration as indicated was undertaken with further resection, and all specimens excised were submitted for frozen section confirmation.

In reviewing the preoperative tests, only 1 of 6 was diagnostically accurate for sonography; for CT, 1 of 5 was a positive result, and 1 was a false-positive test. Celiac angiography was accurate in 43% (6 of 14

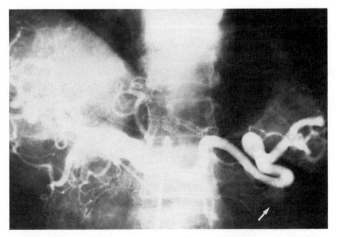

Fig 26–2.—Celiac angiogram demonstrating tumor blush in distal splenic artery. (Courtesy of Katz, L.B., et al.: Surg. Gynecol. Obstet. 163:509–512, December 1986.)

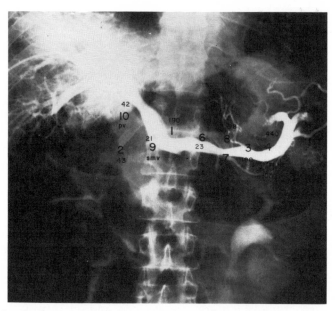

Fig 26–3.—Portal venous sampling, in same patient as in Figure 26–2, with corresponding insulin "step up" in distal splenic vein. The large numbers refer to the multiple sites of venous blood sampling, and the small numbers are the measured insulin levels. *pv*, portal vein, and *smv*, superior mesenteric vein. (Courtesy of Katz, L.B., et al.: Surg. Gynecol. Obstet. 163:509–512, December 1986.)

and 2 false-positive results); and in the percutaneous portal venous sampling, 11 of 13 were positive. In all patients the blood sugar level after successful resection sustained elevation. Preoperative portal venous sampling and intraoperative glucose monitoring complemented each other. Benign insulinoma was pathologically diagnosed in all patients. Tumors ranged from 3.0 mm to 2.5 cm, the smallest found because the results of preoperative percutaneous portal venous sampling led the surgeon to concentrate the search in a limited area. Mean follow-up was 6 years, with no recurrences of hypoglycemia after operation.

Tumors that may have been missed on routine digital palpation and some below the resolving power of operative ultrasonography were able to be excised. All patients with positive angiogram also had positive portal venous sampling (Figs 26–2 and 26–3), but angiograms of 5 patients who had positive venous sampling were negative. The authors found the combination of transhepatic portal venous sampling and arteriography to be the most accurate means of preoperative tumor localization, but they have not found sonography or CT helpful.

▶ This is good demonstration of the value of selective pancreatic venous sampling in the preoperative localization of insulinomas. Results with other endocrine tumors are not nearly so good, and we have had no help at all with preoperative localization of gastrinomas (*Ann. Surg.* 197:594–607, 1983). I am not sure if anyone else has had the consistent good results reported here, and I still believe that the best single study is probably intraoperative ultrasonography (*Lancet* 1:483–486, 1981; *Ann. Surg.* 200:486–493, 1984) by which method a tumor as small as 3 mm has been located (see next paper and *J. Pediatr. Surg.* 21:262–266, 1986).—J.C. Thompson, M.D.

Benign Pancreatic Insulinoma: Preoperative and Intraoperative Sonographic Localization

Brian Gorman, J. William Charboneau, E. Meredith James, Carl C. Reading, Angelo K. Galiber, Clive S. Grant, Jon A. van Heerden, Robert L. Telander, and F. John Service (Mayo Clinic and Mayo Found., Rochester, Minn.)
AJR 147:929–934, November 1986   26–6

Insulinomas are small solitary benign pancreatic tumors. Accurate localization of these tumors allows efficient and safe excision. Intraoperative and preoperative sonography was used to visualize benign pancreatic insulinoma in 29 patients.

Preoperative sonography was performed in 24 patients with solitary insulinomas, and 63% were localized. Intraoperative sonography was performed in 22 of these patients, and 86% of the tumors were visualized. Four of these tumors could not be detected by palpation. All of the solitary tumors could be detected by a combination of palpation and intraoperative sonography. Nonpalpable tumors were visualized in 2 of the 4 patients with multiple insulinomas.

Sonography is a sensitive, noninvasive, inexpensive technique for the detection and localization of insulinoma to facilitate surgical removal.

▶ A success rate of 86% in the localization of insulinomas at operation is an outstanding batting average (see discussion, previous paper). Intraoperative sonography achieved a resolution sufficiently good to allow detection of a 3-mm insulinoma in this series. Preoperative selective pancreatic venous sampling and intraoperative sonography are complimentary and, applied together, should provide for localization of almost any macroscopic tumor.—J.C. Thompson, M.D.

Bone Metastases in Malignant Gastrinoma

James C. Barton, Basil I. Hirschowitz, Paul N. Maton, and Robert T. Jensen (Univ. of Alabama in Birmingham; VA Med. Ctr., Birmingham; and Natl. Inst. of Health, Bethesda, Md.)
Gastroenterology 91:1179–1185, November 1986   26–7

Approximately two thirds of the gastrin-producing islet cell tumors of Zollinger-Ellison syndrome are malignant and have already metastasized upon diagnosis. The tumor usually spreads to regional lymph nodes or to the liver. Six cases of bone metastases of malignant gastrinoma in Zollinger-Ellison syndrome are described in this study.

Four men and two women with malignant gastrinoma developed bone

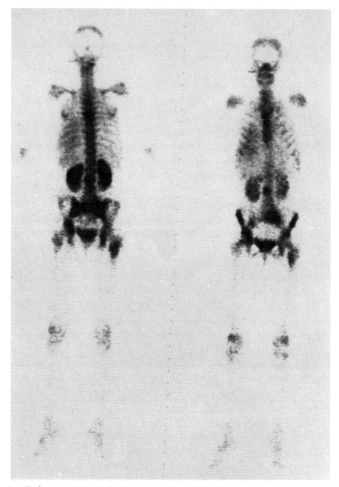

Fig 26–4.—Technetium 99m-Tc-hydroxymethylene diphosphonate bone scintigraph performed before intravenous chemotherapy showing multiple areas of increased radionuclide uptake. (Courtesy of Barton, J.C., et al.: Gastroenterology 91:1179–1185, November 1986.)

metastases, primarily in the central skeleton. Most of the lesions were symptomatic, and some produced vertebral body collapse. Some of the lesions were detected by radionuclide bone scanning (Fig 26–4), and others were identified as osteolytic or osteoblastic, or both, by radiography. Two patients developed hypercalcemia in association with bone metastases. Response to cytotoxic drugs was poor. Two of four patients who received radiotherapy achieved symptomatic relief of bone pain. Peptic ulcer was relieved in all patients by administration of cimetidine with or without anticholinergics or by ranitidine alone. Five of the six patients died after diagnosis of Zollinger-Ellison syndrome with a mean survival of 3.3 years (range, 1–7 years). The poor clinical prognosis for patients with bone metastases in gastrinoma is evident in this study.

▶ Gastrinomas manifest a tremendous variation in biologic aggression. Most patients go along for years having little trouble with their tumor, but in some, the tumors spread rapidly to involve multiple organs and lead to death within a few years. All six patients in this series died (all but one within 4 years of diagnosis). On the basis of finding three patients with bone metastases among 88 sent to the NIH, the authors conclude that bone metastasis is a relatively common occurrence among patients with advanced gastrinoma. Since only seven cases of gastrinoma metastatic to bone (these six plus one other [*Radiology* 118:63–64, 1976]) have ever been reported, that conclusion seems unlikely. Clearly, any gastrinoma patient who develops bone pain should be studied for metastasis. One of these patients was operated upon, and evidence of noncurability of the gastrinoma was secured in the other five patients. It is worth repeating the plea that every patient with a potentially curable tumor should be operated upon. Since gastroenterologists learned to manage the hypersecretory aspects of the Zollinger-Ellison (ZE) syndrome with drugs, many have advocated total nonoperative treatment of ZE patients. Dr. Zollinger (*Surgery* 97:49–54, 1985) has called attention to the fact that gastrinoma is the only endocrine tumor of the pancreas that is not routinely operated upon. All ZE patients should be operated upon for their tumors unless clear evidence of noncurability is present.—J.C. Thompson, M.D.

Progression of a Benign Epithelial Ampullary Tumor to Adenocarcinoma
D.J. Gouma, H. Obertop, J. Vismans, D. Willebrand, and P.B. Soeters (Maastricht Univ., Maastricht, The Netherlands)
Surgery 101:501–504, April 1987   26–8

The high recurrence rate following local resection of benign tumors of the extrahepatic biliary ducts is well known, but the tumors' development from benignancy to malignancy has received little attention. The authors describe a benign periampullary tumor that developed into a well-differentiated papillary adenocarcinoma 4 years after local excision.

Man, 54, had continuous pain in the right upper abdomen, intermittent obstructive jaundice, and pruritus. Percutaneous transhepatic cholangiography showed a filling defect in the distal common duct, and a small tumor was found. Local excision was performed and preoperative biopsy specimens showed papillomatosis and no evidence of malignant disease. He was symptom free for 4 years, until recurrent pain recurred in his right upper abdomen. He had a normal white blood cell count and clotting screen, but abnormal liver function. Dilated bile ducts were revealed, and there was again a filling defect in the distal common duct. A biopsy specimen of a small tumor showed a well-differentiated papillary adenocarcinoma. Celiac angiography showed normal vascular anatomy and no tumor invasion, and computed tomography showed no evidence of liver metastases. No sign of metastases was found at laparotomy, and a pancreatoduodenectomy was performed. The patient was discharged 26 days after the operation.

This is a unique case because of the postoperative 4-year disease-free interval before recurrence and the development into a malignant tumor.

It is highly unlikely that a focus of adenocarcinoma was present during the first laparotomy, but it is possible the benign tumor was incompletely excised and therefore recurred. It is concluded that these benign lesions have a malignant potential. Radical surgery should be considered in managing these tumors, especially in patients aged younger than 70 years, since preoperative and perioperative diagnosis is not always conclusive. Preoperative external biliary drainage is not performed routinely at present, since recent randomized trials have not shown reduction of morbidity and mortality, although it was done before this patient's first laparotomy.

▶ This paper was chosen as a reminder that all ampullary tumors are dangerous, and any time we decide to treat one by local excision, we assume a great responsibility to follow the patient carefully for years. We are particularly apt to get into trouble with carcinoid tumors of the ampulla, which have a high rate of malignancy to begin with, but in which, additionally, malignant change may supervene in apparently benign adenomas. The question is: which course has the greater risk in a benign tumor, a Whipple resection or a wide local excision of the tumor and careful follow-up? Safety of the latter choice would depend upon clear histologic evidence that all the tumor was removed and a mutual decision between surgeon and patient about frequency and diligence of follow-up examination. If both requirements could be met, I would vote for local excision. If not, the tumor should be removed radically.—J.C. Thompson, M.D.

Carcinoma of the Exocrine Pancreas: A Sex Hormone Responsive Tumour?
B.A. Greenway (London Hosp.)
Br. J. Surg. 74:441–442, June 1987   26–9

A new approach in the management of pancreatic carcinoma was suggested in 1981, when the presence of high concentrations of estrogen receptors in both the cytoplasm and nucleus was demonstrated for the first time in human pancreatic adenocarcinoma of ductular origin. With the finding of progesterone receptors within tumor tissue, there was evidence that these receptors were important, since these require the presence of functioning estrogen receptors for their formation. Using improved sensitivity techniques, androgen receptors have been recently demonstrated. Thus, all three sex-steroid receptors have been demonstrated in pancreatic carcinoma tissue. Enzymes distributed in uterine prostate and breast cancer have now been demonstrated in pancreatic carcinoma.

Studies have strongly suggested that pancreatic cancer should now be considered a hormone responsive neoplasm, and that hormone manipulation may offer a new approach to treating pancreatic carcinoma. Results of animal studies have confirmed the inhibiting effect of hormone manipulation on the growth of human pancreatic adenocarcinoma xenografts. Now human studies are urgently required. Two phase II studies demonstrated an increase in median survival and an increased number of patients with long survival using tamoxifen in patients with unresectable pancreatic carcinoma. One preliminary report using an analogue luteinizing hormone-releasing hormone in five patients was encouraging. One of the five patients with stage IV tumor and liver metastases lived 16 months, and all five showed clinical and subjective improvement. As demonstrated in earlier experimental work, this study provided further support for the apparent central role of testosterone in tumor growth. Alteration of the hormonal milieu is not a cure for this tumor, but it may be a major advance in treating what is virtually an untreatable malignancy.

Currently there are a number of phase III trials in progress involving hormonal therapy in pancreatic carcinoma. In one study using cyproterone, there was no difference in survival when compared to the control group, whereas 8 of 37 patients treated with tamoxifen survived more than 1 year. Other hormonal therapies should be investigated in phase II trials. All agents shown to be effective in treating breast or prostatic carcinoma are worthy of study.

▶ Estrogen receptors were first demonstrated in the pancreas in man 15 years ago (*Steroids* 22:259–271, 1973), and 7 years ago, estrogen receptors were found in human ductal cancer (*Br. J. Med.* 283:751–753, 1981). Later studies have demonstrated receptors for both progesterone (*IRCS Med. Sci.* 12:575–576, 1984) and for androgens (*Cancer* 57:1992–1995, 1986) in human pancreatic cancer. This editorial notes that early studies with tamoxifen and an analogue of luteinizing hormone-releasing hormone have been encouraging and pleads for new human studies. When dealing with a tumor that is nearly 100% lethal, any glimmer of hope should be aggressively followed.—J.C. Thompson, M.D.

Cystic Neoplasms of the Pancreas

Stephen G. ReMine, Daniel Frey, Ricardo L. Rossi, J. Lawrence Munson, and John W. Braasch (Lahey Clinic Med. Ctr., Burlington, Mass.)
Arch. Surg. 122:443–446, April 1987   26–10

Neoplastic cysts of the pancreas (cystadenomas and cystadenocarcinomas) are rare and account for 9% to 10% of malignant cystic lesions and 1% of primary malignant lesions. The potential for benign cysts to undergo malignant degeneration is ill-defined, and methods of management are still controversial.

Twenty-six patients with neoplastic cysts of the pancreas were treated during a 20-year period from 1963 to 1983. Fifteen patients had cystadenoma, and 11 had cystadenocarcinoma. The mean age of the 16 women and 10 men was 60.5 years. Ninety-five percent of the patients experienced symptoms, mainly mild abdominal pain. The prodrome of symptoms in more than half of the cystadenocarcinoma group was present for longer than 5 years. The mean size of the cysts was 7.5 cm, and the cysts were evenly distributed among the head, body, and tail of the pancreas (Fig 26–5). The most commonly performed surgical procedure was distal

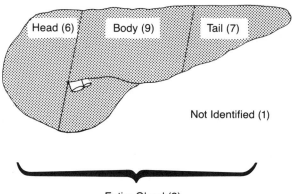

Fig 26–5.—Location of cystic neoplasms of pancreas. Number of patients is given in parentheses. (Courtesy of ReMine, S.G., et al.: Arch. Surg. 122:443–446, April 1987.)

pancreatectomy, performed in 10 patients. Eight of the 11 patients with cystadenocarcinoma were noted to have metastatic disease upon exploration. One patient died postoperatively, for a mortality of 3.8%. Patients with cystadenocarcinoma had a median adjusted survival of 6.0 months after surgery; the adjusted 5-year survival rate was 20% ± 12.6% (mean ± SEM). Patients with cystadenoma had no recurrent benign or malignant disease during follow-up periods lasting from 2 months to 12 years. These data suggest that an aggressive surgical approach is warranted and that complete excision of cystic neoplasms of the pancreas is the treatment of choice.

▶ Anytime we see a cystic lesion of the pancreas we should always consider the possibility of a tumor, even though cystic tumors of the pancreas are rare. They also are curable if they are benign or if they are malignant and discovered early. The long prodrome of symptoms in patients with cystadenocarcinomas (greater than 5 years in more than half) is tantalizing. If they had undergone study by computerized tomography or by ultrasound within the first year or two, they may well have been cured. As it was, the 5-year survival rate was 20%. One cautionary note is that some patients with cystic tumors of the pancreas have been mistakenly treated for pseudocyst, and the patient had later died from metastases. If there is ever any doubt, the wall of any pancreatic cyst should be biopsied for frozen section diagnosis.—J.C. Thompson, M.D.

Gastrojejunostomy: Is It Helpful for Patients With Pancreatic Cancer?
Donald W. Weaver, Robert G. Wiencek, David L. Bouwman, and Alexander J. Walt (Wayne State Univ., Detroit)
Surgery 102:608–613, October 1987   26–11

The efficacy of gastrojejunostomy as a palliative measure for patients with pancreatic cancer remains a controversy. To clarify further, a retrospective review of 81 patients who underwent gastrojejunostomy for pancreatic cancer was conducted. The patients were divided into two groups based on duodenal patency. Group I (n = 45) had no evidence of duodenal obstruction, but gastrojejunostomy was performed as a hedge against future obstruction. Group II (n = 36) had evidence of impingement on the duodenum by the pancreatic cancer and was thought to comprise potential beneficiaries of gastrojejunostomy. Poor outcome was defined as either death during the hospitalization for gastrojejunostomy or death within 30 days of operation even if the patient left the hospital.

Significantly more patients in group II (70%) had poor outcome compared to group I patients (40%) (Fig 26–6). In 21 patients who had significant nausea and vomiting and in whom gastrojejunostomy was judged to be essential, 19 (90%) had poor outcome, including 5 patients who had no evidence of duodenal impingement. Eleven patients with partial or substantial obstruction appeared to have benefited from gastrojejunostomy, but an upper gastointestinal series performed within 30 days of the procedure showed that the stomach emptied preferentially through the duodenum despite a patent gastrojejunostomy.

It appears that gastrojejunostomy has little, if any, role in the management of patients with pancreatic cancer. In addition, effective palliation is

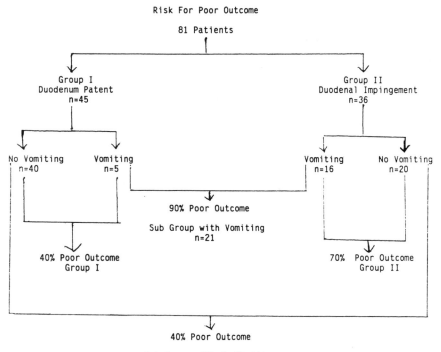

Fig 26–6.—Analysis of data to determine which patients benefited from gastrojejunostomy and risk for poor outcome. (Courtesy of Weaver, D.W., et al.: Surgery 102:608–613, October 1987.)

rarely achieved for patients with significant nausea and vomiting with or without impingement on the duodenum.

▶ This problem was reviewed in this section in 1985, and although I said that the evidence appeared to be against routine addition of gastrojejunostomy to a palliative procedure for a patient with carcinoma of the pancreas, I noted conflicting evidence and concluded that the right answer was not clearly apparent. With time, I have felt even less inclined to advocate gastrojejunostomy. These authors call attention to the paradox that the more a patient seems to need a gastrojejunostomy, the less likely they are to have a favorable course. That is, signs of impending duodenal obstruction are a harbinger of early death. This seems to state the situation well, and I would agree with their conclusion that gastrojejunostomy appears rarely to be helpful. Truth to tell, I am not sure that any palliative surgical effort is worthwhile.—J.C. Thompson, M.D.

Pylorus-Preserving Pancreatoduodenectomy: A Clinical and Physiologic Appraisal
Kamal M.F. Itani, R. Edward Coleman, Onye E. Akwari, and William C. Meyers (Duke Univ.)
Ann. Surg. 204:655–664, December 1986   26–12

Several advantages have been suggested for pancreatoduodenectomy with pylorus preservation. It is believed that the nutritional status of patients would benefit from preservation of the intact stomach, and that jejunal ulceration, perforation, and bile reflux would be less likely to occur following this operation. The authors describe a multicenter study of 252 patients who underwent pylorus-preserving pancreatoduodenectomy.

Forty-five percent (113) of patients underwent surgery for benign conditions. Resection of malignant tumors of the ampulla and periampullary region was performed in the remaining patients, representing a significant change in the application of this procedure. The most frequent postsurgical complication was delayed gastric emptying, which was reported in 76 (30%) patients. Six patients developed jejunal ulceration at the anastomosis site, 2 of whom required vagotomy and antrectomy. Major complications included anastomotic leaks and fistulae (19% of patients), pancreatic fistulae (11%), biliary fistulae (4%), and enteric fistulae (4%). The overall mortality associated with this operation was 2.8%.

A review of data on 252 patients who underwent pylorus-preserving pancreatoduodenectomy showed that this procedure was associated with fewer postsurgical problems than the standard Whipple operation. Delayed gastric emptying, the most commonly reported complication, is probably best treated by placement of a gastrostomy tube for decompression. The results of this study support pylorus preservation as the current technique of choice for gastrointestinal reconstruction after pancreatoduodenectomy. Further studies are needed to determine the physiologic effects of this operation.

▶ This operation was initially designed for patients with benign disease of the pancreas or carefully selected localized duodenal tumors, not for cancer of the head of the pancreas. Initially many felt that retention of the pylorus would lead to compromise of chances for cure of a carcinoma of the head of the pancreas. The authors note that 55% of the patients in their series had carcinoma, including carcinoma of the head of the pancreas and of the distal common bile duct. They suggest that the popularity of the operation is due to a simpler reconstruction after gastrectomy and to the concept that an intact stomach allows for better digestion. I have difficulty with both premises, and the concern that preservation of the pylorus may compromise the chance of curing a pancreatic carcinoma appears valid. Nonetheless, the operation is popular. Gastric retention postoperatively is a problem, and the authors suggest decompression with a gastrostomy tube. Gastrostomy tubes sometimes leak and may cause severe trouble. Nasogastric tubes, although widely condemned by everyone, have led to fewer major complications, and I would certainly decompress the stomach by nasogastric suction. The authors provide a good description of the operation, including a careful assessment of resectability. One final note: this is a strange amalgam of patients. The authors report 7 patients of their own, 188 patients who have previously been reported in the literature, and 57 patients that they gathered by writing to other centers. An interesting pastiche.—J.C. Thompson, M.D.

27 The Endocrine Glands

Thyroid Neoplasia Following Radiation Therapy for Hodgkin's Lymphoma
Christopher McHenry, Harriet Jarosz, David Calandra, Anne McCall, A.M.
Lawrence, and Edward Paloyan (Loyola Univ., Maywood, Ill., and VA Hosp.,
Hines, Ill.)
Arch. Surg. 122:684–688, June 1987   27–1

Patients with Hodgkin's lymphoma often receive radiation in the cervical and mediastinal lymphatic areas, including the thyroid gland. The authors describe the occurrence of thyroid carcinoma following high-dose radiotherapy to the head, neck, and mediastinum in children and young adults.

Five patients developed thyroid neoplasms following cervical and mediastinal radiation for Hodgkin's lymphoma. The patients were aged 19–39 years at the time of surgical excision of their neoplasm. Three patients had papillary carcinomas, and two had follicular adenomas. The latency period ranged from 8 to 16 years.

Because of the high incidence of thyroid dysfunction and the potential for the development of thyroid neoplasia, patients who undergo radiation therapy for Hodgkin's lymphoma should be given suppressive doses of thyroxine before radiation therapy to suppress thyrotropin, and then be permanently maintained on a regimen of thyroid-stimulating hormone suppression. Some of these patients will develop thyroid tumors: they should be screened periodically.

▶ Development of thyroid cancer after irradiation of the head, neck, or upper mediastinum has been recognized for almost 40 years (*J. Clin. Endocrinol. Metab.* 10:1296–1308, 1950). Development of thyroid tumors after irradiation of the neck for Hodgkin's lymphoma was not anticipated: the 20+ Gy dose usually used was assumed to be sufficient to either destroy follicular cells of the thyroid or to prevent their ability to divide. Unfortunately, cancer has developed in a few cases, and the syndrome has been recognized for a decade (*Acta Radiol. Oncol.* 17:383–386, 1978; *Cancer* 45:2056–2060, 1980). All surgeons should be aware of the possibility of development of cancer in patients treated for Hodgkin's disease. The authors' suggestion that all patients who undergo radiation treatment of the neck for Hodgkin's should have thyroid activity suppressed by exogenous thyroxine preoperatively and for the rest of their lives appears sound. Even so, as they suggest, the patients should be informed of the risk, and the cases should be followed up.—J.C. Thompson, M.D.

The Incidence of Thyroid Carcinoma in Solitary Cold Nodules and In Multinodular Goiters

Anne McCall, Harriet Jarosz, A.M. Lawrence, and Edward Paloyan (VA Hosp., Hines, Ill., and Loyola Univ., Maywood, Ill.)
Surgery 100:1128–1132, December 1986   27–2

In patients with multinodular goiters, the incidence of cancer has been reported to be lower than in those with a single cold nodule. Nevertheless, "single cold nodule" has been subjectively defined and is often accompanied by qualifying terminology that implies such a nodule is more likely to be a neoplasm than the multiple nodules that appear to result from colloid changes. A study of the relative incidence of carcinoma was undertaken in patients where criteria were used to strictly define the number of nodules in the thyroid.

A series of patients who had undergone thyroidectomy were evaluated, and the incidence of carcinoma was compared between patients with multinodular goiters and those with operatively and histopathologically confirmed solitary cold nodules. In almost half the patients who had clinically palpable solitary nodules, additional nodules were found at operation. Of the patients with true solitary cold nodules, 17% had thyroid carcinomas. Thyroid carcinomas were found in 13% of patients with multiple nodules.

In this study, there was no significant difference in the incidence of carcinoma between patients with multinodular goiters and those with true solitary cold nodules. Therefore, the decision to recommend surgery or to treat the nodule with thyroid-stimulating hormone suppression should not be determined primarily by the number of nodules.

▶ All thyroid surgeons recognize scant correlation between the number of thyroid nodules felt preoperatively in the neck and the number found at operation. Although I agree with the authors' conclusion that the decision of whether or not to operate upon a patient with a thyroid nodule should not depend primarily upon the number of nodules, I would suspect that the incidence of cancer is much smaller in people with multinodular goiters than in patients suspected of having a single nodule (a suggestion that is counter to the authors' statistics). Most patients with multiple lumps in their thyroid are not referred to surgeons for operation. Only those suspected of having cancer usually reach us. There is probably no field in surgery in which reported association between conditions vary more widely than in the reported incidence of carcinoma in solitary thyroid nodules. Dr. Lahey used to tell people that one of four people with a solitary nodule had cancer. Practitioners in community practice retorted that the incidence was less than 1%. The problem is that patients we see have often been through two or three stages of selection, and only patients with particularly suspicious lesions have been referred to us. The incidences of thyroid carcinoma reported here of 17% in solitary nodules and of 13% in multiple nodules doubtless reflect the concentrating effect of selectivity.—J.C. Thompson, M.D.

Medullary Thyroid Carcinoma: Role of High-Resolution US

Brian Gorman, J. William Charboneau, E. Meredith James, Carl C. Reading, Lester E. Wold, Clive S. Grant, Hossein Gharib, and Ian D. Hay (Mayo Clinic and Mayo Found., Rochester, Minn.)

Radiology 162:147–150, January 1987   27–3

Surgery is required for initial treatment and recurrence of medullary thyroid carcinoma (MTC), which accounts for 10% of thyroid malignancies. Consequently, accurate determination of the extent of the disease is important. The records of 15 patients (20 to 73 years; mean age, 41 years) who had MTC and had been examined with high-frequency, 10-MHz ultrasonography (US) during a 4-year period, and in whom pathologic proof of the extent of the disease was obtained, were reviewed retrospectively.

Nine of the 15 had undergone thyroidectomy but had biochemical evidence of a recurring tumor: in all 9, cervical lymph nodes were detected by US, but only 3 had palpable nodes. The sizes of the nodes detected ranged from 0.5 to 4.0 cm in diameter (mean, 1.7 cm), and all had pathologic confirmation of tumor at surgical reexploration. In 7 of the 9, US showed bright echogenic foci associated with acoustic shadowing within some of the cervical lymph nodes (Fig 27–1), and there was no correlation between the size of the lymph node and the presence of bright echogenic foci. Some of the large nodes did not contain bright foci, and some very small ones did.

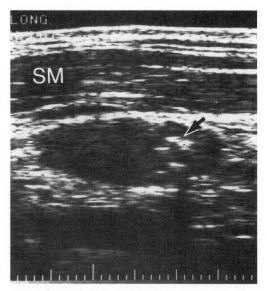

Fig 27–1.—Metastatic medullary thyroid carcinoma in cervical lymph node. Longitudinal sonogram of a 2.0 × 0.7-cm cervical lymph node reveals bright echogenic internal foci *(arrow)*, which cast an acoustic shadow. **SM,** strap muscles. (Courtesy of Gorman, B., et al.: Radiology 162:147–150, January 1987.)

The primary tumor mass was identified with US but was palpable in only 3 of the 6 patients who had not undergone thyroidectomy. All tumors appeared hypoechoic and relatively well defined. None were cystic or hyperechoic or surrounded by a halo. Five were solitary lesions, and 1 patient had two nodules seen with US that were not palpable. In 5 patients bright echogenic foci were seen within the thyroid mass. Three subsequently were found to have metastatically involved cervical lymph nodes at surgery, and in all of them US was used to detect the involvement before surgery. In only 1 of these 3 patients were these nodes palpable.

The authors prefer initiating the search for cervical lymph nodes with high-frequency US, 10-MHz, because it is a sensitive technique for detecting minimally enlarged lymph nodes and enables these nodes to be distinguished readily from vessels. It allows evaluating the internal architecture of nodes and providing real-time guidance for percutaneous aspiration or biopsy of the nodes. It is performed at a lower cost than computed tomography (CT) and does not require the intravenous administration of contrast material. Bright echogenic foci, commonly seen in both the primary tumor and metastatic cervical lymph nodes, appear to be caused pathologically by calcium and amyloid deposition. While they agree with Hajek et al. that benign and metastatic lymph node enlargement cannot be distinguished with certainty, the authors believe the presence of these echogenic foci in the cervical lymph nodes supports nodal involvement by tumor; this is of clinical importance, as cure can be obtained only by surgical excision.

▶ Since these nodes are just under the skin, preoperatively ultrasonography ought to be almost as accurate in detecting metastatic foci in lymph nodes as intraoperative ultrasound is in detecting pancreatic tumors (see Chapter 26, The Pancreas). What about other metastatic cervical nodes (papillary carcinoma, squamous carcinoma from the face or mouth, lymphomas)? The echogenic foci within the lymph nodes apparently are due to collections of calcium. The authors prefer to initiate the search for cervical lymph nodes with ultrasound as opposed to CT scanning because ultrasound is sensitive, allows differentiation from blood vessels, allows evaluation of the internal architecture, and provides guidance for percutaneous aspiration or biopsy. Additionally, it is cheaper than CT and does not require contrast material.—J.C. Thompson, M.D.

Parathyroid Localization
G. Gutekunst, A. Valesky, B. Borisch, W. Hafermann, E. Kiffner, E. Thies, U. Löhrs, and P.C. Scriba (Med. Univ. Lübeck, Lübeck, W. Germany)
J. Clin. Endocrinol. Metab. 63:1390–1393, December 1987   27–4

In patients with primary hyperparathyroidism (pHPT), preoperative localization of the abnormal glands remains a challenge. Ultrasound, sonographically guided fine needle aspiration, cytology, and immunocytochemical parathyroid hormone (PTH) staining were combined to detect enlarged parathyroid glands in 29 patients.

Solitary adenomas were detected in 23 patients, and two enlarged glands were identified in 2 patients. Surgical findings agreed with ultrasonography in both size and location (Fig 27–2). In 4 patients, the abnormal glands were not located prior to surgery. In two of these cases, the adenomas were retrosternal. In 1 patient, detection was blocked by a goiter. One patient with renal osteodystrophy had two enlarged parathyroid glands that were not detected until surgery. Cytologically, parathyroid cells have lighter, foamier, and more narrow cytoplasm with larger nuclei than thyroid cells (Fig 27–3). Positive PTH immunostaining was detected in cells from all aspirates.

Ultrasound should be routinely used for the preoperative localization

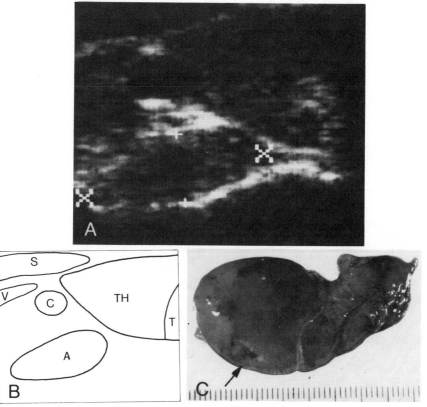

Fig 27–2.—**A,** right transverse sonogram of the thyroid and the typical sonolucent parathyroid adenoma, as indicated in **B,** in patient 17. **B,** schematic drawing of the sonogram. *TH,* thyroid; *C,* carotid artery; *A,* parathyroid adenoma; *S,* sternocleidomastoid muscle; *T,* trachea; *V,* jugular vein. **C,** surgical specimen of the enlarged parathyroid gland (4 cm) with the lesion *(arrow)* caused by preoperative fine needle aspiration. (Courtesy of Gutekunst, G., et al.: J. Clin. Endocrinol. Metab. 63:1390–1393, December 1987.)

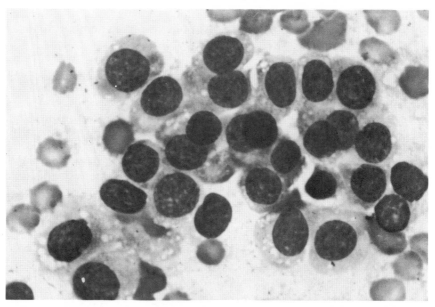

Fig 27–3.—Smear from fine needle aspiration of a parathyroid adenoma (May-Grünwald-Giemsa; original magnification, × 480). (Courtesy of Gutekunst, G., et al.: J. Clin. Endocrinol. Metab. 63:1390–1393, December 1987.)

of abnormal thyroid glands in patients with pHPT. Fine needle aspiration and immunocytochemical PTH staining can provide confirmation.

▶ This is one of four papers selected this year that boost the use of ultrasound in the localization of tumors (see also Abstracts 24–2, 26–6, and 27–3). The glands were localized sonographically and identified by aspiration cytology. In the series reported here of 29 patients, 2 had retrosternal adenomas; of the remaining 27 patients, enlarged glands were accurately located in 25. Could intraoperative application of ultrasonography have facilitated the location of the other two? Preoperative ultrasound is clearly valuable and should be certainly used in any patient with recurrent hyperparathyroidism. Three years ago, we reviewed here a paper from Sweden (*Acta Chir. Scand.* 150:199–204, 1984) in which two thirds of parathyroid adenomas had been successfully located preoperatively by means of ultrasound, and I made the remark that in such studies there was often a Darwinian factor of selectivity operating so that only the best results were reported. Here we have correct localization in 25 of 29 patients: things are getting better all the time.—J.C. Thompson, M.D.

Causes of Failure in Operations for Hyperparathyroidism
Hajo A. Bruining, Jan C. Birkenhäger, Giok L. Ong, and Steven W.J. Lamberts (Erasmus Univ., Rotterdam, the Netherlands)
Surgery 101:562–565, May 1987   27–5

Hyperparathyroidism can be successfully managed with surgical intervention of 95% of cases. Operative failure is indicated by hypercalcemia or recurrence of hypercalcemia after a period of normocalcemia. In an attempt to prevent future failures, which are frustrating to both physician and patient, the authors examined some of the causes of surgical failures in a patient population.

Eight hundred sixty-two patients with hypercalcemia thought to be due to hyperparathyroidism were surgically treated. After a mean follow-up period of 6.1 years, the reasons for treatment failure were evaluated. In 27 patients, incorrect diagnosis was cited as the reason for operative failure. In 89 operative failures, the most frequent causes were physician inexperience, abnormal localization, and multiple tumors. Misjudgment of the tumor site was also given as a reason. Of the 226 patients with multiple gland involvement, failure to remove the affected gland led to persistent disease in 20 patients, and 21 patients had recurrence after 6 months to 17 years.

Due to the possibility of recurrent hyperparathyroidism in patients with multiglandular involvement, a long follow-up period is required. None of the patients in this study with single gland disease had a recurrence.

▶ Although the authors say that hyperparathyroidism can be successfully managed by surgery in 95% of cases, they had 89 operative failures in 835 patients with hyperparathyroidism (10.6% rate of failure). Analysis of this huge series of patients confirms that the real problem is in patients who have more than one enlarged gland; no postoperative recurrence was found in patients with involvement of a single gland. An important finding was that 10 patients were surgically aparathyroid due to removal of all glands (5 of these were operated on by the authors and 5 were operated on elsewhere; the authors state that the 5 aparathyroid patients they operated on were all due to removal of enlarged glands, whereas the 5 aparathyroid patients operated on elsewhere were due to removal of normal glands). The message is clear in any case: one should never remove or damage all four glands. It is far better to reoperate than to render anyone persistently hypoparathyroid.—J.C. Thompson, M.D.

Parathyroid Carcinoma Versus Parathyroid Adenoma in Patients With Profound Hypercalcemia
Kenneth E. Levin, Maurice Galante, and Orlo H. Clark (VA Med. Ctr. and Univ. of California, San Francisco)
Surgery 101:649–660, June 1987   27–6

The differential diagnosis of parathyroid carcinoma is difficult due to similarities to parathyroid adenoma. This study examined 10 patients with diagnoses of parathyroid carcinoma and compared them to (A) 8 patients with atypical benign adenomas and mean serum calcium levels of 13.4 mg/dl, and (B) 13 patients with typical benign adenomas and mean serum calcium levels of 14.2 mg/dl.

The carcinoma patients had a 50% incidence of osteoporosis and osteitis fibrosa cystica, group A patients had a 33% level, and group B patients had a 62% incidence. Renal disease was seen in 70% of carcinoma patients, 38% of group A patients, and 15% of group B patients. Combined bone and renal disease was most common in carcinoma patients.

Patients with parathyroid carcinoma have more profound metabolic abnormalities than patients with primary hyperparathyroidism. However, these changes are similar to those in patients with parathyroid adenomas and hypercalcemia. Atypical adenomas share many features with parathyroid carcinomas. It is often difficult to distinguish between atypical adenomas and parathyroid carcinomas. Therefore, patients with atypical parathyroid adenomas should be carefully monitored.

▶ Reading the case histories of these patients with parathyroid carcinoma, one cannot help but compare them with standard patients with hyperparathyroidism 30–50 years ago, when cases were discovered only when the disease was sufficiently severe to induce renal, bone, or mental pathology. The disease is rare: only 3 years ago a study at Oxford found that fewer than 100 confirmed cases had been reported (*Ann. R. Coll. Surg. Engl.* 67:222–224, 1985, reviewed in the 1986 YEAR BOOK OF SURGERY, pp. 479–480). That report added five cases, and this one adds ten. Since the carcinomas apparently actively secrete PTH and since severe symptoms of hypercalcemia are present, why are the carcinomas not detected earlier? Of the ten patients with parathyroid carcinoma in this series from San Francisco, three are dead, one is alive with disease, and six are well with no evidence of disease 3–19 years after diagnosis. The authors report eight patients with atypical benign adenomas (so classified because the tumors either possess some histologic features of carcinoma or were adherent to adjacent tissues, yet possessed insufficient histologic criteria for diagnosis of carcinoma). Is this a local diagnosis? The authors suggest that these lesions may be premalignant and should be followed up.—J.C. Thompson, M.D.

Elevated Plasma Vasopressin (AVP) Levels During Resection of Pheochromocytomas

Jonathan Kay, Daniel T. Minkel, Anthony B. Gustafson, M. Skelton, Allen W. Cowley, Jr., and Stuart D. Wilson (Med. College of Wisconsin, Milwaukee)
Surgery 100:1150–1153, December 1986   27–7

While evaluating the efficacy of epidural blockade with light general anesthesia in patients undergoing resection of pheochromocytomas, increases in plasma arginine vasopressin (AVP) were documented. Perioperative hemodynamic instability and fluid management problems are thought to be related to excess catecholamines (CA) in these patients; consequently, perioperative AVP and CA concentrations and related hemodynamic changes were measured preoperatively, after epidural placement and blockade, after general anesthesia and intubation, during tumor manipulation, and 24 hours postoperatively in eight consecutive patients undergoing resection of pheochromocytomas.

Extraordinarily high levels of AVP were observed during tumor manipulation and remained elevated for 24 hours postoperatively. Tumor manipulation was associated with maximal AVP levels along with significant increases in norepinephrine, epinephrine, and dopamine levels. Furthermore, tumor manipulation caused an increase in mean arterial pressure, wedge pressure, and systemic vascular resistance. The other perioperative procedures had no effect on AVP or CA levels, while heart rate, mean arterial pressure, and cardiac index fell significantly only during induction of general anesthesia.

This is the first study that documents extraordinarily high levels of AVP in patients undergoing resection of pheochromocytoma. Whether AVP is released centrally by hormonal manipulation or by direct expression from the tumor remains to be investigated.

▶ What is the significance of this paper? Why hasn't this been noted before? Have other investigators simply not measured vasopressin, or is the technique for resection of pheochromocytomas different in Milwaukee? In an understatement in the introduction the authors state that little is known about AVP in patients with pheochromocytomas (they quote the finding of AVP in a single pheochromocytoma [*J. Clin. Endocrinol. Metab.* 58:688–691, 1984]). Vasopressin is supposed to come from the posterior lobe of the hypophysis; what is it doing here? None of the patients developed complications, so what does it all mean?—J.C. Thompson, M.D.

Clinical and Hormonal Effects of a Long-Acting Somatostatin Analogue in Pancreatic Endocrine Tumors and in Carcinoid Syndrome
Jean-Christophe Souquet, Geneviève Sassolas, Jacques Forichon, Pascal Champetier, Christian Partensky, and Jean-Alain Chayvialle (Hôpital Edouard Herriot and Centre de Médecine Nucléaire, Lyon, France)
Cancer 59:1654–1660, May 1, 1987   27–8

Somatostatin-14 suppresses tumoral secretion by pancreatic and gut endocrine tumors, but its short half-life and the necessity of a continuous intravenous administration hampers its clinical usefulness. A recently developed long-acting somatostatin analogue, SMS 201-995, can be administered subcutaneously, and its clinical usefulness has been demonstrated in malignant carcinoid syndrome, in acromegaly due to pituitary adenoma, and on digestive endocrine tumors. In this study, nine patients with pancreatic apudomas and nine with metastasized carcinoid tumors were treated with SMS 201-995, which was administered subcutaneously twice daily for 3 days.

In all six patients with gastrinoma, decreased gastrin levels resulted from the treatment; four patients had normal gastrin levels after 3 days. Treatment inhibited the residual gastric acid secretion under H2-

blockers. In four patients with diarrhea, there was no clear effect, but epigastric pain was improved in two of three. One patient with glucagonoma had decreased plasma glucagon levels, and her skin lesions disappeared. One patient with a tumor secreting a substance P-like component had moderately decreased plasma substance P level.

The patients with carcinoid syndrome had partial and inconstant clinical efficacy. Plasma substance P-like immunoreactivity was increased in six patients with carcinoid syndrome; in all patients it was reduced by SMS. Normalization of 5-hydroxyindole acetic acid did not occur in any patient.

Three patients have been treated for more than 8 months, two with a gastrinoma and one with a carcinoid tumor, with no antitumoral effect as judged by a recent computed tomographic scan. Except for occasional pain at the injection site, no adverse effects have been noticed by the patients.

Somatostatin 201-995 is an easy-to-use and well-tolerated new therapeutic agent that is most useful for controlling symptoms in secreting pancreatic endocrine tumors such as gastrinomas and glucagonomas. Its effects on carcinoid syndrome, although far from dramatic, may be tested systematically at this and higher doses along other treatments to select patients for whom long-term benefit may be expected on symptom severity.

▶ Somatostatin is the great endocrine off-switch, but its clinical usefulness is limited by a short biologic half-life. The long-acting analog of somatostatin (SMS 201-995) has proved to be effective in treating secretory diarrhea as well as the effects of pathologic levels of peptides secreted by endocrine tumors. This paper from Lyon details one of the largest clinical experiences with the long-acting analog. Experience with treating the hypersecretory aspect of the Zollinger-Ellison (ZE) syndrome was good and did not diminish with long-term administration. Its action in treating the ZE syndrome is twofold: it suppresses gastrin release from tumor cells, and it inhibits the action of gastrin on the parietal cell. No side effects were noted. Surprisingly, their results with carcinoid syndrome were not as good (see Abstract 22–6). They found no tumoricidal activity of SMS even on long administration, although they quote several experimental and clinical examples of such action. My colleagues have reported suppression in nude mice of the growth of human malignant carcinoid tumors (*Gastroenterology* 92:1676, 1987) and of two human pancreatic adenocarcinomas (*Am. J. Surg.*, in press). We have found the agent to be wonderfully effective in managing the devastating consequences of massive fluid loss from proximal jejunal or duodenal fistulas.—J.C. Thompson, M.D.

Subject Index

A

Author Index

A

Abouna, G.M., 402
Abston, S., 43
Acinapura, A.J., 263
Addonizio, V.P., Jr., 30
Adler, S., 239
Ahmed, S.W., 255
Ahn, S.S., 400
Akagawa, H., 235
Akins, C.W., 255
Akwari, O.E., 411, 440
Alagaratnam, T.T., 336
Albert, J.D., 37, 51, 52
Alexander, G.J.M., 144
Alexander, J.W., 105, 131
Allmendinger, P., 279
Allo, M.D., 73
Almoguera, C., 174
Al-Nakib, B.M., 402
Alouini, T., 274
Al-Sayer, H.M., 104
Altschule, M.D., 267
Ament, M.E., 313
Anbar, R.D., 109
Andersen, O.B., 337
Anderson, C.B., 288
Anderson, D.L., 58
Andreae, G.E., 246
Andre-Fouet, X., 248
Andrzejak, D.V., 79
Appelman, H.D., 386
Appleton, G.V.N., 360
Aprile, J., 124
Aranha, G.V., 428
Arcidi, J.M., Jr., 256
Askanazi, J., 46
Asselain, B., 192
Au, F.C., 342
Aufses, A.H., Jr., 33, 431
Augenstein, D., 69
Austen, W.G., 280
Avis, F.P., 153
Axelrod, H.I., 270
Axon, A.T.R., 330

B

Babcock, G.F., 131
Bach, M.-A., 136
Bachulis, B.L., 64
Baekgaard, N., 337
Bahnson, H.T., 131, 148
Bailey, B.N., 97
Bailey, J.S., 213
Bailey, M.L., 70
Bailie, F.B., 97
Bains, M.S., 218
Baird, R.N., 293
Baissony, H., 402

Baker, A.R., 418
Balakrishnan, K.G., 276
Balk, R.A., 60
Ballan, A., 374
Barakat, M., 201
Barbot, D.J., 379, 403
Barcelli, U., 105
Barfred, T., 177
Bargeron, L.M., Jr., 237, 238
Barner, H.B., 278
Barratt-Boyes, B.G., 249
Barrett, J., 309
Bartlett, S.T., 301
Barton, J.C., 433
Barttelbort, S., 116
Bashore, T.M., 259
Bashour, T.T., 246
Battey, P.M., 287
Baumann, F.G., 270
Baxter, C.R., 110
Beart, R.W., Jr., 360
Beck, G.J., 372
Beddoe, A.H., 43
Beller, F.K., 132
Benckart, D.H., 269
Bender, H.W., Jr., 234
Bender, J.R., 159
Ben H'Tira, S., 168
Bennett, G., 114
Bennett, G.K., 196
Bennett, K.G., 202
Bennett, W.M., 126
Benson, L.N., 236
Benvenisty, A., 142
Berardi, V.P., 139
Berg, R., 55
Bergan, J.J., 301
Bergelin, R.O., 295
Berger, R.L., 269
Bergström, J.P., 46
Berkowitz, H.D., 30
Berling, J., 166
Bernatz, P.E., 219, 313
Bernhard, W.F., 269
Berquist, W., 313
Bethencourt, D.M., 231
Beutler, B., 51, 52
Beven, E.G., 297
Bhuta, S., 231
Bickell, W.H., 70
Bighardi, M., 206
Birchall, N., 116
Birkenhäger, J.C., 448
Bistrian, B.R., 44
Bitondo, C.G., 74, 78
Björk, V.O., 245
Black, C.T., 314
Blackburn, G.L., 44
Blackstone, E.H., 237, 238
Bladwin, J.C., 125
Bland, K.I., 367
Blazar, B.R., 124

Block, A.V., 107
Bloem, J.J.A.M., 180
Bloom, J.R., 194
Bluett, M.K., 322
Boey, J., 336
Bohle, W., 166
Bonadimani, B., 422
Bone, R.C., 60
Bonnesen, T., 337
Boorman, J.G., 185
Border, D., 66
Border, J.R., 66
Borisch, B., 446
Bornman, P., 395
Borovetz, H.S., 148
Borst, H.G., 273
Bos, J.L., 174
Botet, J., 390
Bouwman, D.L., 438
Boyd, A., 271
Braasch, J.W., 420, 437
Bradley, B.A., 134
Bradley, E.C., 159
Bradley, N., 208
Bradley, S.J., 173
Bramwell, N.H., 147
Branch, H.M., 379
Branson, R.D., 83
Braun, P., 232
Bray, C.L., 234
Brennan, T.G., 417
Brensilver, J., 142
Bridges, M., Jr., 100
Bridges, R.M., 57
Brinton, L.A., 168
Bristol, J.B., 360
Brock-Utne, J.G., 59
Brough, M.D., 208
Brown, J.A., 185
Brown, P.W., 199
Bruining, H.A., 448
Brunner, R.G., 75
Buchholz, B., 132
Buchi, K.N., 393
Buckley, M.J., 280
Bülzerbruck, H., 223
Bunton, R., 242
Burch, J.M., 74, 78
Burchard, K.W., 103
Burcharth, F., 374
Burhenne, H.J., 189
Burhenne, L.W., 189
Burkholder, J.A., 269
Burnett, D.A., 393
Burns, D.K., 38
Burrows, F., 239
Burt, M.E., 228
Burton, G.V., 327
Bush, H.L., Jr., 139
Busuttil, R.W., 400
Butch, R.J., 32

475